Complementary Therapies
Physical Therapists

Edited by

Robert A. Charman FCSP MCSP DipTP
Lecturer in Physiotherapy (part-time)
University of Wales College of Medicine
Cardiff
UK

Chairman
Association of Chartered Physiotherapists in Bioenergy Therapies

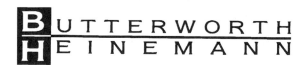
BUTTERWORTH
HEINEMANN

OXFORD   AUCKLAND   BOSTON   JOHANNESBURG   MELBOURNE   NEW DELHI

Butterworth-Heinemann
Linacre House, Jordan Hill, Oxford OX2 8DP
225 Wildwood Avenue, Woburn, MA 01801-2041
A division of Reed Educational and Professional Publishing Ltd

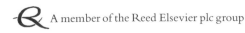 A member of the Reed Elsevier plc group

First published 2000

British Library Cataloguing in Publication Data
A catalogue record for this book is available from the British Library

Library of Congress Cataloguing in Publication Data
A catalogue record for this book is available from the Library of Congress

ISBN 0 7506 4079 0

Typeset by BC Typesetting, Keynsham, Bristol BS31 1NZ
Printed and bound in Great Britain by The Bath Press, Somerset

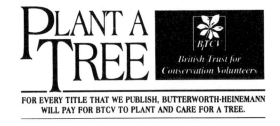

FOR EVERY TITLE THAT WE PUBLISH, BUTTERWORTH-HEINEMANN
WILL PAY FOR BTCV TO PLANT AND CARE FOR A TREE.

Contents

Contents

We are pleased to offer the following chapters
as an additional resource on our website.
The chapters may be found by visiting our
website at http://www.bh.com/companions/
0750640790.

Bioenergetic profiling
Richard J. Atkinson

Reiki healing
Cheryl Ritchie

Applied kinesiology
Ann Childs

The Bowen technique
Richard A. Harries

Polarity therapy
Lesley Finlayson

Zero Balancing for physical therapists
Della Tysall

Emotional therapy
Vivien Nichols

The use of Process Work within
physiotherapy
Judy Hockley

Aura-Soma
Ann Childs

Dowsing for health
Trish Niblock

The placebo phenomenon
Richard J. Atkinson

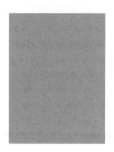

Contributors

Robert A. Charman qualified from the West Middlesex School of Physiotherapy in 1956. After extensive clinical experience in the UK he moved to Cardiff in 1979 and took his physiotherapy teaching diploma in 1971. He was a full-time senior teacher at the School of Physiotherapy, Cardiff, now the Department of Physiotherapy Education, College of Wales University of Medicine, until 1993, when he retired to become a part-time lecturer. In 1994 he was awarded the Fellowship of the Chartered Society of Physiotherapy (FCSP), and also completed the Open University Science Foundation Course in the same year. He is Chairman of the Association of Chartered Physiotherapists in Bioenergy Therapies (ACPBET), and is a member of the Scientific & Medical Network, and the Doctor–Healer Network.

His particular interests are neurophysiology and electrotherapy, and it was through the latter that he became interested in bioelectricity, and discovered the pioneering work of Robert O. Becker, H. Burr, A. A. Marino, and others. This, in turn, led him to an interest in the concept of bioenergy fields, and he has developed a data bank on the research literature concerning healing and related phenomena. His publications include an eight-article series on Bioelectricity and Electrotherapy (*Physiotherapy*, 1990/91), and an article on The Field Substance of Mind (*Network*, 1997). He has contributed chapters for textbooks on the Neurophysiology of Pain, Physiotherapy for Pain Relief, Electrical Properties of Cells and Tissues, and the cybernetic principles of Motor Learning.

Richard J. Atkinson qualified from the Sheffield School of Physiotherapy in 1976. After qualification he began a basic rotation post at Manchester Royal Infirmary, before specializing in Orthopaedics and Manual therapy under Mr David Markum. He left the UK in 1979 to take up a senior post responsible for developing a Physical therapy department in the King Khalid Military City in Saudi Arabia, taking on the responsibility of chief therapist in 1980. Further jobs in Hong Kong and postgraduate study in Australia followed before settling down to marriage, family and private practice in Yorkshire. In 1991 he formed the Worth Healing Company to work alongside the local GPs and hospital trusts. One of its goals is to research and integrate orthodox and complementary medicine in order to centralize and refocus patient care, ensuring a holistic approach to community and family health. In 1995 the Worth Healing Centre was opened as a health research, diagnostic and treatment institute. Richard holds postgraduate diplomas in Acupuncture, Biofeedback, Complex Homoeopathy and Bioresponse therapies, and is currently studying cybernetics. He is presently on the executive committee of the Association of Chartered Physiotherapists in Bioenergy Therapies, and is a member of the Scientific and Medical Network.

Mark F. Barnes' educational background is a Bachelor's degree in exercise physiology from the University of Colorado, Boulder, and a three-year Master's degree in physical therapy with an emphasis in clinical research from Shenandoah University/Winchester Medical Center, Winchester, Virginia. He is in orthopaedic private practice in Boulder, Colorado. In addition to clinical care, Mark Barnes is publishing articles on various topics in manual therapies, including a recent manual on *Equine Myofascial Release*.

Andrea Battermann is a chartered physiotherapist and a registered practitioner and teacher with the Shiatsu Society UK. She is the Principal of the Shiatsu College in Edinburgh and works in private practice and occasionally in the NHS. At present Andrea studies process orientated psychology, a body-orientated psychotherapy.

Her past experience includes several years' professional involvement in social work and alternative education. She qualified as a physiotherapist in Germany in 1992 and gained extensive experience in neurology and outpatients before specializing in Shiatsu. She became interested in Oriental medicine and Shiatsu because she felt a holistic approach is important to enhance the Western medical model and paradigm.

Tessa Campbell trained at the Southern General School of Physiotherapy in Glasgow, and initially worked in Jersey before returning to Scotland to work at the Orthopaedic Clinic in Edinburgh. Here she gained a lot of experience in outpatients and domiciliary physiotherapy before having a career break, during which time she had four children. Tessa returned to physiotherapy 10 years later to find a profession that was changing rapidly, and, after a couple of years, decided it was better to specialize than be a 'jack of all trades'. She felt strongly drawn to massage and other 'hands-on' techniques, so she concentrated on these, taking her Diploma in aromatherapy at the Elisabeth Jones Tuition Centre. She has since built up a successful practice incorporating physiotherapy and aromatherapy treating mainly musculoskeletal problems.

After several years in the field, Tessa was invited by Elisabeth Jones to join her tutoring staff, and now teaches on the ITEC Anatomy, Physiology and Massage Course as well as the Aromatherapy Course. Meanwhile Tessa continues to expand her areas of interest within aromatherapy and physiotherapy, treating the long-term chronic sick both with aromatherapy and hydrotherapy. Tessa also pursues a connection with Riding for the Disabled through her position as Physiotherapist to the Itchen Valley Group.

John D. Chacksfield trained as an occupational therapist at the Welsh School of Occupational Therapy, Cardiff, and qualified in 1989. He has since worked in the field of mental health with a particular interest in work with people who are addicted to alcohol and drugs.

John has been interested in healing energy therapy for many years and trained as a 'contact healer' in the evenings during the years of his occupational therapy training, via the Healer Practitioner Association International (now affiliated to the Institute of Complementary Medicine). He learnt under the guidance of a healer who was also a nurse manager in South Wales.

John is currently Clinical Specialist OT in Forensic Addictive Behaviours at Broadmoor Hospital and a researcher at the Institute of Psychiatry, where he is studying for his MPhil in Psychology. For the last three years John was Chairman of the Association of Occupational Therapists in Mental Health.

He still holds an active interest in healing and other complementary therapies, as well as the fields of parapsychology and consciousness studies.

Ann Childs worked for 16 years as a physiotherapist in a natural therapy clinic, while exploring, developing and teaching many aspects of complementary medicine and the importance of the therapeutic relationship. In 1989, these therapeutic techniques were integrated within an NHS setting at Bassetlaw Hospital, Worksop, with children and adults who experience moderate and severe learning difficulties. Concurrently, Ann held the Senior Physiotherapist post at Rampton Special

Secure Hospital, innovatively combining subtle energy therapies with physiotherapy practice. Since 1996, she has developed physiotherapy in mental health at the Queen's Medical Centre, Nottingham, and is actively involved in teaching students on the Mental Health Module, as part of the Nottingham Physiotherapy BSc (Hons) course. Ann has presented a number of papers and facilitated workshops throughout the country for physiotherapists, nurses, teachers and adult education.

Having observed the integration and enhancement of subtle energy therapies within mind–body medicine, Ann enthusiastically supports the open access and choice of complementary therapies for all patients within the NHS. This has involved membership of the working party to develop policy guidelines for the use of complementary therapies in the Nottingham Healthcare Trust.

Lorraine Cookson qualified from the Leeds School of Physiotherapy in 1980. Specializing in orthopaedics, Lorraine has worked both in the NHS and in private health care. In 1990 she became a member of the Association of Chartered Physiotherapists in Animal Therapy (ACPAT) and began to learn how to utilize her physiotherapy skills in the care of animals. Working alongside veterinarians, she has since been involved in the treatment of a wide range of musculoskeletal problems, using a combination of electrotherapy and manual techniques. Interested in complementary therapy, Lorraine has more recently qualified as a Tteam practitioner. 'Tteam' is the Tellington-Jones equine Awareness Method, incorporating Tellington Touch. This has proved to be a useful means of addressing many of her patients' (horses') problems. In her attempts to understand 'how?', Lorraine has also considered other methods, such as Shiatsu massage and Reiki healing.

Anna Corser has been a chartered physiotherapist for over 30 years, specializing for the last 10 years in mental health. In order to meet the needs of clients with mental health problems, she has gained diplomas in both stress management and aromatherapy. She has recently completed a course on behavioural family therapy, focusing on supporting clients with enduring mental illness within the context of their family and social setting. She uses her skills in stress counselling for the clients and hopes to also expand her involvement in the Trust's Health at Work Initiative to assist in training staff in stress management.

John R. Cross qualified as a chartered and state registered physiotherapist in 1970 while serving in the Royal Navy. In 1972, following a debilitating spinal condition (ankylosing spondylitis) he commenced to study homoeopathy, as this had been the medical approach that had helped him so much. The study of acupuncture followed, as he found that physiotherapy alone was not achieving the desired results he wanted with his patients. He studied acupuncture at the British College in London, achieving his Licentiate in 1978, Bachelor degree in 1982 and an acupuncture Doctorate in 1987, following his thesis and research with the Chakra energy system.

Over his many years of clinical work he has studied several methods of mobilization and manipulation, craniosacral therapy, radionics, biomagnetics and reflexology. He developed an interest in working with the subtle energies, as he wanted to combine his knowledge of Traditional Chinese Medicine with practical physiotherapy. He therefore devised his own system of 'clinical acupressure' and treats acute and chronic conditions alike with it. He founded Moorlands Natural Medicine Teaching Centre in Newton Abbot, Devon, with his wife (also a chartered physiotherapist) in 1975 and taught practical, experiential workshops to physiotherapists, osteopaths and doctors for several years. After a short spell in management he returned to clinical work and teaching last year.

He has served on several physiotherapy committees and is currently President of the Acupuncture Association of Chartered Physiotherapists. He has written scores of articles for lay and professional publications and is writing two books, one on the use of acupressure in the treatment of musculoskeletal conditions and the other on the Chakra energy system in therapy.

Ann M. Davies qualified from Cardiff School of Physiotherapy in 1968. She was awarded a degree from the Open University in 1979 and gained an NVQ Level 3 in Aromatherapy in 1996. She has worked within many specialities over the years, particularly rehabilitation and elderly care. At present she is specializing in learning disabilities. Approximately 20 years ago she realized that patients treated holistically responded to treatment by balancing and healing themselves. This was more effective than a purely physical approach and had longer lasting, if not permanent, positive healing outcomes. She is particularly interested in acupressure, energy balancing and therapeutic massage.

Bernadette Dunne qualified in 1983 from the Withington School of Physiotherapy, and worked for several years in Canada before specializing as a Senior I in Cardiorespiratory.

She became involved in spiritual healing in 1996, with a particular interest in animal healing, and has since worked with the Oxford Spiritual Healing Centre. She is a member of ACPBET (Association of Chartered Physiotherapists in Bioenergy Therapies) and the Scientific and Medical Network.

Hermione Evans qualified as a chartered physiotherapist in 1969, graduating from the Royal London Hospital with distinction. In her early years as a therapist she worked both abroad and at home, covering many physiotherapy specialities including rehabilitation of the neurologically-impaired patient, rheumatology, cardiothoracic surgery, rehabilitation of the amputee, orthopaedics and outpatient work. While her children were small she took time out to study English Literature and French at the University of Reading. Although the value of a language and literature degree to physiotherapy was not immediately obvious, it later became clear that language and literature, explored at depth, gave insight into those often unanswered existential questions that may be at the heart of healing. While studying for her degree she also discovered Christine Jones and the Midland School of Reflextherapy. In spite of initial cynicism she, like so many others, was converted to the idea of 'energy medicine' and the body's potential for self-healing. She later became an associate tutor with the school.

She has explored healing through the Anahata Touch Healing School, Reiki, Yoga, Cranio-

sacral therapy and, more recently, Visceral Manipulation. At present Hermione works as a physiotherapist specializing in musculo-skeletal conditions in a multidisciplinary clinic in Reading. Her speciality is in helping people suffering from chronic pain, and she uses an eclectic mixture of conventional and complementary approaches according to the perceived needs of the patient.

Lesley Finlayson qualified from Bradford Hospitals School of Physiotherapy in 1978. After working in the UK and abroad she gained extensive experience in acute respiratory intensive therapy. She began training at the British School of Reflex Zone Therapy of the Feet in 1986 which opened the doorway to the use of subtle energies. Her Polarity Training was with Anthony Deavin in Surrey and following Mind, Body, Spirit courses she now uses a truly holistic approach when treating her patients.

Richard A. Harries, after six years in industry, trained as a mature student at the Sheffield School of Physiotherapy. In what should have been his final year he was involved in a climbing accident, resulting in a spinal cord injury. After completing his rehabilitation he eventually qualified, from his wheelchair, in 1978. He worked in a District General Hospital, gaining general experience, before specializing in outpatient physiotherapy. As physiotherapy from a wheelchair began to take its toll he started searching for other less physically demanding therapies and, in 1993, was on the first Bowen course to be held in Britain. His interest in light touch therapies continued and he started training in craniosacral therapy under Upledger in 1994. Early in 1996 he left the NHS for private practice and now lives, and works, in West Yorkshire.

Judy Hockley is a locum physiotherapist who enjoys time out to travel and learn. She has been fascinated by Process Work since being introduced to it three years ago, and is also interested in healing energy therapies. Her chapter is dedicated to her father Norman and her friend Juliet.

Christine Jones qualified as a chartered physiotherapist from the Queen Elizabeth Hospital,

Birmingham, in 1961. Intrigued with the philosophy of holism, she continued her training in naturopathy, nutrition, reflexology, metamorphosis, counselling and spiritual healing. In 1976, she founded the Midland School of Reflextherapy (MSR), teaching the holistic approach to patient care and reflextherapy (a development of reflexology adapted to the individual and particularly to the needs of the sensitive, or seriously ill, patient). The MSR course 'Reflextherapy and Associated Studies for the Health Professional' is credited by the University of Coventry and endorsed by the Chartered Society of Physiotherapy. This UK course is also held in Israel.

Christine is a private practitioner who continues to research reflextherapy which she has presented to medical audiences worldwide. She is the author of several publications, including a chapter on Reflextherapy in *Physiotherapy in Mental Health* (Everett, Dennis and Rickette, eds, 1995), and has been commissioned to write a book on the MSR approach. As Founder Chair of the Association of Chartered Physiotherapists and Health Care Professionals in Reflex Therapy (ACPIRT) she continues her commitment to promote the highest standards of practice in the healthcare professions.

In 1994, Christine was awarded a Doctorate of Medicine by the International University of Alternative Medicine and, in 1997, was awarded an Honorary Fellowship of the Association of Reflexologists. The Fellowship of the Chartered Society of Physiotherapy was conferred in 1997 for innovative practice, and for broadening the scope of physiotherapy to encompass holism in the approach to patient care in the widest sense: that of body, mind, and spirit.

Elisabeth Jones is an internationally recognized authority on aromatherapy. She has lectured, broadcast and written many articles on aromatherapy, and has travelled the world on behalf of aromatherapy. She is an accredited tutor for the International Federation of Aromatherapists (IFA), and an accredited tutor for the International Society of Aromatherapists (ISPA). Her work is now centred mainly in the UK, where she established a Training Centre for Aromatherapy in 1978. Many leading names in aromatherapy received their training at the Centre. As well as aromatherapy she has taught anatomy, physiology and Swedish body massage for over 20 years. She is Vice-Chairman of the Association of Chartered Physiotherapists in Massage (ACPIM), and is the spokesperson for the Aromatherapy Subcommittee.

Fiona Mantle has been a nurse, health visitor and teacher for 30 years and has written extensively in the nursing press. She has currently authored three monographs about complementary therapies for the *Nursing Times* and is completing her own book on complementary therapies using a problem-solving approach. She lectures at a number of universities and is a regular speaker at nursing conferences. She is currently undertaking a PhD course investigating the role of hypnosis in the treatment of children suffering from atopic dermatitis.

Sara Mokone gained a BSc degree in physiotherapy at Witwatersrand University in South Africa, in 1966. She worked as a paediatric physiotherapist for 10 years in numerous settings, including child development units. She has a BSc in social science and took training in drama and art therapy, completing an introduction to counselling at the Westminster Pastoral Foundation and a diploma in counselling at the South West London College. All of these courses have been integrated into developing her clinical skills and abilities.

In 1987, she was part of a research team, identifying health needs of residents in Local Authority run homes for the elderly in Southwark. She has taught adult education classes in Islington, and at City University, on Health Promotion and Occupational Health courses, on the theme of Managing stress at work. She has also worked part-time as a teacher and as a counsellor, with MIND in Haringey. In 1992 she completed a three-year diploma in acupuncture, which included a month of travel in China. Her interest in Qigong, Traditional Chinese Medicine and body–mind medicine has continued, and she has spent the past 7 years studying with many teachers.

Sara has organized national and international conferences and is Treasurer of the International Acupuncture Association of Physical Therapists. In 1997 she co-edited a book on acupuncture and related techniques in physical therapy. Her interests include yoga, Qigong, Taichi and health promotion.

At present, Sara works part-time as a senior physiotherapist in a community team for people with learning difficulties, in Haringey, North London. She has a private practice treating women's health problems, and teaches Qigong and acupressure to health workers and adult education groups.

Trish Niblock MCSP Dip Grad Phys, aromatherapist, ElectroCrystal therapist, Reiki practitioner. Trish qualified in physiotherapy from The London Hospital and specialized in rehabilitation, latterly working with children with cerebral palsy. She has a special interest in sensory integrative therapy for children with dyslexia. She qualified in aromatherapy in 1991 and in ElectroCrystal therapy in 1994 and was attuned to Reiki 1 in 1995. She was introduced to dowsing by the late Dr Muriel Mackay of Edinburgh, and Frank Moody from Australia with whom she still studies. She is currently researching Magnet Therapy.

Vivien Nichols qualified at the Liverpool School of Physiotherapy in 1978 and has had an interest in neurology which has led to working with multiple sclerosis (her mother having the disease) and strokes. She qualified as an aromatherapist in 1988 and became interested in mind–body links, body energies and energy interactions.

She has studied healing with NFSH (National Federation of Spiritual Healers) and studied Emotional Therapy in 1991 finding it a useful adjunct to her physiotherapy and healing.

She is now hoping to set up workshops to teach health care workers how to keep themselves bioenergetically healthy.

Her present post is as a Senior I in Elderly Care at the Royal Leamington Spa Rehabilitation Hospital, Heathcote, Leamington Spa.

James L. Oschman received his BS (Biophysics) degree in 1961 and his PhD (Biol) in 1965. He has held a series of Postdoctoral Fellow research posts and assistant professorships in neurobiology, biological chemistry and the biological sciences in the USA, Denmark and Cambridge University (UK). His laboratory research projects have focused upon mechanisms of axon conductivity in the giant squid, the ultrastructure and physiology of epithelia relating to water and ion transport, and the role of calcium in cellular functions. He was a former Director of Research for the World Dolphin Research Society, trying to prevent dolphin mortality during purse seine fishing. He has served as Director, Chairman and Acting President of the Faculty at the New England School of Acupuncture, Watertown, Massachusetts, and has taught physiology and biophysics at the Rolf Institute, Boulder, Co. He is now President of Nature's Own Research Association, Dover, New Hampshire.

He has served on the editorial board of the *Journal of Membrane Biochemistry* and the *Journal of Bodywork and Movement Therapies* and is a member of many scientific societies. His research interests are now to bridge the gap between orthodox and complementary medicine by synthesizing the new insights arising from findings collated from a wide range of scientific disciplines.

Dr Oschman has published over 60 scientific papers, many in major scientific journals, has written two books *The Natural Science of Healing* (1986) and *Readings On The Scientific Basis of Bodywork, Energetic, and Movement Therapies* (1997), and is currently writing a textbook on the scientific basis of energy medicine. He is an international lecturer on energy medicine and bioenergy therapies, including acupuncture, craniosacral therapy, Rolfing, myofascial release and healing.

Lynn Pearce, Grad Dip Phys, MCSP, SRP, LicAc., chartered physiotherapist and licensed acupuncturist. She is an Advanced Member of the Acupuncture Association of Chartered Physiotherapists (AACP) and Senior Lecturer, Acupuncture Association of Chartered Physiotherapists, UK.

Lynn qualified at Addenbrooke's Hospital School of Physiotherapy in 1982, and trained in acupuncture at the Centre for the Study of Complementary Therapies in Southampton in 1989, going on to complete her traditional training at the British College of Acupuncture in 1993. She has worked in the NHS, independent hospitals and at present is in part-time private practice and part-time occupational health at John Lewis, Oxford Street, London. She teaches on the AACP two-year MSc course at Coventry University.

Kirsty Petre Mont Dip, DTM, SP Dip A, aromatherapy teacher, Reiki practitioner. Kirsty studied physiotherapy at the Glasgow Royal Infirmary. She later qualified as a Montessori Teacher with the St Nicholas Montessori School. In 1984 she obtained a Diploma in Therapeutic Massage from the College of Holistic Medicine and subsequently qualified in aromatherapy, eventually becoming a teacher for the Shirley Price School of Aromatherapy. She and her co-author Trish Niblock studied together on the ElectroCrystal therapy course in Edinburgh (1993–4) with Harry Oldfield and Dr Muriel Mackay.

Richard Reoch is the author of *Dying Well: A Holistic Guide for the Dying and Their Carers.* First published in 1997, the book has appeared in eight editions internationally. Richard Reoch is a specialist in Oriental and complementary health systems in which the aged, and the dying, are treated with great respect. He is a member of the Register of the Shiatsu Society for the United Kingdom and a former practitioner in the Hoxton Health Group for the over 60s in East London. He has been a Tai Chi Chuan instructor at the Royal College of Nursing and the European School of Osteopathy, and currently leads Tai Chi classes at the City and Islington College in London.

In 1991, Richard was invited by Master Lam Kam Chuen to collaborate with him to produce *The Way of Energy,* which opened up the Zhan Zhuang system of Chi Kung to the West and, most recently, *The Way of Healing.* Born in Canada in 1948 he grew up in a Buddhist family and was, for many years, a senior official in Amnesty International, working on behalf of the tortured and with the families of the dead and 'disappeared' throughout the world.

Cheryl Ritchie qualified from Queens College, Glasgow in 1981. She has been interested in complementary therapies since 1985. This began with an acupuncture course in Liverpool which made her look at people in a more holistic way. She then did an aromatherapy diploma in Hinckley which was useful in conjunction with

her physiotherapy. She completed a series of courses with the National Federation of Spiritual Healers (NFSH) including parts 1–4 of their healer training programme and she is currently a probationer healer. The NFSH training is long and comprehensive and has provided a sound and very useful grounding. On one of these courses she met a lady who had learned Reiki and this sparked off the interest to find out more. She completed her Reiki I in 1994 and Reiki II in 1995. She finds that once on the path of complementary therapies one thing leads to the next – knowledge of the similarities and differences of various therapies allow her to choose the best method and treatment approach.

She finds more and more people are turning to complementary therapies, becoming more open to the concepts and are becoming spiritually aware.

Linda J. Skellam qualified from the Withington Hospital, Manchester in 1977. She trained in reflextherapy with the Midland School in 1989. Since then she has been developing her practice in Leek, Staffordshire, incorporating reflextherapy with other physiotherapy modalities.

Josephine Smith Oliver qualified at St Thomas' Hospital in 1978. She worked with Dr James Cyriax for two years and has taught extensively for the Society of Orthopaedic Medicine since that time. Jo qualified in reflextherapy with the Midland School in 1995 and now integrates both orthopaedic and complementary approaches at her own practice in Hackney, East London.

Della Tysall qualified from the Middlesex Hospital School of Physiotherapy, London in 1978, gaining general experience at the Whittington Hospital, London, before specializing in the treatment of medical conditions at Guy's Hospital, London from 1981 to 1985. From 1985 until 1991 she worked in the private sector, at the London Clinic, setting up and running the new hydrotherapy unit and working in outpatients. From 1991 she has worked in private practice as sole practitioner.

She became interested in Body/Mind Medicine in the 1980s feeling the holistic approach to be very important, studying a number of alternative therapies in depth. She then trained in Humanistic Psychotherapy from 1989 to 1992, certifying in 1991 at Spectrum, Centre for Humanistic Psychology, London. For eighteen months she ran a private psychotherapy practice alongside her physiotherapy practice. She then moved further into energy medicine, studying healing at the McNeil School of Healing from 1992, receiving her diploma in Therapeutic Healing in 1994. In 1996, in search of a methodology that combined and integrated work with energy and structural systems, she began training in Zero Balancing, certifying in 1997.

She has also been, in 1973, 1974 and 1975, a member of the British Judo Team and British Judo Champion and held a British Record in Weight Lifting in 1983, the experience of which, has also informed her practice.

ZB plays a major role in her current practice, as she finds it an effective, gentle and powerful way of addressing the specific needs of the individual.

To contact the author, or for a list of workshops or Certified Practitioners, please contact the ZBA UK Tel: 01308 420 007 or e-mail: ZBAUK@aol. com.

Jill Wigmore-Welsh qualified from the Royal London Hospital School of Physiotherapy in 1977. Her interest in sport has led to her working for many years with athletes, among them, the British judo and rowing teams. She has explored many movement approaches, including Pilates, Laban, and the Alexander technique. Her complementary therapy training includes acupuncture, auriculotherapy, connective tissue manipulation, NLP, psychology, T-Touch and meditation. She has completed the UK Lewis 2 training, leading to qualification as a Feldenkrais practitioner and for her MSc in health promotion she undertook research into the Feldenkrais method. She practises privately in London and the home counties, incorporating Feldenkrais into her busy practice. She has published a series of ATM (Awareness Through Movement) lessons on audio cassettes entitled *The Thinking Body*, and is currently writing a book to accompany the series. To contact the author, or for a list of classes, please contact: Movement Matters, Tel. 0118 959 4099.

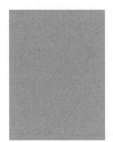

Foreword

Tim Watson

Given the move towards a more general acceptance of 'complementary therapies' over recent years, and given too, the range of knowledge and skills offered by physiotherapists, this is what I would consider to be a timely publication.

Getting this number of authors, all expert in their own fields, to write with a similar target in mind is a significant achievement. I know that Bob Charman has been a strongly encouraging editor, he wanted (quite rightly) for the contributors to consider the evidence for the various approaches. Rather than just another exposition of various complementary therapies for the lay public, this innovative text approaches the subject from a professional point of view. This is not to intimate that other authors and editors have failed to do so, but in this instance, there is a particular audience in mind – the already qualified professional in physical therapy (or physiotherapy). Such individuals have, by virtue of their pre-registration or undergraduate training become familiar with substantial volumes of basic medical science, combined with therapeutic manual skills, and a variety of approaches to patient care, though largely based on the medical model. This knowledge and the commensurate skills acquired provide a sound platform from which to explore this text of some thirty chapters.

Therapies which have at times been labelled 'alternative' are probably better considered to be 'complementary'. This is not just an issue of semantics, but rather one of philosophy.

Practitioners who offer such therapies are appreciated by their patients for their care and concern. Some have argued that this is, in fact, all that they offer. I trust that within the numerous chapters of this multiauthor volume, you will find explanations for both the philosophy and practice of a tremendous range of approaches.

Some approaches, I would imagine you will feel comfortable with, others possibly less so, but whatever your opinion at the end of the day, you should be grateful to the contributors and to Bob Charman for acting as their guide. Agree in part or in total with the contents, this publication offers you the opportunity to explore issues across a range of complementary therapies, to consider the available evidence, its links to the 'established' medical literature and its possible utilization within the therapeutic environment.

Read critically, evaluate against the available evidence and be prepared to change your approach to some extent or another based on what you find. This is fundamental to any evidence based practice such as physiotherapy, and it need not be any different just because there is 'complementary' in the title.

I'll leave it to Bob to introduce the authors and their contributions. I trust that you will be open minded about what you find, reflect on that of which you are currently appraised, and gain insight into therapies of which you have previously been unaware.

Enjoy!

Introduction

Robert A. Charman

In late July 1997 I received an invitation from Mary Seager, Senior Commissioning Editor, Medical Books Division, Butterworth-Heinemann, to be editor of a proposed new book on complementary therapies for physiotherapists. I felt very honoured by the invitation but hesitated for several days before taking a very deep breath to say 'yes'. Acceptance involved responsibility for deciding which therapies should be included and discovering who would be willing to write about each one. I had collected research data into bioelectricity, healing, and related studies, but knew very little about the vast range of complementary therapies now available. Which of them would be considered as most relevant to physiotherapy? Even asking that question led to another problem. Should the title say for 'Physiotherapists', which is a term limited to the UK and the Chartered Society of Physiotherapy? Or should it say for 'Physical Therapists', to include the wider world of our non-UK colleagues? We decided upon the latter, but you will find both terms in interchangeable use.

As for the rest, my worries turned out to be completely unfounded because this new venture could not have come at a better time. I was secretary of the former British Healing Energy Therapy Association (BHETA), now the Association of Chartered Physiotherapists in Bio-energy Therapies (ACPBET), and our directory of members included many physiotherapists who have now contributed to this book. During the autumn of 1997 and spring of

1998 the content took shape, moulded by the interests and clinical expertize of the contributors. By lucky coincidence the new *Journal of Bodywork and Movement Therapies* had commenced publication and was carrying a series of fascinating articles by James Oschman entitled 'What is healing energy?'. Dr Oschman, to my profound relief, readily agreed to contribute the opening chapter on 'Energy medicine – the new paradigm', thus providing the scientific and theoretical foundation upon which much of the book rests. I was in luck, yet again, when the same journal published an article on 'Myofascial release in the treatment of thoracic outlet syndrome' by John F. Barnes. Inquiry soon led me to his son Mark, who is carrying forward this pioneering approach with his father, and Mark has kindly contributed the chapter on 'Myofascial release'. The 'special relationship' forged between the UK and the USA in times of war remains intact in the literary world!

Mary Seager and I were determined to include chapters on the use of complementary therapies at the beginning of life and at the end of life, but we had no idea who to ask. All of my initial inquiries led nowhere and I was becoming rather pessimistic. Then fate, in the form of Jung's well-known Principle of Meaningful Synchronicity at times of crisis, stepped in. While browsing round a dusty little bookshop in Glastonbury I chanced upon a slim volume, half-hidden in the middle of an untidy pile in a corner, entitled *Dying Well: A holistic guide for the dying and their carers*, edited by Richard

Reoch. I knew, instantly, that he was the contributor that we needed. Again, through chance browsing in the college library, I came across some articles on the use of complementary therapies in nursing practice. Two phone calls later and I was led to Fiona Mantle who has written the comprehensive chapter on these therapies for mother and baby.

In retrospect, it has been as if this pioneering new book-to-be was leading me to the authors who would bring it to life – the future writing the present. Not, I may add, without some literary travail in the process!

Well, now that you have opened it, you may ask why this book should be of any interest to you as a busy clinician. The obvious answer to that question is to refer you to the chapters themselves, as no Introduction of mine can do them justice. In brief, I doubt if you can read this book and remain unchanged in the way that you think, for example, about the meaning of life, the processes that support life, and the relationship between body, mind and spirit. You will gain a new perspective concerning the meaning of 'illness' and of 'wellness' and the different ways in which we interact with each other. Even the terms 'therapy' and 'therapist' will take on new meanings as you explore each of the different therapies and the rationale that has guided their development.

The unifying concept that underlies much of the theory and the therapies discussed in this book is 'energy'. Not so much the gross energy of lifting things, but what is often termed the 'subtle energy' or 'bio-energy', the 'chi' or 'prana' or 'vibrational energy' of the life force that is said to inform, guide and maintain all living systems. When this 'energy' is 'blocked' or weakened, the flow of the life force, which is so closely linked to the bioelectrical activity of living processes, becomes distorted and expressed as symptoms of dis-ease. What do you think of this concept?

You will find that the structure and functions of cells and body tissues take on new meanings through the eyes of Dr Oschman and Mark Barnes. We all know about the mechanical and tensile properties of bone and connective tissues because they are our professional 'stock in trade'. But have you considered the clinical implications of the liquid crystalline properties of these tissues? These two authors claim that connective tissue, with its structure of triple helix collagen fibres enclosed within cylinder sheaths of bound water, carries positive currents along proton pathways, connecting everything to everything else in an almost instantaneous informational network system. On the basis of new scientific evidence they claim that the extracellular matrix, the microtrabecular lattice structure of cells that extends its filaments into the matrix through the cell membrane, and the ligaments, tendons, bones and fascia, form an integral tensegrity system with fast conductive properties. They propose, in effect, that we should consider the cells and tissues of the body as forming a three-dimensional, bio-cybernetic feedback system of great sensitivity that operates alongside the very much slower nervous system.

In their recent review of these new findings Ho and Knight (1998) arrived at very similar conclusions. They have proposed that 'memory is dynamically distributed' throughout the body tissues, and that 'a body consciousness, possessing all of the hallmarks of consciousness – sentience, intercommunication, and memory' exists alongside the 'brain consciousness'. They suggest that our 'brain consciousness', which we normally consider to be the only consciousness, is embedded within this 'body consciousness' and coupled to it. This is a truly breathtaking new view of the body and the mind as two major systems: a *bodymind system* that interacts with the familiar *self* of the *brainmind* system. This interaction may occur through the medium of neurohormones as proposed by Pert (1997). The clinical implications of this proposal are profound. Physical therapy procedures may have effects that are more far reaching than we have ever considered previously.

Within the context of such a bodymind system the acupuncture meridians are considered as a specialized information network, based upon embryonically derived liquid crystalline pathways, that carry the 'chi' of living energy along meridian circuits that link body organs to head, trunk and limbs (Chen, 1996; Tsuei, 1996). This provides a rationale for the clinical application of acupuncture and its related therapies as presented so ably by Lynn Pearce.

Dr Oschman also explores the bioelectric properties of the body in relationship to the geomagnetic fields and the 8–10 Hz Schumann wave frequencies. Is the fact that the same frequencies are recorded from the EEGs of healers just chance coincidence? Is it coincidence, again, that the biomagnetic fields emitted from the hands of healers sweep across the same frequencies? Is this frequency band the 'healing harmonic' for body and mind dis-ease?

If body tissues store emotional memories, can past trauma be recalled and released by the physical therapies of tissue mobilization and myofascial release? Are some of the bodily disorders seen in outpatient departments the outward expression of deep mental distress rather than physical trauma? (Motz, 1998, argues very persuasively for tissue memory on the basis of her experiences as a healer working in cardiac transplant units, surgery for cancer and neurosurgery). Does the question 'Why has this accident, or illness, happened to this patient *now*, rather than at some other time?' seem fatuous beyond belief? Or would an answer point to a deeper meaning behind what has happened and what is being experienced? Would awareness of a deeper meaning affect your choice of modalities and objectives of therapy?

The concepts of bodymind, energy flows and energy blockages underlie the touch therapies of shiatsu, craniosacral therapy, reflextherapy and metamorphic technique. Metamorphic technique takes the concept of 'blockage' into the womb. It proposes that experiential development 'blocks' may occur during embryonic to fetal development, and that these 'blocks' are stored as tissue memory, distorting the body structures, especially spinal, that are developing at that time. This may have consequent ill-effect in post-natal life that can be resolved through specialized techniques. What do you think?

Is 'healing' the same as 'curing'? If antibiotics 'cure' by killing the bug, have they also 'healed' in the sense that the body's healing defences are now stronger? Is 'healing' a more fundamental concept than 'curing'? Is Penson (1998) right when she says that 'healing' is about 'wholeness, balance and a sense of wellbeing'? Should we, as physical therapists, incorporate emotional therapy or counselling into our list of therapies to heal both mental and bodily distress as proposed by some experienced clinicians?

Do you think that one person can really affect the physiological, *or* the psychological, *or* the psycho-physiological functioning of another person, across space, purely by directing an intention-to-heal when in a particular mindset? Does the evidence from research, including the 'Maharishi effect', together with the personal experience and concepts explored in the chapters on different systems of healing, really support such a claim? What of the ancient belief in Chakras and the concept of the body as an open energy system that interacts with the universe? Do you think that a physical therapist can assess the state of health of their patient by using their hands as 'antennae' to 'tune into' the 'energy fields' of their patients, and 'rebalance' these energy fields for healing and health? This is what most of the contributors to this book believe, and assert, through their own experience (see Chaitow, 1997, on the palpation skills of bioenergy field assessment, Wisneski (1997), for the intriguing hypothesis that the endocrine system can act as an energy transducer, converting the incoming energy field of the healer into hormones and peptides, and Benor (forthcoming a–d [four volumes]), for a new review of over 175 controlled studies of spiritual healing, and a wide range of related phenomena).

Does the naturopathic approach to assessment, diagnosis and the aetiology of disease offer insights that orthodox physical examination and theory just cannot provide? Does the body, at some hypothetical level of quantum activity, consist of a continuum of interacting vibrational frequencies through which the therapist can act? This is the working hypothesis of vibratory medicine, flower essence and electrocrystal therapies discussed in this book (see Gerber, 1996, for a full presentation of the scientific basis of vibratory medicine and its related therapies). Aromatherapy is definitely coming of age as an accepted therapy, and you will find that Tessa Campbell and Liz Jones have presented you with an authoritative introduction to the use of therapeutic oils in physiotherapy.

Do you think that particular forms of movement, as developed in the Feldenkrais method, and Qigong and Taiji, can rebalance the body, recharge energy and restore psychomotor health, as discussed so persuasively by Jill Wigmore-Welsh and Sara Mokone?

The final two chapters tie the separate threads of the different therapies together, showing how complementary therapies can be combined to serve the mother and the life to come, and help the carers and the life that is ending. They bring the book to a very thought-provoking and satisfying close.

I feel very privileged to be the editor of such a fascinating new book. Why on earth did I hesitate before saying 'Yes'?

References

Benor, D. J. (forthcoming a) *Science Validates Spiritual Healing*, Vol. I. Southfield, MI: Vision.

Benor, D. J. (forthcoming b) *Consciousness, Bioenergy and Healing*, Vol. II. Southfield, MI: Vision.

Benor, D. J. (forthcoming c) *Science, Spirit and the Eternal Soul*, Vol. III. Southfield, MI: Vision.

Benor, D. J. (forthcoming d) *Theory and Practice of Spiritual Healing*, Vol. IV. Southfield, MI: Vision.

Chaitow, L. (1997) *Palpation Skills – Assessment and Diagnosis Through Touch*. Edinburgh: Churchill Livingstone.

Chen, K. G. (1996) Electrical properties of meridians. *IEEE Eng. Med. Biol.*, pt 11, May/June, 58–63, 66.

Gerber, R. (1996) *Vibrational Medicine: New Choices for Healing Ourselves*, 2nd edn. Santa Fe, NM: Bear.

Ho, M. W. and Knight, D. (1998) The acupuncture system and the liquid crystalline collagen fibers of the connective tissues. *Am. J. Chinese Med.*, **26(3–4)**, **1–15.**

Motz, J. (1998) *Hands of Life*. New York: Bantam.

Penson, J. (1998) Complementary therapies: making a difference in palliative care. *Compl. Ther. Nurs. Midwif.*, **4**, 77–81.

Pert, C. B. (1997) *Molecules of Emotion*. London: Simon and Schuster.

Tsuei, J. J. (1996) The science of acupuncture – theory and practice, pt 1, Introduction. *IEEE Eng. Med. Biol.*, May/June, 52–57.

Wisneski, L. A. (1997) A unified energy field theory of physiology and healing. *Stress Med.*, **13**, 259–65.

New science and traditional concepts

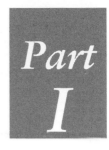

Energy medicine – the new paradigm

James L. Oschman

Introduction

A 'sea change' is taking place in medicine in the USA. A nation-wide survey done in 1993 indicated that patients were increasingly turning to complementary therapies in conjunction with, or even in preference to, conventional medicine (Eisenberg *et al.*, 1993). Now a new survey has shown that visits to complementary therapists in 1997 actually exceeded visits to primary care physicians by an estimated 243 million (Eisenberg *et al.*, 1998).

Accompanying these demographics are dramatic personal stories of the breaking down of barriers between different clinical approaches that have common and worthy goals. In some of the leading research hospitals and clinics, the best methods of cutting-edge Western biomedicine are being combined with both modern and ancient understandings of the roles of emotions, attitude and spirit in the healing process. These are historic developments.

In essence, what has been called alternative or unconventional is becoming the dominant paradigm. The suffering patient benefits from these changes, as documented in books by medical professionals who have opened their hearts and operating theatres to a diversity of methods previously regarded as 'off-limits' (e.g. Oz, 1998; Motz, 1998).

These dramatic changes are creating a favourable climate for advancing an energy paradigm for clinical medicine. For all therapies, regardless of how we name them, have an underlying energetic basis. As a focus, energy gives us a synthetic perspective: we all have much to learn from one another!

> There is this medicine and that medicine, and this method and that method, and then there is the way the body really is. (Kerry Weinstein, pers. com., 1995)

This sentiment is complemented by noted biologist E.O. Wilson (1994), who advocates *naturalism*, a philosophy of realism informed by scientific knowledge of the world as it actually is. Naturalism as applied to medicine is a vigorously honest and hardheaded approach to biological problem-solving that transcends competition, politics, academic promotions, grantsmanship, or the profitability of biomedical technologies.

Inquiring along naturalistic lines can bridge the historic intellectual barriers, fears, scepticism, disparagement and outright ridicule that have separated various approaches that have common and worthy goals. For the marvels of biomedicine and biotechnology are crude in comparison to the ancient evolutionary wisdom of the human body, which still possesses secrets and sophistication beyond our dreams. The future of our medicine depends on our willingness to broaden the scope of our inquiries and investigate the marvellous reality of living systems.

Common goals, common denominators

All providers of health care have in common a deep interest in the human body's inherent systems for self-defence and self-repair. A goal of energy medicine is to explain the energetic processes involved in accomplishing these remarkable tasks. Modern science and complementary therapies are converging on valuable new perspectives on the body's built-in defence and repair systems.

A common denominator to all therapies is two or more living organisms interacting at many different levels and through many different forms of energetic communications. Another common denominator is *living matter*, the pinnacle of evolution, a substance with properties that continue to astonish us.

Remarkable advances in our understanding of biological communications and living matter are changing the landscape of contemporary therapy and biomedical research. To be specific, we are seeing the emergence of:

- softer, gentler, more effective and more cost-effective therapies for both physical and emotional traumas of all kinds
- logical hypotheses for phenomena that have previously seemed inexplicable
- new understandings of chronic and intractable disorders that have been virtually unapproachable in the past
- new possibilities and challenges for basic research
- the winding down of old and emotional controversies and dogmatic attitudes about energy in relation to life and healing.

Introducing an energetic paradigm

In every culture and in every medical tradition before ours, healing was accomplished by moving energy. (Albert Szent-Györgyi, 1960)

Introducing an energy paradigm is not a matter of creating something new, because energy medicines are ancient. Instead, what is being replaced is the confusion, controversy and intellectual bias that has prevented mainstream science from giving serious consideration to energetic therapies.

Part of the paradigm process is to appreciate the pioneers of the field who did brilliant work that was ahead of its time, and therefore did not receive the attention it deserved. Several of these scientists have been particularly influential to the author, and will be referred to in the text: Albert Szent-Györgyi, Harold Saxton Burr, Ida P. Rolf, Herbert Fröhlich, E. Edward Adolph, John Zimmerman, Donald Ingber and Robert O. Becker. For the therapist or biomedical researcher interested in energetics, the writings and discoveries of these individuals are highly recommended. Another aspect of any paradigm is to develop testable hypotheses to guide research. This chapter leads to several such hypotheses. These are presented in the open-minded yet critical spirit of scientific inquiry. Success of any hypothesis is not measured by its acceptance or rejection, but in the new insights that emerge as it is being tested:

One sometimes finds what one is not looking for. (Sir Alexander Fleming, 1932)

A history of controversy and confusion

Historically, energetic approaches to healing have been immensely popular, but have also been surrounded with superstition, fear and controversy. Invisible energies are simultaneously part of competing systems of natural philosophy: scientific, magical, alchemical, religious, metaphysical and mystical. Within science there have been bitter arguments about the existence of 'healing energy' and 'life force'. The resulting debates have engaged leading biologists for centuries, and go to the core of our understanding of life and the nature of the material world (see Oschman, 1996a, for a review).

For various historical and emotional reasons, the words 'energy' and 'touch' continue to be unmentionable in some polite academic circles. There are still some thoughtful persons who regard the whole subject of energy medicine as off limits to science and inquiry. Many serious scholars continue to label any discussion of this kind with words such as 'flaky', 'twilight zone', 'hokum' and 'new age gobbledygook' (Chaitow, 1998). Methods involving energy exchanges between therapist and patient have been given the same credence as voodoo, angels and flying saucers. It is commonly stated, incorrectly, that there is not a shred of evidence for energetic interactions between organisms.

This situation is undergoing rapid change because of a large and growing body of reliable scientific information relating to the biology of energy. This knowledge is clarifying many issues that have been mysterious, confusing and bitterly controversial in the past.

Much of the work has been done by academic scientists, in laboratories around the world, who are seeking answers to basic questions about how the living body works, using conventional logic and methodology. Taken together, their discoveries provide the substance of an energetic paradigm or model of the living state, in health and disease.

Understanding the picture of the living body that is emerging from current research involves contemplating a number of concepts that may not be entirely familiar to those who are not continuously immersed in the biophysical literature. In this chapter an effort is made to present these in a logical manner that makes sense to the non-specialist. In a later section, 'Adding it all up', we attempt to put many of these ideas together with a brief summary. Some of the key concepts that will be presented are:

- the blueprint for the body
- the nature of biological regulations
- communications – chemical, electrical, electronic
- solid-state biochemistry
- continuum
- the cytoskeleton
- integrins
- tensegrity
- physiological integration
- cell crawling
- phase shifts
- crystallinity
- piezoelectricity
- metabolic regeneration
- Wolff's law
- semiconduction
- hydration

- proticity
- the electromagnetic code
- metastability
- solitons
- memory
- cooperativity, collectivity, synergy
- electromagnetic signatures of molecules
- Fourier analysis
- scalar waves.

Stating the problems of defence and repair

A key to the prevention of disease is the ability of the body to defend itself against infectious agents, parasites or inappropriate growths (tumours). A key to the repair of injuries is the intricate cascade of physiological activities and adjustments that take place after any trauma. Even the smallest pin-prick affects millions of cells. Waves of chemical and electromagnetic messages ripple outward in all directions from a site of injury. An intricate web of feedback and feedforward regulatory pathways oversees the repair process, and then winds it down when healing is complete (Marchesi, 1985). Some activities persist for weeks or more after an injury.

Vital processes must be maintained during repair. This may require temporary shifting of functions to other parts or systems or pathways. In terms of the processing of information, tissue repair is even more intricate and impressive than the formation of the organism. For repair requires access to both the organism's original 'blueprint' or structural plan, and to a temporary 'alternative plan' that maintains essential functions while the damaged tissue is being restored.

Cells migrating into a wound or a tumour must be replaced by cell division. If the problem is extensive, clotting, inflammatory reactions or tumour resorption consume cells which must be replaced by proliferation of undifferentiated stem cells in distant organs, such as the lymph nodes, bone marrow or liver. Healing therefore involves an array of dynamic interactions between local and systemic processes. Fever, allergic reactions, and the 'fight or flight' responses are all examples of restorative and life-saving systemic regulations.

Clinicians recognize that the best healing takes place when the body's own systems repair an injury or halt the spread of a disease. Serious problems arise when normal defence and repair mechanisms fail. This can lead to chronic progressive degenerative diseases, which are now the most costly part of the health care budget and the leading cause of death.

Our energetic perspective focuses on the living matrix through which signals move throughout the body, and the kinds of signals that are involved. This matrix is the same matrix through which cells crawl to carry out the essential functions described above. Many complementary therapies have their beneficial effects by opening pathways for both communications and cell migrations.

In the past, the major focus of biological communication has been on chemical factors. It is now being realized that other kinds of messages are involved. Some of these are electrical, analogous to the conduction of electrons through wires. Other messages are electronic or protonic, involving semiconduction through the living fabric and/or its associated layers of water. We shall discuss these phenomena in some detail below.

The blueprint

The concept of a 'blueprint' for the body is important for both biology and for therapeutics. Each wound and each disease is different, and the body's response must be precisely appropriate. When an injury occurs, we watch in amazement while the body restores itself, within certain limits, to the way it was before. This remarkable process implies a relationship between repair mechanisms and the informational systems that define and organize one's unique body structure and features, as well as the detailed architecture of every part. Moreover, damaged tissue is replaced with tissue of the same kind, rather than with tissue of a different kind. Bones are repaired with bone tissue, skin with skin of appropriate thickness, mucous membranes with mucous membranes, etc. Hence wound repair must activate the elusive and controversial 'form-giving' forces that biologists have been debating for centuries.

Concepts of a blueprint in relation to energy fields emerged during the period 1935–56 from the research of a distinguished scientist at Yale University School of Medicine, Professor Harold Saxton Burr. His research indicated that the beginnings of disease can be detected in the energy field of the body *before* physical symptoms appear (Burr, 1972). Moreover, Burr was convinced that the progress of physical symptoms could be reversed by restoring the energy field to its normal or balanced state.

Concepts of balancing energy have been part of acupuncture theory for millennia, but Burr's conclusions were ahead of their time in terms of Western science. Medical researchers around the world are now confirming many of those conclusions. Dozens of medical research groups are using SQUID magnetometers to map the ways diseases alter biomagnetic fields around the body (see Oschman, 1997a). Independently, clinical researchers are applying pulsating magnetic fields to stimulate healing (discussed below). Again, sensitive individuals have long been able to detect and project energy with their hands, but, until recently, science has been sceptical because of a lack of a logical explanation.

Burr was convinced that the 'fields of life' are the basic blueprints for all living things. He described how fields reflect physical and mental conditions. Burr also noted that the fields of organisms are inevitably affected by the larger fields of the planet and other celestial bodies. The mechanisms by which these influences are exerted are not mystical or obscure – they involve well-documented pathways of interaction. For example, sunspots and the cycles of the moon cause changes in geophysical fields which in turn influence living fields. Life on earth is not isolated from the rest of the universe, but is susceptible to forces extending across vast distances of space. This picture, carefully explored by Burr, has been confirmed, and has considerable therapeutic significance (reviewed by Oschman, 1997b).

'Spontaneous' healing

Most of us prefer a medicine that enables us to get over our physical or emotional sicknesses or injuries immediately, if not sooner. The phenomenon of 'spontaneous remission' is a dramatic indication of our innate potential to recover from the most devastating conditions. Clinical experience has shown that rapid and spontaneous remissions can and do happen, even for the most potent cancers or for the most catastrophic of injuries. This fact shows that, under the appropriate conditions, disease fighting and repair processes in the body can be very powerful.

Spontaneous healing is rare and unpredictable, but there are enough well-documented examples of individuals quickly and permanently recovering from 'terminal' and 'uncurable' conditions to stimulate research into how this can happen. Some scientists are attempting to induce spontaneous remissions 'on demand', by triggering the body's own defences against cancer. While there are few answers, it does appear that:

> . . . all the circuitry and machinery is there; the problem is simply to discover how to turn on the right switches to activate the process. (Andrew Weil, 1995)

I have personally seen enough instances of both conventional and complementary practitioners 'turning the right switches' or 'jump starting the healing process' to know that an understanding of spontaneous healing may not be as far away as we might think. Modern research, complemented by the observations of energy therapists, is teaching us about where to look for the 'circuits' and the 'switches'.

Just as exciting as spontaneous healing is the work on the healing of emotional trauma and abuse. Those who suffer from such afflictions can be just as debilitated as those who have a chronic disease. To free a life from emotional pain and agony can be immensely rewarding (e.g. Redpath, 1994).

In the past, the most remarkable success stories of complementary therapists (as well as healings in the religious context) were often dismissed because there was no logical explanation. The practitioners themselves usually could add little in the way of clarification. By bringing recent science into the picture, we are finding the missing links in our images of the human body in health and disease.

Background to the living matrix concept

One of the most important developments in recent science is a better understanding of the structure and energetics of the material substrate of the body – the living substance that is touched and interacted with in all therapeutic approaches. For the hands-on therapist, the energetic properties of this living substance have both conceptual and practical consequences. To understand the new developments, we begin with breakthroughs in our understandings of the cell.

A few decades ago, the living cell was visualized as a membrane-bound bag containing a solution of molecules. Figure 1.1(a) shows a cell as it is often illustrated in texts. Note that the cell is embedded in a fibrous material, called the connective tissue or extracellular matrix. This matrix contains large amounts of a fascinating protein called collagen. Most of the cell interior appears 'empty' in the drawing. Illustrations like this are still widely used today, even though they omit one of the most important attributes of cell structure.

The main reason the image shown in Figure 1.1(a) has persisted, and can still be found in modern texts, is that most biochemists were in agreement that life consists of a sequence of chemical reactions taking place in a 'soup' or solution within the cell. For example, consider glycolysis, the sequential breakdown of sugar molecules by 10 'soluble' enzymes (Figure 1.1(b)). Glycolysis and other biochemical pathways were discovered with techniques in which tissues and cells are broken apart. Centrifugation was then used to separate the dissolved molecules from the solids, which were discarded, because they were not considered important.

The biochemical image of life is as follows: there are 'particles', the enzymes, proteins, amino acids, sugars, etc., that randomly diffuse about within the enclosed volume of the cell. When appropriate molecules chance to bump into each other, they interact, and chemical bonds are formed or broken. In this way, chemical energy is liberated, living structures are assembled or taken apart, toxins are broken down, and life's activities are carried out. Figure 1.1(c) represents this 'random walk' image of the steps in glycolysis.

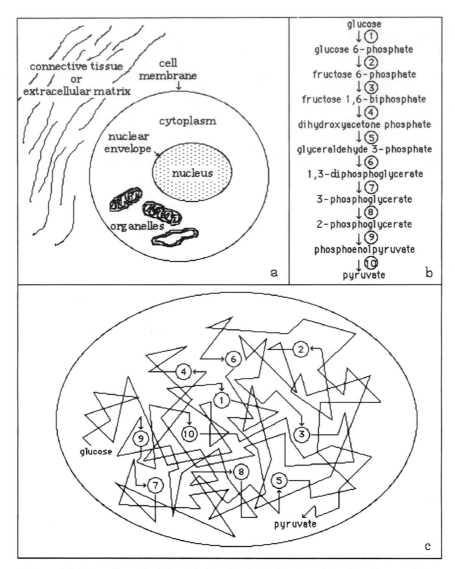

Figure 1.1 The cell and 'solution biochemistry'. (a) A cell as it is often illustrated in texts. Most of the cell interior appears 'empty'. Illustrations like this are still widely used today, even though they omit some of the most important attributes of cell structure. Note that the cell is embedded in a fibrous material, called the connective tissue or extracellular matrix. This matrix contains large amounts of a fascinating protein called collagen. (b) An enzymatic pathway, glycolysis, as it is usually depicted in texts. The 10 glycolytic enzymes convert glucose into pyruvate in a series of steps. (c) The 'bag of solution' model of the cell. The 10 enzymes of glycolysis float about in the solution, and reactants randomly diffuse about until they chance to bump into the next enzyme in the sequence. The probability of locating the next enzyme is enhanced because there are many copies of each enzyme floating about. However, the delays built into system make it a relatively slow process

Early electron microscopy confirmed that cells contain substantial amounts of 'empty' space. It was assumed that this is where metabolism takes place.

The torrent of information and clinical applications developed from this 'molecular soup' view of the cell led to an attitude that 'there are only a few problems remaining, and we will soon be able to answer all of them, using this same, incredibly successful, approach'. Physiologists seized the 'bag of solution' model of cell structure, and conducted decades of research in which an underlying assumption was that substances crossing a layer of cells, such as the intestinal wall, simply diffuse through the fluid compartments inside the cells.

The cell is not a bag

This picture is changing slowly but dramatically because of the discovery that the cell is *not* a

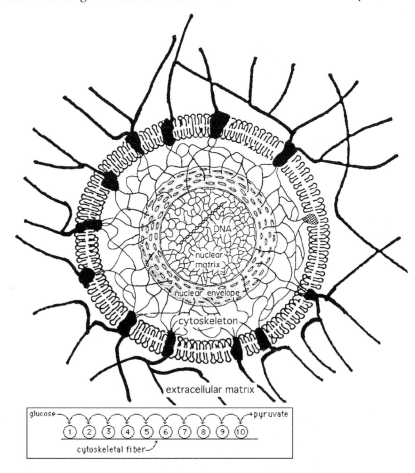

Figure 1.2 Contemporary image of a cell and its relations: *the living matrix.* Modern cell biology has recognized that the cell interior is virtually filled with fibres and tubes and filaments, collectively called the cytoskeleton or cytoplasmic matrix. Likewise, the nucleus contains a nuclear matrix that supports the genetic material. Linkers called integrins extend across the cell surface, connecting the cytoskeleton with the extracellular matrix. The entire system is termed *the living matrix.* The inset shows a more realistic model of a biochemical pathway, glycolysis, in which the enzymes are organized in sequence along the cytoskeletal structure. The reaction sequence can proceed very rapidly because reactants are passed from one enzyme to the next to the next, as in an assembly line.

bag of solution. The more closely biologists and microscopists looked at cells, the more structures they found. With better preparation techniques, electron microscopists began to see within cells the material that the biochemists had been discarding when they purified the 'soluble' enzymes.

We now know that the cell is so filled with filaments and tubes and fibres and trabeculae, collectively called the cytoplasmic matrix or cytoskeleton, that there is little space left for a solution of randomly diffusing 'billiard ball' molecules (Figure 1.2). Moreover, there is very little water inside cells that can dissolve the 'soluble' enzymes. Virtually all the cell water is bound in particular ways to the cellular framework (e.g. Cope, 1967; Corongiu and Clementi, 1981).

Many of the enzymes that were previously thought to be 'floating about' within the cytoplasmic soup are actually attached to structures within the cell and nucleus (see the inset to Figure 1.2; Oschman, 1984; Ingber, 1993b). These attachments are delicate, however, and biochemical homogenization techniques detach enzymes and other proteins from the cellular and nuclear scaffolds that support them in actual living cells. 'Solution biochemistry', while quite instructive, is an artefact:

. . . the empirical fact that a given molecule appears primarily in the 'soluble' fraction may divert attention from the cataclysmic violence of the most gentle homogenization procedure. (McConkey, 1982)

Most textbooks still show metabolic pathways as a sequence of steps (Figure 1.1(b)), without mentioning the essential *structural* or *solid state* context in which the chemistry of life takes place.

Continuum

Soon after the cytoskeleton became a popular subject for research, it was realized that the cellular matrix is connected, across the cell surface, with the connective tissue system or extracellular matrix (also shown in Figure 1.2). A whole class of 'transmembrane' linking molecules, or 'integrins', has been discovered.

Likewise, it is now recognized that the cytoplasmic matrix also links to the nuclear envelope, nuclear matrix and genes.

Conceptually, these discoveries are profoundly important. The boundaries between the cell environment, the cell interior and the genetic material are not as sharp or impermeable as we once thought. As a hands-on therapist, what you touch is not merely the skin – you contact a continuous interconnected webwork that extends throughout the body. Indeed, the skin is one of the first tissues in which this continuity was documented (see Figure 1.3; Ellison and Garrod, 1984).

The entire interconnected system has been called the connective tissue/cytoskeleton (Oschman, 1994), the tissue–tensegrity matrix (tensegrity will be taken up in a later section; Pienta and Coffey, 1991), or, simply, *the living matrix*. A popular acupuncture text refers to 'the web that has no weaver' (Kaptchuk, 1983).

The living matrix is a continuous and dynamic 'supramolecular' webwork, extending into every nook and cranny of the body: a nuclear matrix within a cellular matrix within a connective tissue matrix. In essence, when you touch a human body, you are touching a continuously interconnected system, composed of virtually all of the molecules in the body linked together in an intricate webwork.

The living matrix has no fundamental unit or central aspect, no part that is primary or most basic. The properties of the whole net depend upon the integrated activities of all of the components. Effects on one part of the system can and do spread to others.

This is an important image of the structure of the living body. Our images shape our therapeutic successes because they can give rise to specific intentions. Intentions are not trivial, because they give rise to specific patterns of electrical and magnetic activity in the nervous system of the therapist that can spread through their body and into the body of a patient (for a summary of this fascinating subject, see Oschman, 1998).

While it is obviously useful to study the various parts and systems of the body, each component can be regarded as a local domain or subdivision of a continuous web. The shape, form, mechanical, energetic and functional characteristics of every cell, tissue or organ

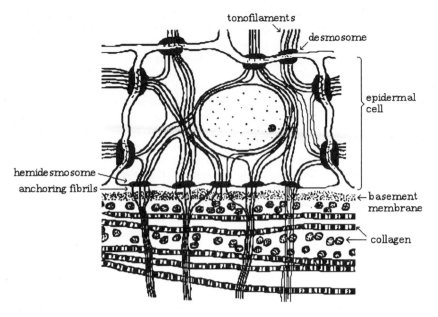

Figure 1.3 The epidermal–dermal continuum. Ellison and Garrod (1984) and others cited by them have described the epidermal–dermal junction in detail. Adjacent epidermal cells are attached to each other by desmosomes, and are anchored to the dermal connective tissue by hemidesmosomes. All of the anchors are traversed by tonofilaments, which form a continuous fibrous matrix joining together all epidermal cells, throughout the skin. Anchoring fibrils link the cellular matrix with the connective tissue. The dermal connective tissue in part of a continuous integrated system extending throughout the body. The cytoskeletons of all other cells in the body are similarly linked to the connective tissue system. Reproduced by permission of the *Journal of Cell Science* and the Company of Biologists Ltd

arise because of local variations in the properties of the matrix. The genome, within the nuclear matrix, is a subdivision of this network.

We shall see that an even more profound realization is emerging. The entire living matrix is simultaneously a mechanical, vibrational or oscillatory, energetic and informational network (Pinta and Coffey, 1991; Oschman, 1994). Hence the entire composite of physiological and regulatory processes we refer to as 'the living state' take place within the context of a continuous living matrix.

A sensible design for a living system is one in which every cell receives information on the activities taking place in every other part of the body (Adolph, 1982):

The integrated human body is the sum of thousands of physiological processes and traits working together. Each breath and each heartbeat involves the working together of countless events. Huge numbers of functions are carried on simultaneously. The parts and processes within an organism are woven together with great intricacy. Coordination occurs at a thousand points. If there were no integration of activities, life would be a random jumble of physical and chemical events that reaches no known accomplishment. In actuality, each process is of consequence to the whole.

Physiological integration is possible because every cell and every molecule fine-tunes its activities appropriately. While the diffusion of chemicals from place to place is one important means of communication, it is too slow a process to account for the rapid and subtle aspects of the living process. We are now discerning that the living matrix itself is a high-speed communication network linking every part with every other.

Matrix dynamics: signalling and cell crawling

Recently there has been tremendous excitement in the research community about the properties of the living matrix. The excitement arises because the matrix has key roles in defence and repair. Moreover, it is through this matrix that nutrients, hormones and other signal molecules, toxins and waste products diffuse to and from all cells.

The molecules that link the cell interior with the extracellular matrix have come to be called *integrins*. From the introduction to a recent review of the subject, by Horwitz (1997):

> Integrins are a class of adhesion molecules that 'glue' cells in place. Surprisingly, at a fundamental level, they also regulate most functions of the body. The author reveals the hidden role of integrins in arthritis, heart disease, stroke, osteoporosis and the spread of cancer.

The living matrix is a dynamic rather than a fixed system. The connections between adjacent cells, and between the cells and the substrate, are labile rather than permanent. Connections form, break and reform as cells change shape and/or crawl about. Specific connectors, called tonofilaments, desmosomes, hemidesmosomes, integrins, connexins and anchoring filaments, are all labile structures that can disconnect, retract, dissolve and reform (Krawczyk and Wilgram, 1973; Gabbiani *et al.*, 1978). These reversible adhesions enable epidermal cells, fibroblasts, osteoblasts and other 'generative' cells to move about when necessary to repair (re-epithialize) damaged skin and restore other tissues. Amoeboid motions enable leukocytes to migrate to sites of infection, or into tumours for resorption of 'non-self' material.

Treating the matrix rather than the symptoms

There are two ways to approach a disease or disorder. One is to focus on the observable problem, and try to fix it; the other is to work upon the context or matrix in which the natural restorative processes are carried out. Many complementary therapies focus on the matrix rather than on the symptoms.

For example, researchers have studied the vital cytoskeletal links joining the cell surface and the nucleus. The cellular framework carries essential information from the cell surface to the genome, and in the opposite direction. If this information transfer is compromised, by disrupting the cytoskeleton, cells lose many important controls and 'social' restraints, and can become autonomous from the organism. When cells lose proper cell contact, recognition and positional controls, and escape from immune surveillance, they can multiply in unregulated fashion, producing unlimited growth and tumours (Nicolson, 1976; Puck, 1977).

Many of the seemingly miraculous consequences of hands-on bodywork arise because of the capacity of the entire living matrix to undergo dramatic changes or 'phase shifts'. These changes are possible, in part, because of the energetic properties of the living matrix. To understand these energetic properties, we need to introduce solid state biochemistry.

Solid state biochemistry

As we discussed above, biochemistry was founded on the study of reactions taking place in solution. The discovery of the cytoskeleton, with its dynamic interconnections with the nuclear and connective tissue matrices, has advanced our understanding of *solid state biochemistry*.

The development of this field obviously does not reject the beautiful and profoundly important work done by biochemists and molecular biologists on the 'soluble' enzymes and their activities. Instead, solid state biochemistry opens up the study of additional processes taking place on and in the solid fibres and filaments that constitute living cells and tissues. This approach also opens up a deeper understanding of the effects of hands-on, structural, energetic and biomechanical therapies on processes taking place throughout the body.

Solution biochemistry required that the molecules within the cell diffuse about more or less randomly until they bump into appropriate enzymes (Figure 1.1(c)). Solid state biochemistry recognizes that chemical reactions proceed in a much more orderly and rapid manner if they are organized on a structural framework (inset of Figure 1.2). Moreover, the living matrix concept opens up the possibilities for global control: signals travelling *in* the matrix can regulate or fine-tune matrix-associated enzymes throughout the organism. Here we distinguish between messages that travel *through* the matrix, as by diffusion through the interstitial fluid lying between its fibres, and messages travelling *in* the matrix itself, as by electronic conduction along the protein backbone, or by hopping of protons in the layers of water associated with the protein surface (Ho and Knight, 1998). We shall detail the mechanisms involved in matrix communication in the next sections.

A mechanism for matrix control of protein conformation has been proposed by Fröhlich (1988b): oscillations set up in particular regions of the DNA (regions referred to as 'junk' or 'selfish' DNA) give rise to informational signals that spread throughout the body, and energize particularly effective conformations of the various enzymes attached to the living matrix. This is a fascinating concept with enormous implications for the theory and practice of hands-on therapies and for our understanding of spontaneous healing.

To understand the therapeutic significance of solid state biochemistry and matrix regulation, we begin with an examination of the high degree of order, or regularity, or crystallinity present in cells and tissues.

Crystalline arrays in cells and tissues; piezoelectricity

Form, in contradistinction to random shape, contains parts or elements in a definite, characteristically recurrent array in space. Thus form is the result of the orderly manner in which those elements are combined and arranged. Form of a higher order of complexity accordingly can emerge from the ordered assembly of simpler formed elements of mutual fit. (Weiss, 1965)

We do not intuitively consider biological materials to be crystalline, because when we think of crystals we usually think of hard materials, like diamond or agate. Living crystals are composed of long, thin, pliable molecules, and are soft and flexible. To be more precise, they are liquid crystals (e.g. Bouligand, 1978). Crystalline arrangements are the rule and not the exception in living systems. Figure 1.4 gives some important examples.

Physicists know a great deal about the properties of crystals. The information they have obtained is of considerable medical importance. For example, certain kinds of crystals are piezoelectric, i.e. they generate electric fields when they are compressed or stretched. Physiologists are aware of this, and have studied the generation of electricity by bone. Each step you take compresses bones in the legs and elsewhere, and generates characteristic electrical fields.

The piezoelectric effect is not confined to bone. Virtually all of the tissues in the body generate electric fields when they are compressed or stretched (see Oschman, 1981). The piezoelectric effect is partly responsible for these electric fields. Another source of such fields is a phenomenon known as streaming potentials. The relative contribution of these two ways of generating electric fields in tissues is under investigation (e.g. MacGinitie, 1995).

The important point is that when a bone or cartilage is compressed, when a tendon or ligament stretches, or when the skin is stretched or bent, as at a joint, minute electric pulsations are set up. These oscillations, and their harmonics, are precisely representative of the forces acting on the tissues involved. In other words, they contain *information* on the precise nature of the movements taking place. This information is electrically and electronically conducted through the surrounding living matrix. One of the roles of this information is in the control of form.

The control of body structure

The therapeutic and physiological importance of the piezoelectric and other electronic properties of tissues is that they provide a framework for understanding how the body adapts to the ways it is used (Oschman, 1989). It has long been recognized that bones and other elements of connective tissue are constantly remodelling

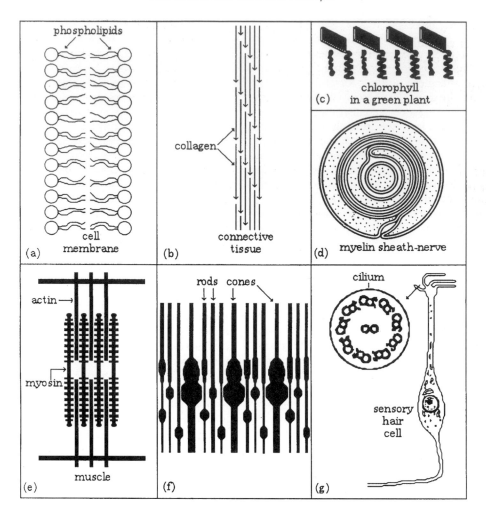

Figure 1.4 Crystalline arrangements in various tissues. Crystalline arrangements are the rule and not the exception in living systems. (a) Arrays of phospholipid molecules form cell membranes. (b) Collagen arrays form connective tissue. (c) Arrays of chlorophyll molecules in the leaf. (d) The myelin sheath of nerves. Each layer is composed of membranes such as shown in (a). (e) The contractile array in muscle, composed of actin and myosin molecules organized around each other. (f) The array of sensory endings in the retina. (g) Arrays of microtubules, microfilaments and other fibrous components of the cytoskeleton occur in nerves and other kinds of cells. Here are the cilia of sensory organs such as those responsible for detecting odours and sound

in response to the loads imposed upon them. From the biochemical perspective, this is referred to as 'metabolic regeneration', a process discovered and documented by Schoenheimer and colleagues over half a century ago (Schoenheimer, 1942; Ratner, 1979).

The electric fields produced during movements are widely considered to provide the information that directs the activities of 'generative' cells (e.g. Bassett *et al.*, 1964; Bassett, 1971). These are the osteoblasts, myoblasts, perivascular cells, fibroblasts and other 'stem' cells that lay down or resorb collagen and thereby reform tissues so they can adapt to the ways the body is used. This regulatory concept dates to Wolff, in 1892 (see Bassett, 1968):

Wolff's law: The form of the bone (or other connective tissue) being given, the bone elements (collagen) place or displace themselves in the direction of the functional pressure and increase or decrease their mass to reflect the amount of functional pressure.

Again, these concepts are highly relevant to the hands-on, energetic or movement therapist. They provide the basis for progressive changes in body structure that take place because of the ways an individual uses their body in relation to gravity, because of habits or injuries. They also provide a basis for the restorative measures that can be used to correct gravity-related disorders (Rolf, 1962; Oschman, 1997c).

Solid state properties of molecular arrays

The beginnings of solid state biochemistry and the continuum concept can be traced to a landmark paper published simultaneously in *Science* and *Nature* by Albert Szent-Györgyi (1941a, 1941b):

If a great number of atoms be arranged with regularity in close proximity, as for example in a crystal lattice, single valency electrons cease to belong to one or two atoms only, and belong instead to the whole system. A great number of molecules may join to form energy continua, along which energy, namely excited electrons, may travel a certain distance.

Many years later, Szent-Györgyi (1963) summarized how he reached the above conclusion:

It was at an early date that I began to feel that the wonderful subtlety of biological reactions could not be produced solely by molecules, but had to be produced partly by much smaller and more mobile units which could hardly be anything else than electrons. The main actors of life had to be electrons whereas the clumsy and unreactive protein molecules had to be the stage on which the drama of life was enacted. Electrons, to be mobile, need a conductor, which led me to the conclusion that proteins have to be electronic conductors. Toward the end of the 1930's theories began to appear about the submolecular structure of condensed matter. This opened the possibility of electronic mobility in proteins, and thus in 1941 I proposed that proteins may be conductors.

The importance of Szent-Györgyi's prophetic statement is that it recognizes a fundamental process taking place within the crystalline domains of cells and tissues and throughout the body. The process involves certain electrons that are free to move about within crystal lattices. These electrons are therefore capable of conducting energy and information throughout the whole system.

The continuous fabric described above, the living matrix, then, becomes an energetic and informational continuum. The preventive and restorative effects of many hands-on therapies result from improving the flow of energy and information throughout the body. This is a concept that is part of the theory underlying a variety of approaches, from acupuncture to zero balancing. The dramatic and progressive benefits of these approaches have been ignored by the biomedical sciences because it appeared that they lacked any underlying scientific logic. Szent-Györgyi's prophetic statement of semiconduction, and the work on electronic biology that followed, has led to an enlightened and sophisticated explanation of the significance of energy and information flows in living systems.

Solid state physics recognizes several types of materials in relation to how well electronic energy flows through them. There are conductors, which can conduct electricity well; there are insulators, which cannot; and there are intermediate materials, the semiconductors, that can conduct electricity to some extent.

After a period of great scepticism, during which it appeared that Szent-Györgyi's 1941 statement was entirely wrong, there emerged a new field of research on the electronic and other solid state properties of molecules. This research continues to gather momentum today. While Szent-Györgyi suggested that the proteins in the body are *conductors*, research soon revealed that they are actually *semiconductors*. Virtually all of the molecules in the body are semiconductors (Rosenberg and Postow, 1969).

Moreover, it has been found that electrons are not the only entities that travel about within the molecular arrays in living systems. A variety of other charge or energy or information carriers are probably present as well. Some of them are listed below:

- electrons
- holes
- phonons
- photons
- excitons
- protons
- solitons
- polarons
- conformons.

The importance of water

In considering the living matrix as a whole system, it is profoundly important to recognize that its constituents are everywhere coated with layers of water. This water is not ordinary liquid water, because its properties are modified in important ways by the close association with the molecules comprising the living matrix continuum. This hydration layer is organized in part by electrical fields surrounding the charged groups on the various matrix molecules. The water film is several layers thick, and each layer has different properties. Some water molecules are trapped within the protein, and are so tightly bound that they cannot be removed by any method. The next water layer, close to the surface of a molecule, is highly ordered, and subsequent layers are less structured.

There is evidence that the chain-like layer of water associated with the living matrix forms a continuous system of its own, with important roles in regulation and communication. The 'messages' conducted through the water system are carried by protons. This is called '*proticity*' to distinguish it from *elec*tricity (Mitchell, 1976). The importance of these forms of signalling has been summarized (Feigelson, 1969; Oschman, 1994; Ho and Knight, 1998) but has not been widely appreciated.

Discussions of the important discoveries about water and information conduction are found in technical journals of physics and electronics. Biologists who are aware of this research have learned a great deal about the ways living systems process energy and information at the molecular and atomic levels.

Solid state biochemistry is developing new and important explanations for aspects of systemic regulation that have been difficult to explain in the past. Robert O. Becker is one of the scientists who has confirmed the presence of semiconduction in living systems, and applied the information to the study of injury repair (Becker, 1990a, 1991; Oschman, 1996a).

The challenge:

> What is urgently needed is to be able to read the language of electromagnetic biocommunication to complement our understanding of the genetic code. (Smith, 1994)

We now know some of the 'letters' in the electromagnetic or energetic language or code (see list above), and the next step is to determine how they are organized into words and sentences. An important key comes from research on biological coherence.

Biological coherence

For those who are interested in the science behind energetic therapies, there is no recent literature that is more significant than that of Herbert Fröhlich and the scientists who have followed in his footsteps. This research is of such importance for therapists that we have written a 'review and commentary' on a book edited by Fröhlich (1988a), *Biological Coherence and Response to External Stimuli*. Our summary explains the important work of Fröhlich and his colleagues in terms that can be comprehended by therapists who may not have an extensive background in biophysics (Oschman and Oschman, 1994).

Fröhlich was widely recognized in the physics community for the development of modern theories of crystalline or highly ordered non-living materials. Based on his expertize on the physics of crystals, Fröhlich was quite impressed by the living cell membrane. Membranes are very thin liquid crystal arrays, and have enormous electrical fields across them (Figure 1.5).

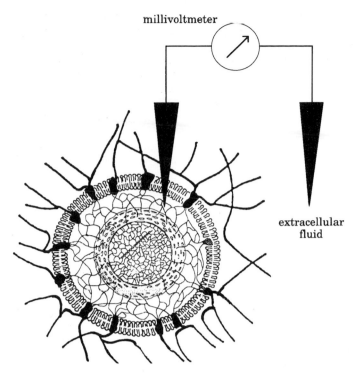

millivoltmeter

extracellular
fluid

Figure 1.5 Electrical field across the cell membrane. The potential across
the cell surface can be measured between two microelectrodes connected
to a millivoltmeter. Both the extracellular fluid and cell interior are excellent
conductors, while the membrane is an insulator. The potential between
the extracellular fluid and the cell interior is typically 5–150 mV, with the
cytoplasm negative. The actual potential depends upon cell type and
cellular activities, and averages between 70 and 90 mV (Charman, 1990).
Since the membrane is very thin (of the order of some 7.5–10 nm), the field
strength amounts to some millions of volts per meter. Fröhlich's interest in
the application of coherence in biological systems was stimulated by the
realization that the liquid crystalline dipolar cell membrane molecules exist
in the context of this enormous electrical potential. That sparks or lightning
flashes do not jump across cell membranes attests to the ability of the
phospholipid bilayer to act as an electrical insulator. For many ordinary
insulating materials (e.g. transformer oil, paraffin, rubber, glass and
plastics) such a field strength would cause electrical breakdown.
Remarkably, nature has manufactured cell membranes with a dielectric
material that is charged very close to the electrical breakdown point, yet
continues to orchestrate electrical and non-electrical events in a controlled
and specific manner (Pethig, 1979)

On the basis of quantum mechanical calculations, Fröhlich predicted that the molecules
in a highly ordered system such as the cell membrane, under the influence of a very strong
electrical field, would vibrate strongly, and
would therefore radiate particular kinds of
signals. His calculations indicated that these
energies would be in the range of 10^{11}–10^{12}
cycles per second, which is in the microwave
and near infrared parts of the electromagnetic
spectrum. Moreover, the high degree of regularity of the components of the membrane
should give rise to an energy radiation that is
highly organized, or coherent. Likewise, a
system that generates coherent signals will
acquire much of its structural stability as a consequence of its coherent vibratory or oscillatory
nature.

A consequence of Fröhlich's analysis is that cell membranes should produce large coherent or laser-like oscillations that will move about within the organism and that will be radiated into the environment.

Coherence as a general property of living systems

Fröhlich's predictions have been confirmed by a number of investigators for a variety of living systems. In laboratories around the world, scientists are studying the roles of Fröhlich oscillations in a wide range of biological processes. In addition to the book edited by Fröhlich, there are a number of other monographs that can be consulted for this literature (Popp *et al.*, 1981, 1992; Rattemeyer and Popp, 1981; Ho, 1993, 1998; Allen *et al.*, 1994).

At the same time, cell membranes and other highly regular or crystalline systems such as those shown in Figure 1.4 can also display great sensitivity to energies present in the environment. The mechanism proposed by Fröhlich (1968a,b, 1970, 1974, 1975) involves the establishment of a finely-tuned, metastable energized state within a molecular array. Figure 1.6 defines what is meant by a metastable state, and distinguishes it from the stable and unstable conditions.

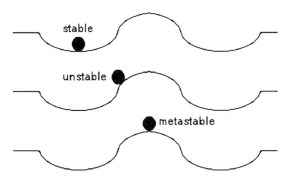

Figure 1.6 The metastable state. The dictionary defines metastable as marked by only a slight margin of stability. Consider a round ball in a bowl that has a convex bump in the centre. The *stable* configuration is with the ball in the lowest part of the 'valley'. If the ball is placed on the side of the bump, it is *unstable* – it will roll down into the valley. If the ball if balanced on top of the bump, it is *metastable* – it is temporarily stable, but will roll off if its balance is even slightly disturbed

This concept of metastability is of interest to therapists, who sometimes find that the tissues of their client are poised for a rapid and overall change (the 'phase change' mentioned earlier). A complementary concept is that of the *singular point* or *organizing centre*, a place on the surface of the body where a small input of energy will produce a large change (Chang, 1989).

An exceedingly weak signal of the appropriate frequency, applied to the appropriate area, disturbs the balance or equilibrium within a metastable array so that its components flip or rotate in space, releasing an amount of energy within the organism that is far in excess of that contained in the original signal. Hence, a crystalline macromolecular array can be a delicately-tuned and extremely sensitive detector, amplifier and processor of electromagnetic signals coming from other parts of the organism or from the environment. Such systems are able to detect minute signals, even when they are embedded in much stronger 'noise'.

Fröhlich's conclusions regarding cell membranes have been of great value to scientists attempting to understand how cells 'whisper' to one another, and pick up information from their environment (e.g. Adey, 1993).

Solitons

Occasionally, therapists notice a slow wave, a sort of shudder or vibration, that begins under their hands and spreads throughout the body. This is probably another coherent phenomenon known as a soliton wave.

A soliton is a fascinating type of wave. It is a solitary or singular wave that can occur on the ocean or in any other medium. An example is the tsunami or tidal wave produced by a submarine earthquake or volcanic eruption. These waves can carry a large amount of energy over a long distance without loss. In other words, in contrast to normal waves, solitons do not disperse or dissipate their energy by spreading out.

In the body, soliton waves appear to have beneficial effects, including the release and/or resolution of traumatic memories (Oschman, 1993). This is a fascinating subject, often experienced in the therapeutic setting but seldom discussed. We have presented a detailed model of how traumatic memories may be stored in tissues, accessed by coherent vibrations and released by solitons (Oschman and Oschman, 1995a,b).

A cooperative, collective or synergetic system

It is becoming fashionable to look at living systems as cooperative or collective or synergetic non-linear systems (e.g. Haken and Wagner, 1973; Haken, 1983; Fröhlich, 1988a). For the hands-on therapist, this may seem like a lot of fancy talk. It is not, for these concepts have direct and profound implications for clinical practice. It is the difference between a linear approach, in which the harder one presses, the more the effect, and a non-linear method, in which 'less is more' to use the homoeopathic principle. In essence, new and unexpected properties, or phase changes, can arise in non-linear systems after a small input of energy. This may occur as a consequence of the assembly of parts to produce structures and properties that cannot be predicted by looking at the parts. Again, Szent-Györgyi (1963) stated the situation in a memorable fashion:

> If Nature puts two things together she produces something new with new qualities, which cannot be expressed in terms of qualities of the components. When going from electrons and protons to atoms, from here to molecules, molecular aggregates, etc., up to the cell or the whole animal, at every level we find something new, a new breathtaking vista. Whenever we separate two things, we lose something, something which may have been the most essential feature.

Therapeutic and scientific approaches usually begin with a focus at the level of parts, and the practical understandings of the body that arise from studying their relations. After some experience, when techniques have been mastered, the 'breathtaking vistas' begin to open up.

Tensegrity

Tensegrity is a useful architectural and energetic concept developed by R. Buckminster Fuller (see Pugh, 1976). Tensegrity concepts underlie geodesic domes, tents, sailing vessels, and various stick-and-wire sculptures and toy models (Figure 1.7(a)). Tensegrity also provides a valuable perspective for therapists who work with the body from a structural, movement, biomechanical or solid state perspective.

A tensegrity system is characterized by a continuous tensional network (tendons) supported by a discontinuous set of compressive elements (struts). One might be inclined to place bones in the strut category, but this would be incorrect because bones contain both compressive and tensile fibres, and are therefore tensegrity systems unto themselves (Figure 1.7(b)). Attach tendons and muscles to the bones, and one has a three-dimensional tensegrity network that supports and moves the body (Figure 1.7(c)).

Tensegrity provides a conceptual link between the structural systems and the energy-informational systems we have been discussing. The body as a whole and the various parts, including the interiors of all cells and nuclei, can be visualized as tensegrity systems (Oschman, 1996b, 1998; Ingber, 1998).

Tensegrity accounts for the ability of the body to absorb impacts without being damaged. Mechanical energy flows away from a site of impact through the tensegrous living matrix. The more flexible and balanced the network (the better the tensional integrity), the more readily it absorbs shocks and converts them to *information* rather than *damage*.

This concept is useful for practitioners who work with athletes and other performers: flexible and well-organized fascia and myofascial relationships enhance performance and reduce the incidence of injuries.

Tensegrity also accounts for the fact that inflexibility or shortening in one tissue influences structure and movement in other parts. While a therapist may focus on improving flexibility and/or mobility of a particular part of the body, the effects can and do spread to other areas. This is, in part, due to the tensional

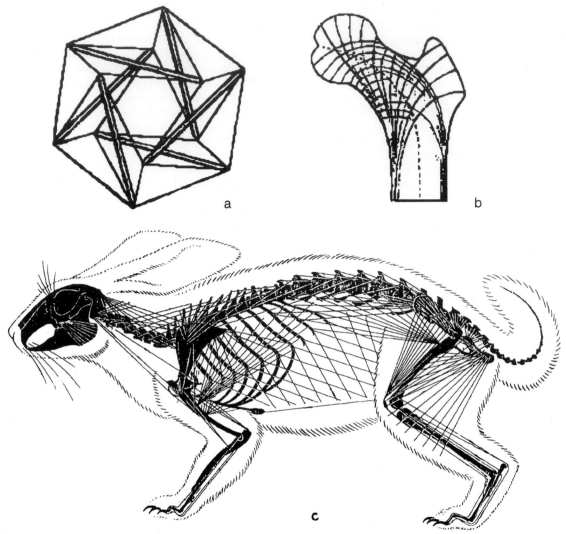

Figure 1.7 Tensegrity. A tensegrity system consists of a continuous network of tensile elements (called tendons) and a discontinuous system of compression members (called struts). Reproduced with permission of Oxford University Press from *The Life of Mammals* by J. Z. Young.

integrity of the system, but it is also due to the fact that the tensional system is a vibratory continuum. This can be demonstrated with a tensegrity model by plucking one of the tendons. This will cause the entire network to vibrate.

Since the living tensegrity network is simultaneously a mechanical and a vibratory continuum, restrictions in one part have both structural and energetic consequences for the entire organism. Structural integrity, vibratory integrity and energetic or informational integrity go hand in hand. One cannot influence the

structural system without influencing the energetic/informational system, and vice versa. Again, the highly trained athlete or other performer can describe what it feels like, energetically, to have a body that has tensional integrity.

Ingber and his colleagues have brought both tensegrity and solid state biochemistry concepts into biomedicine by describing how physical forces exerted on tensegrous molecular scaffolds regulate the biochemical pathways involved in determining biological patterns (the 'blueprint' mentioned earlier; Ingber, 1993a,b; Wang *et al.*,

1993). This work is important to the therapist because it describes how various kinds of manipulative methods can influence biochemical processes in important ways.

Finally, some of the most exciting therapeutic work the author is aware of involves establishing a conscious and deeply nourishing connection between the energy system of the therapist and the living matrix of the patient. These approaches can be invaluable in resolving chronic physical problems, but they are even more profoundly significant for the resolution of deeply repressed emotional trauma and abuse (e.g. Redpath, 1994).

Normal looking tissue can be compromised

Conventional medicine has a remarkable track record for correcting a wide range of problems. In spite of this, complementary practitioners have daily encounters with patients who are in pain or discomfort, and who have been told by their physician that nothing appears to be wrong. Often these patients have been probed with the full range of modern medical diagnostic technology. Many have been treated with a variety of drugs or surgery, with no change or even a worsening of their conditions, and with the development of side-effects that must also be treated.

What many complementary methods have in common is a recognition that tissue that appears to be 'normal' from the biomedical perspective can nevertheless be compromised in a variety of subtle but profoundly important ways. The reason for this is that complementary therapists can often perceive the 'quality' of the living matrix, and locate the places where the matrix is not functioning optimally. A variety of interventions can open up the network to the communications and cell migrations so essential to defence and repair processes. This is beneficial, regardless of the patient's problems.

Example

According to Western biomedicine, a broken leg is healed when the fracture has mended. The fact of a successful treatment can be confirmed with an X-ray. Many years after the injury, the patient may develop back problems that seem to have no immediate cause. The physician is unable to detect any pathology, and therefore prescribes a muscle relaxer or a pain medication in the hope that the condition will go away. In some cases, this works. In others, the condition persists or worsens, and more elaborate tests are ordered. These may lead to more invasive measures, such as surgery.

Energetics and treatment for back pain

The complementary therapist may take a quick look at the patient with low back pain, cited above, and ask when they broke their left leg. The therapist is not psychic, but has simply noticed a slight aberration in the individual's gait. This perception has an energetic basis. It may be visual, involving a sensitive awareness of how the patient moves in relation to the gravitational field. Or it may be an electric or magnetic field interaction, such as that documented by Schwartz *et al.* (1996).

The practitioner is detecting a remnant of an imbalanced movement pattern that arose many years ago, in part because the muscles in the injured leg became hypotoned while it was in a cast and/or while crutches were being used. And the muscles in the more active leg became hypertoned because of the extra loads imposed during the healing process.

When one leg is called upon to carry most of one's body weight, as well as the weight of a cast on the opposite, broken leg, the entire erector musculoskeletal system, from the feet to the top of the head, is affected, including the muscles that pass through and around the pelvis and attach to the vertebrae. Subtle remnants of such compensations can be retained in the tissues for decades, and give rise to problems at a much later date (Myers, 1997a,b).

Compensations accumulate and are 'remembered'

The back pain example documents an important concept that is relatively obvious and comprehensible to conventional medicine, but that is understood and applied far more widely in complementary therapies. A traumatic physical and/or emotional experience can force the body to compensate in various ways, such as by subtly altering posture and/or movement patterns.

A classic example is the limp that is activated after spraining an ankle. Pain is the teacher, and a new and temporary way of walking is the lesson. From the biological perspective, the limp is an appropriate and adaptive response that reduces motion and loading of the injured part while it heals. The neurophysiologist might describe the limp as a temporary change in a reflexive neuromuscular pattern, a response that is possible because of the plasticity of the nervous system.

While limps, casts, canes, crutches, braces and splints are temporary measures, they can leave subtle records in the body's structure and patterns of movement in the gravity field. The conventional physician recognizes this, and may recommend exercises to restore muscle strength in the affected area. While this may be beneficial, it can be a slow and discouraging process, because attention is focused on strengthening the injured part, and the overall biomechanics may not be addressed in a systematic manner. The success of Rolfing/structural integration lies in part from the systematic manner by which the overall biomechanics and energetics are addressed.

Complementary methods employ various ways of identifying subtle structural and functional imbalances that accumulate from injuries that appeared to heal but that nevertheless left subtle imprints upon the tissues. Imbalanced structure and function impact the circulation, lymphatics, immune, nervous and endocrine systems, and physiological processes involved in defence, repair and organization of structure.

One of the physiological lessons documented by the experiences of complementary medical practitioners is that tissues seem to 'remember' what has happened to them. A problem such as back pain can be the result of an accumulation of factors some time and some distance away from the place that hurts, rather than a single, reducible, isolable cause.

From the emotional perspective, traumatic injuries leave their marks in the form of repressed memories, and reduced physical or emotional flexibility that results from those

memories. Autonomic systems are inevitably affected. These are not trivial phenomena. Traumatic events can produce long-term compensations that can become debilitating and even life-threatening decades after they took place. Hence, our first hypothesis:

> Stresses, imbalances, and compensations that are not revealed by medical laboratory tests can nevertheless accumulate and compromise the body's ability to defend and repair itself.

While this hypothesis is not a major focus of biomedicine, it is reasonable and testable, and can contribute to our understanding of chronic degenerative and untreatable disorders. Energetic approaches to diagnosis can help resolve this situation. Here is a second hypothesis for consideration:

> The conundrum of chronic, progressive and intractable disorders arises in part because conventional medicine has no diagnostic measures for the properties of the living matrix. Diagnostic procedures based on energetics can help improve this situation.

Here we see one of the most costly (in terms of human suffering) consequences of the traditional bias that biomedicine has had against exploring energetic approaches. For example, acupuncture, in its tried and tested theory and practice, has a variety of diagnostic procedures for determining the health of the living matrix. The medicine of the future will integrate this ancient wisdom with emerging concepts of bioelectromagnetics.

As an organism develops, ages and experiences, the network of physiological compensations and adjustments becomes more intricate. There is a continuous range in ability to respond to genetic problems or injury or disease. Each life experience produces multiple rearrangements of the living matrix. This intricate situation cannot be understood as the sum of the behaviours of isolated parts:

> The reality (of disease) is the inability of one person's homeostasis, conditioned by his genotype and a lifetime of special

experiences, to maintain equilibrium; neither genes nor environment 'cause' disease, it is simply that the organism is unsuited for adaptive action in one, or several environments. (Childs, 1970)

Energy and diagnosis

Energetic approaches can revolutionize diagnostic procedures. This is possible because, as Harold Saxton Burr stated many years ago (see p. 6), every activity taking place within the organism broadcasts detailed energetic messages into the space around the body. The rationale behind this is straightforward: diseases and disorders alter the electromagnetic properties of molecules, cells, tissues, organs and the body as a whole.

The use of energy diagnosis at the level of organs is well known. The electrocardiogram, electroencephalogram, electromyogram and related recordings are widely used in medical diagnosis. These methods are now being complemented with biomagnetic recordings: magnetocardiograms, magnetoencephalograms and magnetomyograms.

At a finer level, every molecule in the body has a unique structure and a unique pattern of energy emission and absorption. Internal motions of each molecule enable it to carry out its function, e.g. as a hormone, receptor, second messenger or enzyme (Oschman, 1997b). A spectrum of different frequencies is given off while a molecule is coiling, twisting, vibrating or bending to carry out its task. Likewise, a corresponding set of frequencies can be *applied* to a molecule, to enhance or inhibit the internal motions involved in the molecule's functioning.

The new energetic diagnostic methods being developed complement and verify what energy therapists have been saying for millennia. Specifically, spectroscopy is a branch of science that involves measuring the electromagnetic emissions and absorptions of molecules. The basis for these processes has been explored in depth for many years (e.g. Sauer, 1955).

Every molecule in the body, and every homoeopathic, herbal or aromatherapy preparation, oscillates in specific ways and emits a characteristic energy spectrum. Complex molecules contain thousands or even millions of atoms, and their spectra can be quite intricate. The spectrum is an electromagnetic 'signature' or 'fingerprint' of a molecule that is an extremely precise representation of the motions of the particles within it. So characteristic are these fingerprints that a chemist can use them to identify an unknown substance.

One of the key techniques for analysing intricate electromagnetic signatures, whether from molecules or distant stars, is Fourier analysis. This is a form of calculus that makes it possible to analyse the most complex wave and determine the individual simple waves that comprise it. Likewise, the simple wave forms can be converted mathematically back into the original pattern. The equations are known as Fourier transforms. Fourier transforms are the language of holography, and it is likely that living systems use this kind of signal processing to store and interpret information (see Oschman and Oschman, 1995a,b).

When molecules in the body 'misbehave' because of some pathological situation, the story of their aberrant activities is broadcast into the living matrix and into the environment as electromagnetic signals. Biomedical scientists are beginning to use spectroscopic methods to detect these signals (Jackson and Mantsch, 1966). Their results confirm what energy therapists have known for a long time: the human body emits vibratory information that precisely specifies the activities taking place within. Science is also confirming that health can be restored by applying the appropriate fields from outside the body, as Burr predicted (see p. 6).

'Jump starting' healing with electric and magnetic fields

Some of the physicians who use energy fields for healing have begun to use the phrase 'jump starting the healing process'. For example, see a recent paper by C. Andrew L. Bassett (1995), a pioneer in the use of energy fields in medicine.

We will look closer at the basis for the concept of jump starting injury repair, as it will give us a possible basis for the effects of hands-on energy therapies. Remarkably, we shall see that the energy fields that can be projected naturally from the hands of therapists correspond closely to those that are produced by successful medical devices.

Healing bone fractures

The focus of Bassett's work was jump starting healing in individuals suffering from a debilitating condition known as 'nonunion of fracture'. In the USA there are some 2 million long-bone fractures every year, of which about 5% do not heal normally within 3–6 months. Some of these never heal, leading to disability or amputation.

Modern use of electricity to stimulate healing in nonunions dates from 1812, with a report by a surgeon at St. Thomas's Hospital in London. 'Electric fluids' were passed through needles inserted into the fracture gap. By the mid-1800s, electrical stimulation was the accepted method for treating slow-healing fractures.

In the late-1800s, electrical and magnetic healing devices had become extremely popular for treating virtually any ailment, from cancer to colds. This situation eventually created a backlash. The Pure Food and Drug Act was passed in 1906, and the 'Flexner Report' was published in 1910. The latter established science as the basis of medicine and clinical education. Soon all electrotherapies, including electrical bone stimulation, were declared scientifically unsupportable. They were legally excluded from clinical practice (summarized by Becker and Marino, 1982).

From quackery to acceptability

Bassett and his colleagues were instrumental in taking energy therapies from the realm of quackery to acceptability (Brighton et al., 1981). This was an enormous undertaking, for several reasons. It involved the prodigious amount of research and documentation required by the US Food and Drug Administration to approve a method as 'safe and effective'. Adding to the difficulty was a widespread but mistaken belief that the only forms of non-ionizing electromagnetic energy that could affect living systems were those intense enough to actually *heat* tissues.

This misguided perspective was, and continues to be, promoted by those with a vested interest in promoting the idea that modern electrical and electronic technologies cannot possibly harm living systems. Not only did this totally erroneous concept slow the progress of energetic therapies, it created great difficulties for biologists who were discovering that living organisms of all kinds, from bacteria to sharks to homing pigeons, are exquisitely sensitive to remarkably minute electromagnetic fields in their environment.

The tides turned solidly against the 'thermal effects' concept in the late 1970s with the publication of an important report by the prestigious Neurosciences Research Program (Adey and Bawin, 1977). The 'paradigm shift' signalled by this article:

'. . . a striking range of biological interactions has been described in experiments where control procedures appear to have been adequately considered. . . .' The existence of biological effects of very weak electromagnetic fields 'suggests an extraordinarily efficient mechanism' for detecting these fields and discriminating them from much higher levels of noise. 'The underlying mechanisms must necessarily involve ever increasing numbers of elements in the sensing system, ordered in particular ways to form a cooperative organization and manifesting similar forms and levels of energy over long distances.'

This conclusion complemented the reintroduction of electric and magnetic fields in clinical medicine, which also stimulated much valuable research on the mechanisms by which energy fields influence cells and tissues. It was also complemented by Fröhlich's discoveries about how the remarkable sensitivity of living systems may be achieved (see p. 18). All of this research has direct application to the various hands-on therapies.

Pulsed electromagnetic field therapy

In an effort to bypass the need for surgical implantation of electrodes into non-healing bones, a less risky and less costly procedure was sought. In 1977, Bassett and his colleagues at Columbia University introduced a non-invasive method involving pulsed electromagnetic fields (PEMFs) (Bassett *et al.*, 1977).

In practice, a small battery-powered pulse generator provides low energy and extremely low frequency (ELF) signals that are introduced into an external coil placed near the fracture site (Figure 1.8). The resulting fields are applied to the fracture site for 8–10 h/day. It is thought that the magnetic fields induce current flows at the fracture site that mimic natural electrical fields. These are the fields created in intact bone when it is dynamically deformed during normal physical activities, such as walking.

The phenomenon of induction is well known in physics, and it is therefore not a surprise that a magnetic field generated by a coil near the body will cause currents to flow in conducting tissues inside the body.

Pulsing magnetic fields trigger a cascade of events in bone, from the cell membrane to the nucleus and on to the gene level, where specific changes take place. Soft fibrocartilage then forms at the fracture site, and is induced to calcify. Blood vessels grow into the region, enabling bone-forming cells to enter the area and convert the rubbery union into a solid bony union.

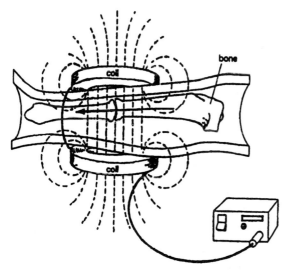

Figure 1.8 Pulsed electromagnetic field therapy. Currents are passed through coils adjacent to an injury such as a bone fracture. The magnetic fields (dashed lines) induce a current flow in the bone (horizontal arrow) that 'jump starts' the healing process (After Bassett, 1995)

The use of pulsing electromagnetic fields for treating nonunions was approved by the FDA in 1979. Over the subsequent 15-year period, more than 300 000 ununited fractures were successfully treated with pulsing magnetic fields. In Bassett's words:

> Jump starting a car with a dead battery creates an operational machine; exposure of a nonunion to PEMF's can convert a stalled healing process to active repair, even in patients unhealed for as long as 40 years! (C. Andrew L. Bassett, 1995)

This work is profoundly important for a number of reasons. First, after a long period of neglect and virtual hostility toward energetic therapies, researchers began to turn their attention to the possibilities of electromagnetic non-drug interventions. Bassett and his colleagues also helped correct the widely-held belief that living tissues can only be influenced by electromagnetic fields that cause ionizing or thermal effects. Finally, inquiry into the mechanisms of electromagnetic field effects is providing a scientific basis for hands-on energy therapies.

The similarity between PEMFs and 'hands-on' energy therapies

In the early 1980s, John Zimmerman began a series of important studies on therapeutic touch (TT), using a SQUID magnetometer at the University of Colorado School of Medicine in Denver. Zimmerman discovered that a pulsating biomagnetic field emanated from the hands of a TT practitioner. Figure 1.9 shows one of Zimmerman's recordings.

Zimmerman's findings were confirmed in 1992, when Seto and colleagues, in Japan, studied practitioners of various martial arts and other healing methods. The 'Qi emission' from the hands is in the range of 2–4 mGauss, which is more than 10 times stronger than the magnetocardiogram. The signal is sufficiently robust that it can be detected with a simple magnetometer consisting of two coils of wire. A SQUID is not needed. Since the Seto report, a number of studies of QiGong practitioners and others have extended these investigations

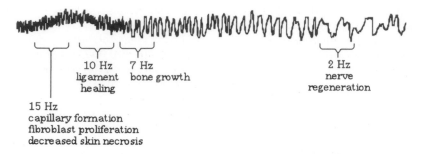

10 Hz
ligament
healing

7 Hz
bone growth

2 Hz
nerve
regeneration

15 Hz
capillary formation
fibroblast proliferation
decreased skin necrosis

Figure 1.9 Therapeutic touch signal. Signal recorded by Dr John Zimmerman from the hand of a therapeutic touch practitioner. The frequency is not steady, but 'sweeps' up and down, from 0.3 to 30 Hz, with most of the activity in the range of 7–8 Hz. The 1-second wide brackets show portions of the 'sweep' that approximately correspond to the 'frequency windows of specificity' for the healing of different tissues, discovered independently by medical researchers

to the sound, light and thermal fields emitted by healers (Sancier, 1998).

What is particularly interesting is that the frequency of the biomagnetic pulsations emitted by the hands varies from moment to moment (Figure 1.9). The biomagnetic pulsations recorded by Zimmerman, and by Seto and co-workers, are similar in this regard, and are in the same frequency range as brain waves.

Correlations between PEMFs and the earth's fields

We would like to know why the biomagnetic pulsations emitted by the hands of energy therapists vary in frequency, as shown in Figure 1.9. A variety of lines of investigation, summarized by Oschman (1997a), indicate that brain waves can be entrained or synchronized by the pulsing magnetic fields of the earth, known as the Schumann resonance. This resonance arises from standing waves in the earth-ionosphere cavity created by the energy of lightning (Schumann, 1952). Micropulsations of the geomagnetic field are thousands of times stronger than brain waves. It has been suggested that these micropulsations are detected by the pineal gland and possibly by other magnetite-bearing tissues associated with the brain (Becker, 1990b). The geomagnetic pulsations tend to entrain the brain waves to the earth's resonance, which varies from moment to

moment, but averages about 7.8 Hz. The fields set up by the brain waves are then conducted throughout the body by the perineural and vascular systems. The signals projected from the hands can be stronger than the brain waves (Seto *et al.*, 1992), indicating that an amplification takes place somewhere in the body. Alternatively, the body may simply act as an effective antenna for the Schumann micropulsations.

This fascinating concept of resonant interactions between the fields of the earth and living systems has important evolutionary implications (e.g. Direnfeld, 1983). The term 'atmospherics' refers to the range of electromagnetic energies produced by lightning. Atmospherics have a number of biological effects, particularly for 'weather-sensitive' individuals (Schienle *et al.*, 1998). Geomagnetic activity has been correlated with a wide range of pathologies (e.g. Rajaram and Mitra, 1981).

Correlations between the energy output from the hands and the output of medical devices

Perhaps the most illuminating realization from reviewing the recent literature is that medical devices are being developed that emit signals in the same frequency range as those emitted from the hands of energy therapists, meditators and practitioners of the martial arts. A recent summary of the relevant medical literature is in a book edited by Martin Blank of Columbia University (Blank, 1995).

Medical researchers are now asserting that pulsating magnetic fields can 'jump start' healing in a variety of soft and hard tissues. Of course, energy therapists, and their patients, have daily experiences of the healing process being jump started, but academic medicine has been suspicious because there was no logical explanation. Clinical evidence for the effectiveness of pulsating magnetic fields is now being published in medical journals. Specific frequencies stimulate the growth of nerves, bones, skin, capillaries, ligaments and fibroblasts. This medical research provides direct support for the phenomena taking place in the various energetic therapies.

Remarkably, the emissions from the hands of therapists are not confined to any specific frequency, but 'sweep' up and down through the same range that is being employed in therapeutic devices. In Figure 1.9, we show portions of one of Zimmerman's recordings from the hand of a TT therapist that correspond to the 'healing frequencies' for specific tissues discovered by medical researchers. On the basis of this, we propose a definition for 'healing energy', whether produced by medical devices or projected from the human hand:

'Healing energy', whether produced by medical devices or projected from the human body, is energy of a particular frequency or set of frequencies that 'jump starts' the repair of one or more tissues.

The experiences of energy therapists and modern medical researchers are converging: tissue healing can be facilitated by the application of appropriate energy fields. For a severe injury, with damage to a number of different kinds of tissues, several medical devices, each with a specific pulsation frequency, could stimulate healing. In contrast, the biomagnetic pulsations from the human hand appear to naturally sweep back and forth through a range of therapeutic frequencies.

The mechanism of pulsed magnetic field therapy

The theoretical problem faced by medical researchers is the same as that of energy therapists. How can minute magnetic pulses jump start the healing process? Bassett's 1995 paper, 'Bioelectromagnetics in the service of medicine', is one of his last publications, and summarized his conclusions from a lifetime of research. Bassett pointed out that bone is formed by myriads of cells known as osteocytes. Figure 1.10(a) shows a single osteocyte. Note that it consists of a central nucleus and a large number of slender processes or extensions of its cell surface.

Figure 1.10(b) is a micrograph showing the relations between a number of osteocytes. Notice that the slender processes from the various cells extend in various directions, and appear to touch the processes from neighbouring osteocytes. While the details vary, this extensive contact is a characteristic of 'generative' or 'stem' cells in a variety of tissues: connective tissue, muscle, nerve, skin, blood vessels, etc. What these cells have in common is that each is responsible for forming, maintaining and repairing a particular type of tissue.

Images such as those shown in Figure 1.10(b) are obtained with the light microscope. The higher magnifications of the electron microscope reveal details of the cell–cell contacts. What the electron microscope shows is that these contacts are *gap junctions* (Holtrop and Wenger, 1971). This is important, because gap junctions allow for electrical coupling or continuity from one cell to another (Gilula *et al.*, 1972; Lowenstein, 1972; Staehelin, 1974). Hence, the cells shown in Figure 1.10(b) can be said to form an electrical and electronic *continuum* – the osteocytes are an energetically interconnected *system*, much like the skin system shown in Figure 1.3.

Figure 1.10(c) is from Bassett's paper, and shows an osteon, the cylindrical unit of compact bone. Each osteon has a blood vessel running through its centre, surrounded with an *array* of electrically interconnected osteocytes. Many osteons pack together to form the bulk of the bone structure. The biological/physics problem is to explain how the osteocyte *system* is so incredibly sensitive to the minute fields

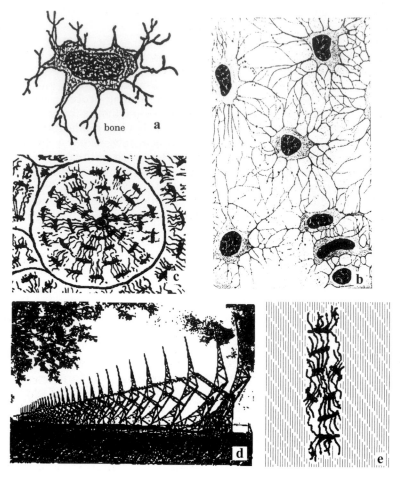

Figure 1.10 Osteocytes. (a) A single osteocyte. There is a central nucleus and a large number of slender processes or extensions of the cell surface. (b) The relations between a number of osteocytes in a bone, as seen in the light microscope. The slender processes from the cells extend outward and appear to touch the processes from neighbouring osteocytes. (c) An osteon, the cylindrical unit of compact bone. Each osteon has a blood vessel running through its centre, and this is surrounded by an array of electrically interconnected osteocytes. Many osteons pack together to form the bulk of the bone structure (After Bassett, 1995). (d) A phased array of radiotelescope antennas such as those at Jodrell Bank in England. To explain how bone cells respond to tiny magnetic fields, Bassett (1995) makes the analogy between the array of osteocytes in the osteon and the phased radiotelescope array. (e) The liquid crystal collagen arrays in bone and other forms of connective tissue consist of collagen molecules that are precisely offset, like the elements of a radiotelescope array

produced by a PEMF device or from the hand of a therapist.

Bassett (1995) made a fascinating analogy between the *arrays* of bone cells in the osteon and the *phased arrays* of radiotelescope antennas, such as those at Jodrell Bank in Cheshire, England. Radiotelescope antennas are used by astrophysicists to detect extremely weak electromagnetic signals from nebulae thousands of millions of light years away in distant space (Figure 1.10(d)). Phased arrays are also used in radar systems to produce a beam that sweeps back and forth, and to detect the echoes returning from distant objects.

By *phased array* we are referring to a set of transmitting or receiving antennas that optimizes the projection or detection of a particular frequency of electromagnetic energy in a particular direction. This is accomplished by placing the antenna elements in a particular spacing and geometry, and by utilizing electronic circuitry that delays energy input into each element by a precise amount. This delay, or phase delay, controls the direction of the beam. Comparable detection circuits can determine the delay between signals arriving at adjacent receiving elements, and thereby determine the direction of an incoming signal.

Bassett's fascinating idea is that tissues detect information from pulsing magnetic fields by a physical process akin to that involved in radioastronomy. Perhaps this concept can teach us about energetic communication with cells and tissues.

'Seeing' into tissues

We can carry the analogy between the phased arrays of bone cells and those of radioastronomy a step further. Radiotelescopes can 'see' into deep space and reveal features that can never be revealed by light telescopes. The reason for this is that optical telescopes are limited by the unsteadiness of our atmosphere and by the deflection of light by interstellar clouds of small dust particles. The long wavelengths detected by radiotelescopes are much less affected by these disturbances than is light.

We cannot 'see' very deeply into the living body, because the skin is relatively opaque to light. But another way to find out what is happening inside the body is to study the patterns of electric fields generated by the activities of the various organs and tissues. These fields can be detected with electrodes on the skin surface (electrocardiography, electroencephalography, electromyography, etc.). However, these electric fields are modified and distorted as they pass through the intervening tissues to the skin surface, much like the light from distant galaxies is distorted by its encounters with dust particles in deep space.

For example, the electrical brain waves recorded in encephalography must pass through a layer of connective tissue (the dura), then

through the skull and scalp before they reach the surface of the head. In contrast, living tissue is transparent to the long wavelength magnetic and electromagnetic pulsations produced during living processes. It is therefore easier to detect what an organ inside the body is doing by recording its magnetic rather than its electrical emissions. Likewise, the introduction of electric currents into specific tissues can be done much more precisely if magnetic fields are used to *induce* the current flows (e.g. Figure 1.8), rather than by electrical stimulation at the skin surface.

Bassett could have taken his *phased array* analogy a step further. The array of osteons is embedded in another array, the collagenous matrix shown in Figure 1.4(b). In Figure 1.10(e) we show an array of osteocytes embedded in an array of collagen molecules: an array within an array. Add to the picture the array of phospholipid molecules in the osteocyte cell membranes, and the array of water molecules associated with all of the elements in the circuit.

We conclude with another hypothesis: perhaps the collagenous array is the antenna, and the cellular array contains the phase-delay circuitry for transmitting and receiving electromagnetic information. Perhaps evolution has provided all of us with a built-in electromagnetic 'radar' array that can both detect disorders in those around us, and project energy that can stimulate the body's repair systems. This is certainly an hypothesis worthy of further study.

Adding it all up

The ideas presented here are leading to a new image of the way the organism functions in health and disease. The abstract of a 1991 paper by Pienta and Coffey, entitled 'Cellular harmonic information transfer through a tissue tensegrity-matrix system', combines the concepts of the living matrix, vibratory and resonant interactions, cellular and tissue continuity, piezoelectricity, solid state biochemistry, coherence and tensegrity to paint a picture of the regulation of living systems:

Abstract – Cells and intracellular elements are capable of vibrating in a dynamic manner with complex harmonics, the frequency of which can now be measured and analyzed in a quantitative manner by Fourier analysis [and by other methods]. Cellular events such as changes in shape, membrane ruffling, motility, and signal transduction occur within spatial and temporal harmonics that have potential regulatory importance. These vibrations can be altered by growth factors and the process of carcinogenesis. It is important to understand the mechanism by which this vibrational information is transferred directly throughout the cell [and throughout the organism]. From these observations we propose that vibrational information is transferred through a tissue tensegrity-matrix which acts as a coupled harmonic oscillator operating as a signal transducing system from the cell periphery to the nucleus and ultimately to the DNA.

The vibrational interactions occur through a tissue matrix system consisting of the nuclear matrix, the cytoskeleton, and the extracellular matrix that is poised to couple the biological oscillations of the cell from the peripheral membrane to the DNA through a tensegrity-matrix structure. Tensegrity has been defined as a structural system composed of discontinuous compression elements connected by continuous tension cables, which interact in a dynamic fashion. A tensegrity tissue matrix system allows for specific transfer of information through the cell by direct transmission of vibrational chemomechanical energy through harmonic wave motion. (Parts in brackets were added)

This picture is by no means complete. Each aspect is the subject of ongoing research. However, Pienta and Coffey's paper provides a concise summary, and a foundation for further exploration, both by the scientist and the therapist.

Local vs. non-local healing: scalar waves?

This chapter has focused on the molecular, architectural and energetic design of living sys-tems that enables them to respond in beneficial ways to electric, magnetic and electromagnetic fields. In terms of electronics, we are dealing with near-field interactions. These occur when the interacting elements, such as the therapist and patient, are close enough to one another so that their energy fields, which abruptly drop off in strength with distance, can interact.

What about other healing modalities that seem independent of distance? A large and growing body of reliable evidence shows that intercessory prayer is effective, even when the patients and those praying for them are sepa-rated by great distances (Dossey, 1988, 1993).

The idea of subtle interactions at a distance is embodied in the 'synchronicity' concept of Jung (Peat, 1987), and is also part of the daily practice of radionics (e.g. Fellows, 1997). While these and related phenomena, such as telepathy and clairvoyance, are too far-fetched for some scien-tists, there is now too much evidence to ignore them (see Woodhouse, 1996).

Some scholars seriously look to the peculiari-ties of quantum mechanics for explanations, such as 'quantum non-locality', that seem to fit with the laws of physics. It is often stated that non-local phenomena are mediated by unknown forms of energy, sometimes vaguely referred to as 'subtle energies'. Some look to these phenom-ena for clues about the nature of consciousness and the structure of the physical universe. Others suggest the word 'energy' is inadequate, and its use in relation to healing should be dis-continued. The philosophical and metaphysical implications are the subject of ongoing discus-sions (e.g. exchanges between Dossey and Woodhouse in *Network*, **64**, 1997).

Key studies of non-local interactions have been published by Grinberg-Zylberbaum *et al.* (1992, 1994). Pairs of subjects who achieve a feeling of emotional connection (empathy) can develop correlated electroencephalographic (EEG) patterns that are not attenuated by spatial separation or by electromagnetic shielding (Faraday cages). When one of the subjects was stimulated, as with a flash of light, the evoked brain wave was 'transferred' to a non-stimulated subject in another electromagnetically shielded room. The researchers assert that these findings represent a genuinely non-local, macroscopic manifestation of consciousness that is physio-logically relevant.

Studies like this, using shielded rooms, seem to rule out electromagnetic interactions, but do they? Few scientists realize that associated with all electromagnetic fields are electrostatic scalar potentials and magnetic vector potentials. The physics of these phenomena was developed a long time ago.

Briefly, in a situation where coils are set up in a geometry such that the vectors (the directions and magnitudes) of the electric and magnetic fields destructively interfere or cancel each other, there nevertheless remain electrostatic scalar potentials and magnetic vector potentials. Even though the classical fields are cancelled, energy and information are still present, and radiate outward as waves. These waves have spherical symmetry. According to theoretical physics, these waves do not diminish with distance, and are therefore ideally suited to explain non-local interactions. The waves appear to interact with atomic nuclei rather than with electrons. They are not blocked by Faraday cages or other kinds of shielding, they are probably emitted by living systems, and they appear to be intimately involved in healing (e.g. Jacobs, 1997; Rein, 1998).

Potential waves were discovered by Tesla (1904), who called them non-Hertzian waves. The classical electromagnetic field is in fact derived from two potential waves interfering with each other. The mathematics for this interconvertibility concept was worked out by Whittaker (1903, 1904). The quantum basis for scalar and potential waves was described by physicists Aharonov and Bohm (1959). These authors concluded that potential waves, and not fields, are primary. The quantum mechanics of scalar and potential waves was further elaborated by Olariu and Popescu (1985).

Much more is known about electric and magnetic fields than potential waves, because fields are easy to measure. It is widely assumed that it is the electric and magnetic fields that interact with organisms, but we are beginning to see that scalar and potential waves actually underlie these effects.

For the evolution of energy medicine, there are a number of important consequences. For each bioelectric and biomagnetic field produced by the human body, whether emitted by the brain, the heart, the eye, the muscles, an organ, or by the hand of a therapist, there will also be potential components. Moreover, the energy fields in the environment, whether natural or created by technology, also contain potential waves.

For example, the Schumann resonance, discussed earlier, is described by five quantities: velocity of propagation, electric field, magnetic field, electric scalar potential and magnetic vector potential. Further research needs to be done to determine the extent to which the biological effects of the Schumann resonance and other atmospherics are actually due to potentials rather than to fields. An interesting speculation is that long-range biological interactions may be due to modulation of Schumann resonance potential waves. In this respect, it is fascinating that well-documented 'telepathic experiences' are systematically associated with global geomagnetic activity (Persinger and Krippner, 1993). Moreover, there are correlations between the onset of various pathologies and geomagnetic activity (Venkataraman, 1976; Rajaram and Mitra, 1981).

In the 1980s, several personal electromagnetic shielding devices were developed, based on the use of self-cancelling coils (Möbius design) that emit scalar waves, which were said to be safe for living systems. One of these devices was a watch containing a microchip that produced a Schumann-type signal at about 8.0 Hz. This device purportedly stabilized a person's brain waves at a frequency that was considered safe and beneficial. Many of these devices were sold, and there were reports of benefits from wearing them, including reduction of 'jet lag', more energy, lower blood pressure, feelings of well-being, etc.

Rein (1998) has summarized the biological effects of scalar waves. They can inhibit neurotransmitter uptake into nerve cells and stimulate the growth of human lymphocytes. There are indications that the effects are in part mediated by effects on the properties of cell and tissue water.

Recently, far more powerful emitters of potential waves have been developed (Abraham, 1998). The devices emit potential waves at the average Schumann frequency, 7.83 Hz. Preliminary tests indicate that potential waves at this frequency are safe, and protect those who suffer from electromagnetic field sensitivity.

Moreover, clinical trials in progress are indicating a variety of health benefits to these scalar waves.

The existence of a reliable and powerful source of potential waves opens up many possibilities for studies of the clinical effects of this form of energy, and, possibly, for resolving some of the mysteries and variability of local and non-local biological effects.

Some conclusions

The aim of this chapter is to document a convergence of clinical and scientific perspectives that is leading to a logical paradigm for energy medicine. When freed of the historical biases and confusions, an inquiry into energy can help us understand more about the regulation of vital physiological processes, such as wound healing and disease resistance.

The author also believes that fascinating topics such as memory and consciousness cannot be understood without a better picture of the energetics of cells and tissues. As an interesting example, Charman (1997) logically views what we refer to as 'mind' as a brain-generated neuromagnetic field. To paraphrase:

> When the mosaic of neurons resonates at preferred frequencies, so will their associated microfields. These will interact with each other to form a complex, neuromagnetic whole that permeates through the magnetically 'transparent' physical structure of the brain as if it was not there.

Add to this concept of 'mind', the biomagnetic fields of the peripheral neurons and the cell and tissue structures associated with them, and we begin to see a dynamic picture of the biomagnetic body as a whole.

Exploring energy medicine is challenging because it cuts across many different disciplines. It is also rewarding, because it brings together the biology, physics, biophysics and technology of energy and of living processes.

Our health system has much to gain from unbiased, interdisciplinary, and open-minded inquiries into energetic and other forms of complementary medicine. It will be particularly valuable to continue exploring the energetic emissions from the hands of therapists, and the mechanisms by which these emissions affect the living matrix of molecules, cells and tissues. Investigations of the potential waves that give rise to electromagnetic fields open up new possibilities for locating the 'circuits and machinery and switches' that trigger 'spontaneous' healing. Energy research obviously has many therapeutic and technological implications. The future of our medicine and our species depends on our willingness to broaden the scope of our inquiries and investigate the reality of living systems.

Acknowledgements

The author is indebted to Robert Charman for inviting this chapter, for providing a variety of valuable references, and for stimulating questions on aspects of the manuscript. I also thank Guy Abraham, M.D. and Rolfer Deborah Stucker for comments on portions of the manuscript. I especially thank Dr Abraham for introducing me to the physics literature on scalar waves, and for providing scalar wave generators for research purposes.

References

Abraham, G. (1998) *Synchroton*® *Scalar Synchronizer: Potential Shields Against Electro-magnetic Pollution.* Optimox Corporation, P.O. Box 3378, Torrance, CA 90510-3378.

Adey, W.R. (1993) Whispering between cells, electromagnetic fields and regulatory mechanisms in tissue. *Frontier Perspect.*, **3**, 21–25.

Adey, W.R. and Bawin, S.M. (1977) Brain interactions with weak electric and magnetic fields. *Neurosci. Res. Prog. Bull.*, **15**(1), 1–129.

Adolph, E.F. (1982) Physiological integrations in action. *The Physiologist*, **25**(2), 1–67.

Aharonov, Y. and Bohm, E. (1959) Significance of electromagnetic potentials in the quantum theory. *Phys. Rev.*, **115**(3), 485–91.

Allen, M.J., Cleary, S.F. and Sowers, A.E. (eds) (1994) Proceedings of the 1994 International Symposium on Charge and Field Effects in Biosystems – 4. Singapore: World Scientific.

Bassett, C.A.L. (1968) Biologic significance of piezo-electricity. *Calcified Tissue Res.*, 1, 252–72.

Bassett, C.A.L. (1971) Effect of forces on skeletal tissues. In *Physiological Basis of Rehabilitation Medicine* (Downey, J. and Darling, R. C., eds) Philadelphia: W.B. Saunders, pp. 283–316.

Bassett, C.A.L. (1995) Bioelectromagnetics in the service of medicine. In *Electromagnetic fields. Biological Interactions and Mechanisms* (Blank, M., ed.). *Adv. Chem. Ser.*, 250, 261–75.

Bassett, C.A.L., Pawluk, R.J. and Becker, R.O. (1964) Effects of electric currents on bone formation *in vivo. Nature* (Lond.), 204, 652.

Bassett, C.A.L., Pilla, A.A. and Pawluk, R.J. (1977) A non-operative salvage of surgically-resistant pseudarthroses and non-unions by pulsing electromagnetic fields. *J. Clin. Orthopaed.*, 124, 128.

Becker, R.O. (1990a) The machine brain and properties of the mind. *Subtle Energies*, 1(2), 79–97.

Becker, R.O. (1990b) *Cross Currents. The Perils of Electropollution. The Promise of Electromedicine.* Los Angeles: Jeremy P. Tarcher, p. 80.

Becker, R.O. (1991) Evidence for a primitive DC electrical analog system controlling brain function. *Subtle Energies*, 2(1), 71–88.

Becker, R.O. and Marino, A.A. (1982) *Electromagnetism and Life.* Albany: State University of New York Press.

Blank, M. (ed.) (1995) *Electromagnetic Fields. Biological Interactions and Mechanisms* (Blank, M., ed.). *Advances in Chemistry Series*, 250, American Chemical Society.

Bouligand, Y. (1978) Liquid crystals and their analogs in biological systems. *Solid State Phys.*, suppl. 14, 259–94.

Brighton, C.T., Black, J., Friedenberg, Z.B. *et al.* (1981) A multicenter study of the treatment of nonunion with constant direct current. *J. Bone Joint Surg. Am.*, 63, 1–13.

Burr, H.S. (1972) *Blueprint for Immortality.* Saffron Walden, UK: C.W. Daniel.

Chaitow, L. (1998) The critical mind and 'energy'. Editorial in *J. Bodywork Move. Therapies*, 2(1), 1.

Chang, C. (1989) Singular point, organizing center and acupuncture point. *Am. J. Chinese Med.*, 17(3–4), 119–27.

Charman, R.A. (1990) Bioelectricity and electrotherapy – towards a new paradigm? Part 1: The electric cell. *Physiotherapy*, 76(9), 502–16.

Charman, R.A. (1997) The field substance of mind – a hypothesis. *Network*, 63, 11–13.

Childs, B. (1970) Persistent echoes of the nature–nurture argument. *Am J. Human Genetics*, 29, 1–13.

Cope, F.W. (1967) A theory of cell hydration governed by adsorption of water on cell proteins rather than by osmotic pressure. *Bull. Math. Biophys.*, 29, 583–96.

Corongiu, G. and Clementi, E. (1981) Simulations of the solvent structure for macromolecules. I. Solvation of

B–DNA double helix at $T = 300$ K. *Biopolymers*, 20, 551–71.

Direnfeld, L.K. (1983) The genesis of the EEG and its relation to electromagnetic radiation. *J. Bioelectricity*, 2, 111–21.

Dossey, L. (1988) *Space, Time, and Medicine.* Boulder, CO: Shambhala.

Dossey, L. (1993) *Healing Words. The Power of Prayer and the Practice of Medicine.* Harper Collins: San Francisco.

Eisenberg, D.M., Davis, R.B., Ettner, S.L., Appel, S. *et al.* (1998) Trends in alternative medicine use in the United States, 1990–1997. Results of a follow-up national survey. *J. Am. Med. Ass.*, 280, 1569–75.

Eisenberg, D.M., Kessler, R.C., Foster, C., Norlock, F.E. *et al.* (1993) Unconventional medicine in the United States. *New Engl. J. Med.*, 328(4), 246–52.

Ellison, J. and Garrod, D.R. (1984) Anchoring filaments of the amphibian epidermal–dermal junction traverse the basal lamina entirely from the plasma membrane of hemidesmosomes to the dermis. *J. Cell Sci.*, 72, 163–72.

Feigelson, P. (1969) Electronic aspects of biochemistry. *Ann. N.Y. Acad. Sci.*, 158, 1–438.

Fellows, L. (1997) Opening up the 'black box.' *Int. J. Altern. Complement. Med.*, 15(8), 9–13.

Fleming, A. (1932) Quoted from *People's Almanac*, 2.

Fröhlich, H. (1968a) Bose condensation of strongly excited longitudinal electric modes. *Phys. Lett.*, 26A, 402–3.

Fröhlich, H. (1968b) Long-range coherence and energy storage in biological systems. *Int. J. Quantum Chem.*, 2, 641–49.

Fröhlich, H. (1970) Long-range coherence and the action of enzymes. *Nature* (Lond.), 228, 1093.

Fröhlich, H. (1974) Possibilities of long- and short-range electric interactions of biological systems. In *Brain Interactions with Weak Electric and Magnetic Fields* (Adey, W.R. and Bawin, S.M., eds). *Neurosciences Research Program Bull.*, 15, 1–129.

Fröhlich, H. (1975) Evidence for bose condensation-like excitation of coherent modes in biological systems. *Phys. Lett.*, 51A, 21–22.

Fröhlich, H. (ed.) (1988a) *Biological Coherence and Response to External Stimuli.* Berlin: Springer-Verlag.

Fröhlich, H. (1988b) The genetic code as language. In *Biological Coherence and Response to External Stimuli.* Berlin: Springer-Verlag, pp. 191–204.

Gabbiani, G., Chaponnier, C. and Hüttner, I. (1978) Cytoplasmic filaments and gap junctions in epithelial cells and myofibroblasts during wound healing. *J. Cell Biol.*, 76, 561–68.

Gilula, N.B., Reeves, O.R. and Steinbach, A. (1972) Metabolic coupling, ionic coupling, and cell contacts. *Nature* (Lond.), 235, 262.

Grinberg-Zylberbaum, J., Delaflor, M., Attie, L. and Goswami, A. (1994) The Einstein–Podolsky–Rosen paradox in the brain: the transferred potential. *Physics Essays*, 7(4), 422–28.

Grinberg-Zylberbaum, J., Delaflor, M., Sanchez Arellano, M.E., Guevara, M.A. and Perez, M. (1992) Human communication and the electrophysiological activity of the brain. *Subtle Energies*, 3(3), 25–43.

Haken, H. (1983) *Advanced Synergetics. Instability Hierarchies of Self-Organizing Systems and Devices*. Berlin: Springer-Verlag.

Haken, H. and Wagner, M. (1973) *Cooperative Phenomena*. New York: Springer-Verlag.

Ho, M-W. (1993) *The Rainbow and the Worm: The Physics of Organisms*. Singapore: World Scientific.

Ho, M-W. (1998) *The Rainbow and the Worm: The Physics of Organisms*, 2nd edn. Singapore: World Scientific.

Ho, M-W. and Knight, D.P. (1998) The acupuncture system and the liquid crystalline collagen fibers of the connective tissues. *Am. J Chinese Med.*, 26(3–4), 1–13.

Holtrop, M.E. and Wenger, M.J. (1971) Proceedings of the 4th Parathyroid Conference, International Congress Series, No. 243, Amsterdam: Excerpta Medica.

Horwitz, A.F. (1997) Integrins and health. Discovered only recently, these adhesive cell–surface molecules have quickly revealed themselves to be critical to proper functioning of the body and to life itself. *Scientific Am.*, 276(5), 68–75.

Ingber, D.E. (1993a) Cellular tensegrity: defining new rules of biological design that govern the cytoskeleton. *J. Cell Sci.*, 104, 613–27.

Ingber, D.E. (1993b) The riddle of morphogenesis: a question of solution chemistry or molecular cell engineering. *Cell*, 75, 1249–52.

Ingber, D.E. (1998) The architecture of life. *Scientific Am.*, 278(1), 48–57.

Jackson, M. and Mantsch, H.H. (1966) Biomedical infrared spectroscopy. In *Infrared Spectroscopy of Biomolecules* (Mantsch, H.H., ed.). New York: Wiley-Liss, pp. 311–40.

Jacobs, R. (1997) 21st century medicine. *Kindred Spirit*, 3(10), 37–40.

Kaptchuk, T.J. (1983) *The Web that has no Weaver. Understanding Chinese Medicine*. New York: Congdon and Weed.

Krawczyk, W.S. and Wilgram, G.F. (1973) Hemidesmosome and desmosome morphogenesis during epidermal wound healing. *J. Ultrastruct. Res.*, 45, 93.

Lowenstein, W.R. (1972) Cellular communication through membrane junctions. *Arch. Intern. Med.*, 129, 299.

MacGinitie, L.A. (1995) Streaming and piezoelectric potentials in connective tissues. In *Electromagnetic Fields. Biological Interactions and Mechanisms* (Blank, M., ed.). *Adv. Chem. Ser.*, 250, 125–42.

Marchesi, V.T. (1985) Inflammation and healing. In *Anderson's Pathology*, 8th edn (Kissane, J.M. and Anderson, W.A.D., eds). St. Louis, MO: C.V. Mosby, pp. 22–60.

McConkey, E.H. (1982) Molecular evolution, intracellular organization and the quinary structure of proteins. *Proc. Nat. Acad. Sci. USA*, 79, 3236–40.

Mitchell, P. (1976) Vectorial chemistry and the molecular mechanics of chemiosmotic coupling: power transmission by proticity. *Biochem. Soc. Trans.*, 4, 399–430.

Motz, J. (1998) *Hands of Life. From the operating room to your home, an energy healer reveals the secrets of using your body's own energy medicine for healing, recovery, and transformation*. New York: Bantam Books.

Myers, T.W. (1997a) The 'anatomy trains'. *J. Bodywork Move. Therapies*, 1, 91–101.

Myers, T.W. (1997b) The 'anatomy trains': Pt 2. *J. Bodywork Move. Therapies*, 1, 134–45.

Nicolson, G. (1976) Trans-membrane control of the receptors on normal and tumor cells. II. Surface changes associated with transformation and malignancy. *Biochim. Biophys. Acta*, 458, 1–72.

Olariu, S. and Popescu, I.I. (1985) The quantum effects of electromagnetic fluxes. *Rev. Mod. Phys.*, 57, 339–436.

Oschman, J.L. (1981) The connective tissue and myofascial systems. In *Readings on the Scientific Basis of Bodywork, Energetic, and Movement Therapies*. New Hampshire: N.O.R.A., P.O. Box 5101, Dover, NH 03821, USA, e-mail: joschman@aol.com., web page: www.bodywork-res.com.

Oschman, J.L. (1984) Structure and properties of ground substances. *Am. Zool.*, 24, 199–215.

Oschman, J.L. (1989) How the body maintains its shape. *Rolf Lines*, the news magazine for Rolf Institute members, beginning at volume 17(3), 27.

Oschman, J.L. (1993) Sensing solitons in soft tissues. *Guild News*, the news magazine for members of the Guild for Structural Integration, Boulder, CO, 3(2), 22–25.

Oschman, J.L. (1994) A biophysical basis for acupuncture. Proceedings of the First Symposium of the Society for Acupuncture Research, Rockville, MD, January 23–24, 1993.

Oschman, J.L. (1996a) Healing energy, Pt 1: Historical background. *J. Bodywork Move. Therapies*, 1(1), 34–43.

Oschman, J.L. (1996b) The nuclear, cytoskeletal, and extracellular matrices: a continuous communication network. Poster presentation for *The Cytoskeleton: Mechanical, Physical and Biological Interactions*. A workshop sponsored by the Center for Advanced Studies in the Space Life Science at the Marine Biological Laboratory, Woods Hole, MA, November 15–17.

Oschman, J.L. (1997a) What is healing energy? Pt 3: Silent pulses. *J. Bodywork Move. Therapies*, 1(3), 179–94.

Oschman, J.L. (1997b) What is healing energy? Pt 4: Vibrational medicines. *J. Bodywork Move. Therapies*, 1(4), 239–50.

Oschman, J.L. (1997c) What is healing energy? Pt 5: Gravity, structure, and emotions. *J. Bodywork Move. Therapies*, 1(5), 297–309.

Oschman, J.L. (1998) What is healing energy? Pt 6: Conclusions, is energy medicine the medicine of the future? *J. Bodywork Move. Therapies*, 2(1), 46–60.

Oschman, J.L. and Oschman, N.H. (1994) *Book Review and Commentary: Biological Coherence and Response to External Stimuli* (Fröhlich, H., ed.). Berlin: Springer-Verlag, N.O.R.A., P.O. Box 5101, Dover, NH 03821, USA, e-mail: joschman@aol.com., web page: www.body-work-res.com.

Oschman, J.L. and Oschman, N.H. (1995a) Somatic recall. Pt I: Soft tissue memory. *Massage Therapy J.*, American Massage Therapy Association, 34(3), 36–46; 111–116.

Oschman, J.L. and Oschman, N.H. (1995b) Somatic recall. Pt II: Soft tissue holography. *Massage Therapy J.*, American Massage Therapy Association, 34(4), 66–67; 106–116.

Oz, M. (1998) *Healing from the Heart. A Leading Heart Surgeon Explores the Power of Complementary Medicine*. New York: Dutton/Penguin.

Peat, F.D. (1987) *Synchronicity. The Bridge Between Matter and Mind*. Toronto: Bantam Books.

Persinger, M.A. and Krippner, S. (1993) Dream ESP experiments and geomagnetic activity. In *Silver Threads. 25 Years of Parapsychology Research* (Kane, B., Millay, J. and Brown, D., eds). Westport, CT: Praeger, pp. 39–53.

Pethig, R. (1979) *Dielectric and Electronic Properties of Biological Materials*. Chichester, UK: John Wiley, p. 213.

Pienta K.J. and Coffey, D.S. (1991) Cellular harmonic information transfer through a tissue tensegrity-matrix system. *Med. Hypotheses*, 34, 88–95.

Popp, F.A., Li, K.H. and Gu, Q. (eds) (1992) *Recent Advances in Biophoton Research and its Applications*. Singapore: World Scientific.

Popp, F.A., Ruth, B., Bahr, W. *et al.* (1981) Emission of visible and ultraviolet radiation by active biological systems. *Collective Phenomena*, 3, 187–214.

Puck, T.T. (1977) Cyclic AMP, the microtubule-microfilament system, and cancer. *Proc. Nat. Acad. Sci.*, USA, 74(10), 4491–95.

Pugh, A. (1976) *An Introduction to Tensegrity*. Berkeley, CA: University of California Press.

Rajaram, M. and Mitra, S. (1981) Correlation between convulsive seizure and geomagnetic activity. *Neurosci. Lett.*, 24, 187–91.

Ratner, S. (1979) The dynamic state of body proteins. *Ann. N.Y. Acad. Sci.*, 325, 189–209.

Rattemeyer, M. and Popp, F.A. (1981) Evidence of photon emission from DNA in living systems. *Naturwiss.*, 68, 572–73.

Redpath, W.M. (1994) *Trauma Energetics. A Study of Held-Energy Systems*. Lexington, MA: Barberry Press. Available from the Guild for Structural Integration, Boulder, CO; tel. (1)800-447-0150.

Rein, G. (1998) Biological effects of quantum fields and their role in the natural healing process. *Frontier Perspectives*, 7(1), 16–23.

Rolf, I.P. (1962) Structural integration. Gravity: an unexplored factor in a more human use of human beings. *J. Inst. Comparative Study Hist., Philos. Sci.*, 1, 3–20. Available from the Rolf Institute, Boulder, CO; tel. (1)800-530-8875.

Rosenberg, F. and Postow, E. (1969) Semiconduction in proteins and lipids – its possible biological import. *Ann. N.Y. Acad. Sci.*, 158, 161–90.

Sancier, K.M. (1998) *Qigong Database*. Available from the Qigong Institute, East West Academy Healing Arts, 450 Sutter Street #2104, San Francisco, CA 94108; tel/fax: 415-323-1221; e-mail: matsu@nanospace.com.

Sauer, K. (1955) Biochemical spectroscopy. *Meth. Enzymology*, 246.

Schienle, A., Stark, R. and Vaitl, D. (1998) Biological effects of very low frequency (VLF) atmospherics in humans: a review. *J. Scientific Explor.*, 12(3), 455–68.

Schoenheimer, R. (1942) *The Dynamic State of Body Constituents*. Cambridge, MA: Harvard University Press.

Schumann, W.O. (1952) On the characteristic oscillations of a conducting sphere which is surrounded by an air layer and an ionospheric shell (in German). *Z. Naturforschung*, 7a, 149–54 (for a summary of Schumann's research in English, see Konig, H.L. (1974) ELF and VLF signal properties: physical characteristics. In *ELF and VLF Electromagnetic Field Effects* (Persinger, M.A., ed.). New York: Plenum Press, pp. 9–34.

Schwartz, G.E.R., Nelson, L., Russek, L. and Allen, J.J.B. (1996) Electrostatic body-motion registration and the human antenna-receiver effect: a new method for investigating interpersonal dynamical energy system interactions. *Subtle Energies Energy Med.*, 7(2), 149–84.

Seto, A., Kusaka, C., Nakazato, S. *et al.* (1992) Detection of extraordinary large biomagnetic field strength from human hand. *Acupunct. Electro-Therapeutics Res. Int. J.*, 17, 75–94.

Smith, C.W. (1994) Biological effects of weak electromagnetic fields. In *Bioelectrodynamics and Biocommunication* (Ho, M-W., Popp, F-A. and Warnke, U., eds). Singapore: World Scientific, pp. 81–107.

Staehelin, A. (1974) Structure and functions of intercellular junctions. *Int. Rev. Cytology*, 39, 191.

Szent-Györgyi, A. (1941a) Towards a new biochemistry? *Science*, 93, 609–11.

Szent-Györgyi, A. (1941b) The study of energy levels in biochemistry. *Nature (Lond.)*, 148, 157–59.

Szent-Györgyi, A. (1960) *Introduction to a Submolecular Biology*. New York: Academic Press.

Szent-Györgyi, A. (1963) Lost in the twentieth century. *Ann. Rev. Biochem.*, 32, 1–14.

Tesla, N. (1904) Transmission of energy without wires. *Scientific Am.*, Suppl. 57, 237.

Venkataraman, K. (1976) Epilepsy and solar activity – an hypothesis. *Neurol. India*, 24, 148–52.

Wang, J.Y., Butler, J.P. and Ingber, D.E. (1993) Mechanotransduction across the cell surface and through the cytoskeleton. *Science*, **260**, 1124–27.

Weil, A. (1995) *Spontaneous Healing. How to discover and enhance your body's natural ability to maintain and heal itself*, New York: Alfred A. Knopf.

Weiss, P.A. (1965) From cell dynamics to tissue architecture. In *Advanced Study Institute on Structure and Function of Connective and Skeletal Tissue, St. Andrews, Scotland, 1964*. London: Butterworths, pp. 256–63.

Whittaker, E.T. (1903) On the partial differential equations of mathematical physics. *Math. Annalen*, **57**, 333–55.

Whittaker, E.T. (1904) On an expression of the electromagnetic field due to electrons by means of two scalar potential functions. *Proc. Lond. Math. Soc.*, **1**, 367–72.

Wilson, E.O. (1994) *Naturalist*. Washington, D.C.: Island Press/Shearwater Books.

Woodhouse, M.B. (1996) *Paradigm Wars. Worldviews for a New Age*. Berkeley, CA: Frog.

Zimmerman, J. (1990) Laying-on-of-hands healing and therapeutic touch: a testable theory. *BEMI Currents*, Journal of the Bio-Electro-Magnetics Institute, **2**, 8–17. Available from Dr John Zimmerman, 2490 West Moana Lane, Reno, Nevada 89509-3936.

2

A guide to assessment and diagnosis in naturopathic medicine

John R. Cross

Introduction

It is said that physiotherapy is the 'natural alternative'. To a certain extent this is true, but there is much more to the basics of 'natural medicine' that falls within the boundaries of physiotherapy than is generally understood. In this chapter we shall briefly examine the various naturopathic principles and then look at all the many and varied types of assessment and 'natural' diagnosis that it is possible for the physiotherapist (with some training) to undertake.

Naturopathy (natural or complementary medicine)

This is a system of medicine which seeks to facilitate and promote the body's inherent physiological self-healing mechanisms by means of exercise, massage, hydrotherapy (in various forms), nutrition and diet and manipulative therapy. Naturopathy is one of the oldest forms of medicine in the world and is based on four main principles:

- **Recognition of the individuality of the patient.** Allopathic (orthodox) medicine has a tendency to 'clump' patients with similar symptoms as being the same and they are often ordered the same treatment. Each person is an individual with different physical, chemical, emotional and spiritual make-ups. We each live in different environments and have varied external stimuli. Each of these factors is important in determining the treatment.

- **That one should attempt to establish and treat the *cause* of the condition, not just treat or palliate the symptoms.** Allopathic medicine, in part, can also state this. Naturopathic medicine, however, goes much deeper into the possible causes which are not always apparent, because of the different basic philosophy from allopathic practitioners. An example of this would be the treatment of 'frozen shoulder'. Allopathically this would be treated with analgesics, physiotherapy and exercise, naturally assuming that the cause of the condition is a 'mechanical' one. Natural medicine would give the cause of a 'frozen' shoulder as possible dietary imbalance (too much refined foods, thus causing constipation), emotional upsets such as anxiety and lack of free expression, as well as the obvious ones such as a cervical nerve referral or a sequelae to a shoulder injury.

- **That everyone has the ability within the body to heal themselves (vis medicatrix naturae).** Naturopaths take care not to suppress symptoms but to allow the person to heal themselves by their own built-in energy system (this will be explained later).

- **The need to treat the whole person and not just the local area which may be affected.** This means that we have to look at the patient in a holistic way – mind, body and spirit – and appreciate that a symptom is simply an expression of an imbalance within the whole.

Naturopaths recognize that dis-ease may be due to inherited congenital and developmental factors as well as infection, trauma, nutritional, structural and emotional imbalances. Naturopathy is an approach to health rather than a specific therapy. Its origins and antecedents in natural hygiene and nature cure emphasized a way of life which is in harmony with nature. Modern naturopathic medicine is based on a philosophy which emphasizes the unity of life and sees health and dis-ease very much as the product of human physiological, biochemical and emotional harmony or disharmony.

Figure 2.1 shows that in naturopathic medicine the human body is considered to be made up of equal measures of mechanical, mental or emotional and chemical parts – the Healing Triad (Figure 2.1). The practitioner should always remember this basic fact. One should always ask oneself, during the initial consultation with one's patient, where the root cause of the imbalance lies. Just because we may be dealing with a seemingly obvious mechanical imbalance, it does not mean that the **cause** is mechanical; it may be chemical or emotional. As we shall see later in the chapter and throughout this book, there are scores of examples of this, where a symptom such as pain may be caused by an emotional cause (long-term stress, anger, tension, jealousy, etc.), a chemical imbalance (eating foods or taking chemicals or toxic drugs that cause stomach or liver imbalance), as well as the commonly conceived mechanical cause. As therapists, we should strive to think a little more laterally. For example, a spondylosis of the sixth and seventh cervical vertebrae that has no obvious traumatic aetiology could be caused by a large bowel problem (constipation) or the person's inability to express themselves emotionally. Conversely, the emotion of **fear**, without apparent reason, could be caused by a kidney imbalance due to a cortisone imbalance or a long-term mechanical irritation of L2–3.

Hippocrates was the first physician to say that symptoms are golden pearls that should be used to attempt to reach the true cause of a condition. Symptoms are merely the patient's **expression**; they are like a flag being waved in the direction of the therapist, saying 'this is what my body is attempting to express, but please find the cause'. Symptoms should **never** be suppressed with chemical drugs or such like. Andrew Taylor Still, the founder of osteopathy, recognized this and gave us that wonderful expression, 'structure governs function'.

We have to take the **whole** person into account with our treatments. We are not just a jumble of dissimilar organs and tissues that need a specific medical approach to each; instead, we are a wonderful blend of togetherness. If one part of our body starts to fail, it will cause others to fail. This topic of **holism** is nicely answered in the many **laws** and **fixed principles** that complementary medicine gives us. Such laws as the 'Mother–Son' and 'Five Elements' fall into the bailiwick of Chinese medicine. Constantine Hering spent his life examining the human body in a naturopathic way and gave us his 3 laws of cure. He states that cure takes place from the upper extremities downwards, from the internal towards the external and that, during cure, symptoms appear in a reverse order than they did with the formation of the disease. Quite simply, he was saying that when a patient is being treated with naturopathy, whether by fasting, acupuncture, homoeopathy, herbs, reflexology, healing or 101 other types of natural medicine, they take the opportunity to **self-heal** and do it in specific ways according to the laws.

An example of the 'top to bottom' law would be the migraine that eases with the correct treatment only to present an upper dorsal tension

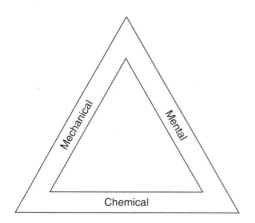

Figure 2.1 The Healing Triad

which, in turn, gives way to low back pain, which then resolves with treatment. An example of the 'interior–exterior' law would be the asthma that eases with treatment to become ezcema, which is possibly the easier of the two diseases to treat successfully. In both of these cases would be hints of the third law which is beloved of naturopaths. Given the correct treatment, the person will exhibit the symptoms in a reverse order to that which came in the first place. These return symptoms may be transient or long lasting. They are often called a 'healing crisis', and are simply the body's **vital force** self-healing to attempt to produce homeostasis within.

The so-called 'unitary' theory has stemmed from Hering's third law of cure. This states that disease is a **force** (of energy) and proceeds from organ to organ and from system to system throughout our lives, always getting deeper and producing more chronic symptoms. When self-healing commences, the patient's healing energy is called into action and the symptoms reappear and proceed towards the superficial from the deep. This is why, when after a couple of treatments, the patient will remark that they **feel** better in themselves, even though symptomatically they may be the same.

'Natural' analysis and diagnosis

One must never forget the fact that practitioners can assess and diagnose what system of the body is in a state of imbalance just by correct and sympathetic questioning, listening and palpation. It does not necessarily need a specialist to do this. The human body is a wonderful and complex thing, but when it comes to assessment we use **what the patient is trying to tell us** by the signs and symptoms of the many reflected pathways (reflexes) that we all have. There are 13 areas of **diagnosis** and 10 areas of **treatment**, using our many disciplines. The areas of diagnosis are:

- iris
- face
- skull
- ear
- foot
- abdomen (2)

- tongue
- temple
- pulse
- hand
- spine
- listening posts.

The areas of treatment that follow are:

- skull
- hands
- feet
- face
- reflexes and acupoints
- abdomen
- ears
- spine
- meridians
- Major and Minor Chakras.

There is an eleventh, the aura, which is covered extensively in Chapter 4.

Areas of diagnosis

All the areas of diagnosis that we shall discuss can be likened to a microcosm within the macrocosm. Each of the reflected areas represents the whole body in miniature and when there is some imbalance in the whole or in an individual organ or body area, this imbalance is reflected into the localized area. The study of each individual area can take a practitioner a lifetime to master (pulse, iris, etc.), but we as physiotherapists can just learn enough to be able to analyse and diagnose correctly. Each area of diagnosis will confirm the findings of the other areas and it should not take long for the practitioner to be able to recognize where the imbalance and disharmony lies and, more importantly, what to do about it!

Many of the foregoing areas come under the umbrella of traditional Chinese medicine (TCM). The main criteria of TCM is that the vital force, mentioned previously, is called **Ch'i** and that there are two components of Ch'i called **Yin** and **Yang**. They are the bi-polars of Ch'i and are opposite and yet complementary to each other. Yang energy covers the **acute** side of disease, whereas Yin covers the **chronic**. Table 2.1 gives a few Yang and Yin equivalents.

Table 2.1 Some Yang and Yin equivalents

Yang	Yin
Summer	Winter
Heat	Cold
Male	Female
Light	Dark
Acute	Chronic
Spastic	Flaccid
Mobility	Stiffness
Inflammation	Oedema
Hypertension	Hypotension
Hollow organ	Vital organ

The well-known symbol known as the **Pakua** (Figure 2.2) or the **Chinese Monad** shows **wholeness**, which according to the Chinese is simply Ch'i. The shaded area is Yin and the light area is Yang. Note that there is not a straight-line division but a curved line – nothing in nature or the human frame is straight, nothing is black and white, but all is various shades of grey. Note also that there is a little Yin in the Yang and a little Yang in the Yin. Put in therapeutic terms, one can never have a wholly Yin or Yang condition. Total Yin is, of course, death of the physical body.

The traditional Chinese doctor (or 'barefoot' doctor as they were known) would make a thorough and comprehensive examination of the patient and take a case history, approaching his patient gently and considerately. He first observed and listened to the patient. He then touched, palpated the body, read the pulses, looked at the tongue, looked at the eyes and palpated the abdomen. The findings of the clinical examination are put under the eight key-symptoms or approaches of TCM, which are: Deep and Superficial; Cold and Heat; Emptiness and Fullness, and finally Yin and Yang. These differentiations enabled the doctor to ascertain the energic imbalance and determine the severity of the ailment.

Emptiness indicated an energy deficiency and included such symptoms as lack of appetite, night sweat and lassitude. Symptoms of Fullness are excess phlegm, flatulence and constipation, indicating an acute disorder. If the patient does not feel thirsty or prefers hot drinks, there is a Cold disorder, whereas thirst for cold drinks, dry lips, red eyes and general restlessness are symptoms of Heat. Pains in the peripheral joints are called Superficial and pains in the chest and abdomen are called Deep. Yin and Yang are the basic principles for the functioning of the whole organism and also describe the others, hence Yang covers Superficial, Heat and Fullness, and Yin covers Cold, Deep and Emptiness. Quite often, as in Western medicine, the object of the treatment is to convert that which is chronic into acute to make it easier to treat; hence we attempt to turn Cold into Heat, Deep into Superficial, Emptiness into Fullness and Yin into Yang.

The iris

Iris diagnosis (iridology) represents a fascinating study and one that can take several years to perfect. Dr von Peckzely, of Budapest, discovered nature's records in the eye, quite by accident, when he was a boy of 10 years of age. Playing one day in the garden at his home, he caught an owl. While struggling with the bird, he broke one of its limbs. Gazing straight into the owl's large bright eyes, he noticed, at the moment when the bone snapped, the appearance of a black spot in the lower central region of the iris, which he later found to correspond to the location of the broken leg. The boy put a splint on the limb and kept the owl as a pet. As the fracture healed, he noticed that the black spot in the iris became overdrawn by a white film and surrounded by a white border (denoting the formation of scar tissue formation at the fracture site).

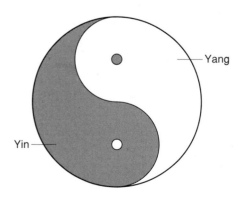

Figure 2.2 The Chinese Monad

In iris diagnosis, there are three basic constitutional types, from which we can narrow down certain organic imbalances. These are **lymphatic**, **haematogenous** and **biliary**:

- *Lymphatic* is found in 62% of the UK population. The iris is always blue or blue/grey. There is random structure with a white ring around the inner wreath. Often associated with blond hair and pale skin. Patients of this type may be prone to immune system problems such as allergies, asthma and ezcema, upper respiratory tract infections, tonsillitis, catarrh and arthritis.
- *Haematogenous* is deep brown, like a velvet carpet with few iris fibres showing. Can have the occasional 'bright' zones which can appear to be yellow. Disease indications suggest lowered blood cell counts, aneamia, glandular and circulatory disorders.
- *Biliary* is where the iris contains both blue and brown fibres. Even though it has its own disposition it can be influenced by lymphatic or haematogenous disposition, depending on the amount of blue/brown showing. The disease indications involve the biliary system, i.e. the liver and gall bladder plus the digestive system. There could be frequent problems with the blood sugar metabolism.

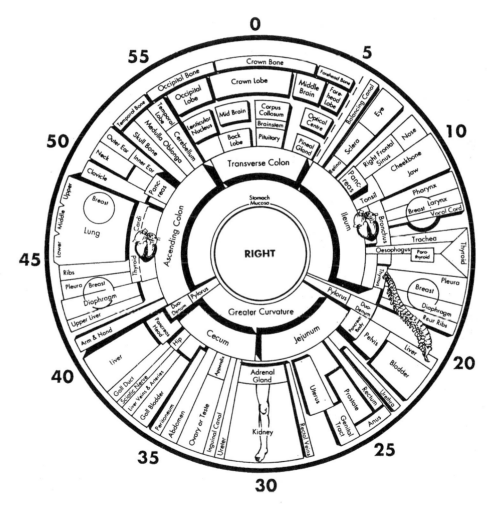

(a)

Figure 2.3(b) and caption on page 42

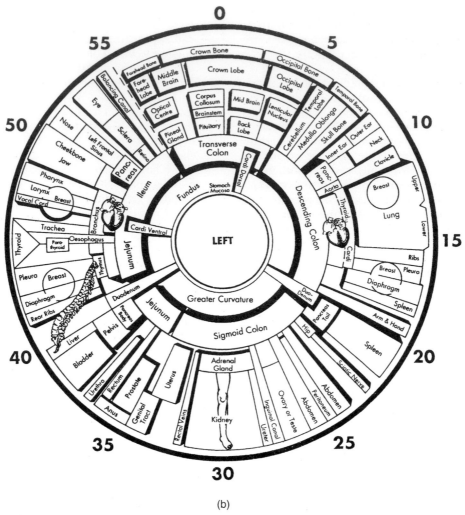

(b)

Figure 2.3 The iris map: (a) right eye (looking at another person's right eye); (b) left eye (looking at another person's left eye)

As with all the reflected pathways in the body, the centre of the iris represents the centre of us and the outside represents the outside, i.e. the area just around the pupil represents the stomach and the very outside represents the skin. Just further out from the stomach 'ring' there is the small intestine and large intestine. Any irregularity with these organs, such as allergic syndromes or inflammation, shows up as yellow or orange in the form of a 'corona'. The remainder of the iris represents the remainder of the body which can easily be identified by looking at the relevant position of the hands of the clock. Brown, blue , black or grey markings

in the exact area corresponding to an invidual body part signifies some state of imbalance in that area of the body. This can range from acute to chronic. With the correct treatment these spots disappear. Figure 2.3 shows a map of the iris, with its reflected pathways.

The tongue

The tongue has represented a useful diagnostic tool for centuries and is one of the chief tools used in traditional Chinese and Japanese medicine. It is said that the tongue in general terms is the outward expression of the stomach. This means that any imbalance with the digestive system can easily be detected in the tongue. The tongue will remain furred with white or yellow coating so long as the stomach remains in a state of imbalance. When we fast, as the body attempts to get rid of accumulated toxins and poisons, the tongue will slowly change from being of a very white and 'yucky' appearance to that of being nice and pink. Traditionally, we are supposed to fast for as long as the tongue remains furred – not many of us are that brave though! The tongue also represents the areas of the body, as with the iris. It is a most reliable indicator and changes often appear in the tongue prior to physical symptoms. By observing the tongue, the practitioner can observe the disease progression. The description below represents just a summary of what tongue diagnosis has to offer; it takes many years to master all the secrets that the tongue holds. The description includes terms based upon TCM, as previously mentioned:

- **Colour.** Pale white represents an empty cold condition with insufficient Yang Ch'i to push the blood up. Scarlet or dark red indicates heat in the body: the more red, the hotter the condition. A purple tongue is a serious condition that involves stagnant blood due to weak Ch'i.
- **Coating.** A white coating indicates excess water internally; if greasy it indicates damp heat with problems with the stomach or spleen. A yellow coating indicates a worsening of the disease process or an infection in the part represented by the area of yellowing. A black or grey coating is a more serious disease. This involves kidney Ch'i and is said to be a cold disease. Figure 2.4 shows the various body associations.

The face

Facial diagnosis represents another facet of traditional diagnosis that has been with us for centuries. It is amazing how much information we can glean from carefully examining the face.

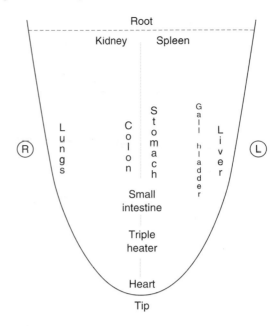

Figure 2.4 Tongue diagnosis, showing areas controlled by particular organs

Facial colour. Chalky white complexion means a general deficiency of Ch'i and coldness, possible condition with the respiratory system. A generalized red colour (not just the cheeks) means a lot of Yang or heat in the system; it may also indicate circulatory imbalance. A yellow appearance means there is a deficiency of Ch'i in the stomach and spleen, with or without dampness. A greenish tinge indicates liver disharmony, internal cold or pain. A blackish tinge, especially under the eyes, indicates a 'water' imbalance and a kidney condition. Please note that the different colours associated with the imbalances follow the colours used in the Law of the Five Transformations or Elements. This law is dealt with in Chapter 9.

Facial diagnostic areas

There are several different interpretations of this. They differ according to the traditional philosophy), i.e. Chinese, Japanese or Ayurvedic. Figure 2.5 represents those correspondences and associations that are borne out by personal experience.

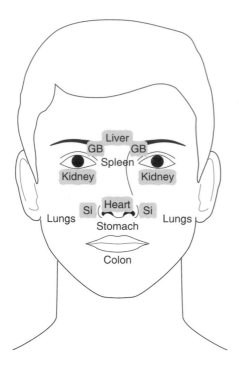

Figure 2.5 Facial and nasal diagnosis (see text for colour representations)

Lungs. Located on the cheeks. A white discoloration indicates Ch'i deficiency, whereas a reddish colour represents heat or inflammation. The more chronic the respiratory condition, e.g. emphysema, the whiter will be the colour.

Bronchi. Situated on the nostrils: white nostrils indicate a chronic complaint, whereas redness indicates heat and inflammation.

Large intestine. This organ is represented on the lower lip and the jaw. Swelling of the lower lip may indicate weakness of Ch'i in the large bowel and its capability of ridding the body of toxins. Dryness indicates a lack of fluid in the bowel. Red indicates heat and inflammation. Most problems with the large bowel that are indicated in the face can usually be cleared with correct dietary advice.

Stomach. This is located midway along the bridge of the nose and on the upper lip. Swelling of the upper lip indicates disharmony in the stomach, in that there is probably toxins that

the stomach is attempting to deal with, or that there may be an imbalance in the protein–fat relationship. Dryness and cracking indicates stomach Ch'i deficiency. Yellowing indicates a general weakness in the digestive system, with particular emphasis on the possibility of allergies.

Spleen. This is located on the bridge of the nose up towards the eyes. Yellowing in that area almost certainly indicates allergies and a weakness in the immune system. Serrated lines along the bridge of the nose indicate a long-term (chronic) imbalance and could mean severe immune disease. A darkish colour would indicate weak spleen Ch'i.

Liver. This is located between the eyebrows around the 'third-eye' point. Furrows and lines there may indicate a chronic organic imbalance and/or allergy of the non-food variety, e.g. hay fever. A redness indicates inflammation of the more acute type.

Gall bladder. Located on the eyelids. Redness here indicates a Yang condition, e.g. cholecystitis. The writer has also occasionally been able to tell the patient of the possibility of calculi in the gall bladder, as there appears tiny hard nodules on the eyelids, not to be confused with either styes or localized lymphatic obstructions.

Nervous system. This is represented as a large area on the forehead. A large number of vertical lines in this area could indicate a weakness in the nervous system such as worry and stress-related problems. The patient's age, obviously, has to be taken into account. As with every other area of diagnosis, facial analysis should *not* be taken out of context but used as just one part of the *whole* picture.

The temple

The 'trigger' points on the temple or, more correctly stated, the temperosphenoidal line (TS) (Figure 2.6) are only used for diagnostic purposes of pain and general imbalance along the spinal column. This is not to be confused with certain aspects of cranial osteopathy that uses similar points (and many others) but also

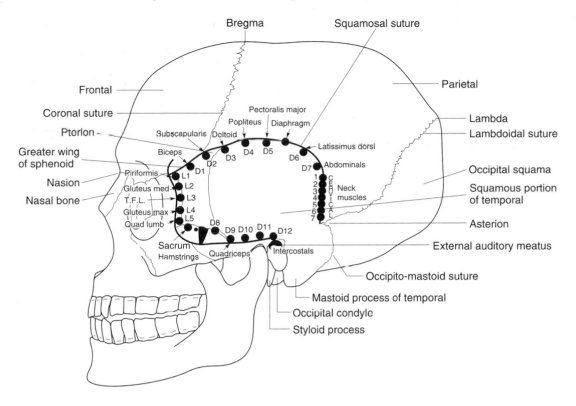

Figure 2.6 The temperosphenoidal line

has a treatment role. Acute tenderness of one or more of the points along the TS line indicates that there is a 'lesion' in the corresponding vertebra *or* the overriding muscle. It could be an acute spondylitis, chronic spondylosis or localized muscular spasm due to a hundred and one vertebral abnormalities. The therapist will use this information as a *guide* only and pool the information together with all other data available from all the other reflected pathways and points to ascertain an accurate symptom picture. Once the spinal condition is successfully dealt with, the tenderness on the TS line will disappear. The more chronic the spinal and muscular condition is, the more will be the tenderness of the point on the TS line, possibly accompanied by a slight swelling or nodule. Palpation is done with a very light touch. On older people the TS line can actually be seen, whereas in younger and more obese individuals, the TS line is more difficult to palpate and requires some experience.

The skull

There are several interpretations of the reflexes that appear on the skull (Figure 2.7) and these have formed the basis of many approaches and disciplines, namely cranial osteopathy, Tibetan head massage, applied kinesiology and craniosacral therapy. The aspect chosen to be highlighted in this chapter is the muscular association which is associated with applied kinesiology, but has correlations with traditional acupressure. Several areas of the skull are associated with certain muscles and by palpating these areas the therapist can tell which muscles are in a state of imbalance (pain, spasm, etc.). Once the analysis has been made, the therapist can immediately go into treatment 'mode' by using a stretching technique along the area of the skull. This is done with a very light, gentle force and is held until there is a discernible heat felt underneath the fingers. When the area of the skull feels relaxed and warm, the

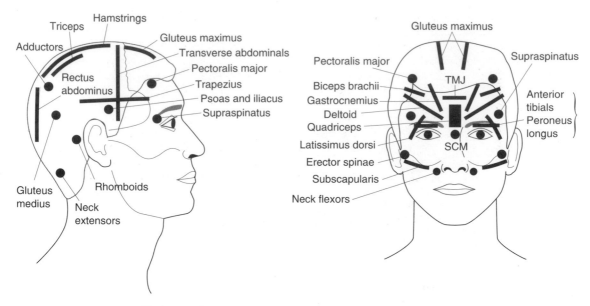

Figure 2.7 Stretch reflexes on the scalp with muscle association

associated muscle will also be eased, thus allowing more in-depth therapy to be done locally to the muscle.

The pulse

The pulse diagnosis (Figure 2.8) represents one of the oldest types of traditional diagnosis. It is extremely complicated if learnt in detail, but can be learnt slowly over the months and years until it is mastered. The physiotherapist is used to the knowledge of having just *one* pulse at the distal end of the radial artery by the wrist. To be told that there are *twelve* interpretations of this one pulse can go against one's basic beliefs, and when one commences to try and find these pulse differences, one is 'all thumbs'. Slowly but surely, however, these subtle differences can be felt. Reading the pulse according to traditional Chinese and Japanese medicine can provide information about the patient's entire constitutional condition. So-called acupuncturists who are only wedded to Western beliefs and who mainly perform 'symptomatic pinpricking' do not know what they are missing without this extra knowledge.

To take the pulse, ensure the patient's arm is horizontal with the wrist lower than the heart.

The therapist should use three fingers placed on the patient's pulse just above the wrist crease. The left hand pulse is usually stronger in men and the right hand pulse is stronger in women. The fingers should, one by one, be pressed down to almost occlude the flow of blood and then released slightly – this gives the deeper or the Yin pulse. The superficial or Yang pulse is felt by a gentle touch of the finger on the radial artery. At each of the six sites there is a Yin and Yang association which is coupled with the energic quality of the corresponding internal organ.

If it is just about acceptable to the sceptical orthodox therapist that there are *twelve* pulses not *one*, it really stretches credulity to the limit to think that there are as many as *twenty-seven* variations of each of these twelve. The pulse can be Superficial, Floating, Deep, Slow, Rapid, Empty, Full, Slippery, Choppy, Thready, Fine, Thin, Tight, Wiry, Weak, etc. Each one of these different variations is significant in the overall picture of the patient's condition. They are far too elaborate and complicated to discuss in this short chapter. Even when the information about the patient has been gleaned via the pulse, the therapist has to take into account the time of day, time of year and general weather conditions. These factors, coupled with a knowledge

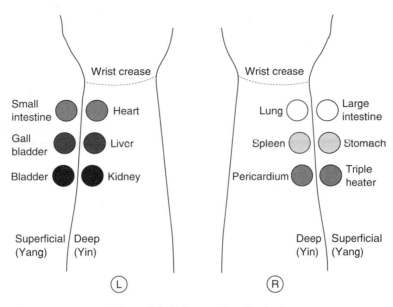

Figure 2.8 Chinese pulse diagnosis

of the natural flow of energy through the body and the Law of Five Elements, should give the therapist a complete picture.

The ear

The study of the ear for diagnostic and treatment purposes is a fascinating one, and one that can occupy the therapist's mind and brain for several years in order to attain true knowledge. It is again based upon the theories of reflected pathways, in that one can map out the whole of the body within the ear, with the centre of the ear representing the centre of the body, i.e. the stomach and the periphery of the ear representing our periphery (Figure 2.9). It represents a whole branch of acupuncture and is known as **auriculotherapy**. There are several acupuncturists that use *only* ear points for their treatments. For practitioners who have a more diverse practice, the use of the ear over and above the use of peripheral points is significantly high in the field of both analgesia and addiction.

The author remembers about 25 years ago, covering an athletics meeting at Crystal Palace as one of the physiotherapists to the Great Britain team against a Soviet team, being confronted by a Soviet athlete with acute pain in the right knee. She was due on track for the 5000 metres in 10 minutes' time and speed was of the essence. My sparse knowledge of ear acupressure came in handy and the 'knee' point of the (R) ear was pressed, along with localized pressure points around the knee. It was an instant success. The athlete competed and won the race. There had been no verbal dialogue between us, as neither spoke the other's language. In hindsight, it must have been very strange to her for some foreigner to stick a finger in her ear after she had complained of knee pain. The story made the popular press and a great deal of interest was aroused. In some small way it could have helped spread the word that physiotherapists were capable of doing such things.

The therapist can use finger pressure, the end of a 'baby bud', a tiny seed pellet held on by micropore or a little magnet. Just do what is comfortable for you. As with each and every reflected pathway of the body, when the body part or organ is in a state of imbalance, it will show in the reflex. We therefore will have the symptoms of localized tenderness, redness and swelling in the ear. Be careful not to press too hard.

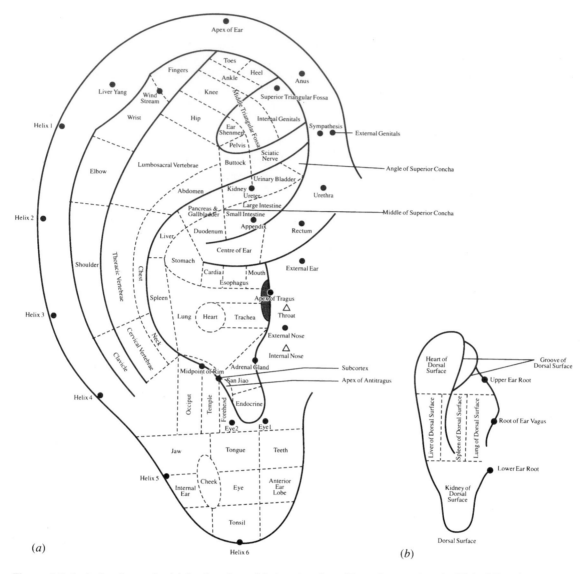

Figure 2.9 Auricular diagnosis: (a) front surface; (b) dorsal surface (From *Acupuncture in Clinical Practice*, Butterworth-Heinemann, 1996 by permission)

The treatment of addictions is more complicated and one that this short chapter cannot possibly go into in any detail about. There has been much research carried out into auriculotherapy and its use in addiction, both the mainstream addictions of alcohol, drugs, nicotine, etc., as well as the treatment of 'cravings' such as food intake. The author has also found auriculotherapy to be extremely good in the treatment of hypertension and anxiety. The points that are mostly used are the ones on the helix for hypertension and point 'Shenmen' in the ear.

The hand and foot

The assessment and treatment of a patient using foot and hand reflexes (reflexology) is given in Chapter 14.

The abdomen

The study of abdominal diagnosis can be divided into two types – the **Hara** diagnosis and the **Alarm** points.

Hara diagnosis

The abdomen is divided into reflected areas or reflexes that correspond with the associated organs. There have been several different interpretations of the abdominal chart and the one shown in Figure 2.10 gives a composite view. If the therapist presses the associated area with a gentle touch and elicits pain or discomfort in the area, there is usually an acute inflammatory state in the associated organ. Pain and discomfort with a much deeper palpation indicates a more chronic situation with the organ. Remember, these are only guidelines and, as has been said before, represent only part of the jigsaw puzzle in the holistic assessment of the patient. There is often some obvious changes to the abdominal areas that show readily that there is some type of imbalance, namely, tension of the tissue, heat and redness, inflammation both on the skin and beneath the skin, swelling of the area. When the patient shows an absolute hatred of the abdomen being touched at all, this often shows a deep-seated emotional imbalance.

Alarm points

Alarm points (Figure 2.11), often called the Front Collecting points, represent acutely painful 'trigger' spots when the associated organ is in a state of inflammation or acute imbalance. These points can also be used as treatment as well as analysis. Do not press heavily, but use a gentle but firm constant pressure with a short rotational massage technique.

The spine

Assessment, analysis and diagnosis through the spine is probably the most common form that physiotherapists deal with in their everyday work. The orthodox therapist is used to dealing with referred spinal pain and parasthesia, dermatomes, sclerotomes and myotomes, but there are more 'energy'-based considerations that we can learn. We owe a great debt of gratitude to a few American chiropractors who, in the 1960s, founded a wonderful form of analysis and therapy called applied kinesiology. The simpler form of this called 'Touch For Health' has been learnt by literally thousands of professional and lay practioners alike to enhance their appreciation and knowledge of the human body and psyche. In 30 short years the science of applied kinesiology, which is based on muscle testing for body energy imbalances, has made huge advances and has incorporated several ancient Chinese and Japanese concepts that are used in acupressure, Tsubo and Shiatsu. It has been shown that each and every muscle in the body is associated with a particular organ, meridian, neurolymphatic point (or Chapman's reflex) and a neurovascular point. There is also a spinal segmental level that can give certain symptoms of pain and spasm around the vertebrae if the organ is in a state of imbalance. In traditional Chinese medicine these tender points around the vertebrae are known as Associated

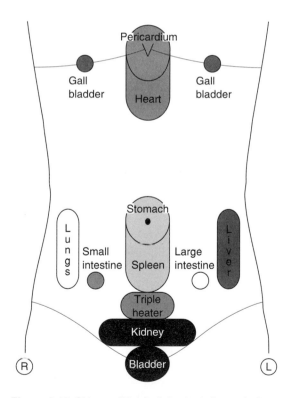

Figure 2.10 Chinese (Hara) abdominal diagnosis (see earlier section of text for colour representations)

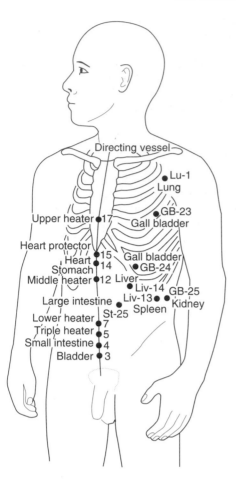

Figure 2.11 Abdominal Alarm points

Effect points (Figure 2.12). They are also called Yu points or Shu points, also the Back Transporting points in kinesiology and Shiatsu. These tender points are *not* to be confused with Neural Trigger points or even the tender points that are on the outer aspect of each vertebra due to spinal misalignments. The latter are usually associated with inflammatory processes in the sympathetic nervous system.

The Back Transporting points lie on the meridian called the inner bladder line and become tender when the associated organ is in a state of imbalance. The more acutely sick the organ, the more acutely tender is the point. They can also be of use both in diagnosis and treatment of chronic organic and spinal maladies. Firm and yet gentle pressure massage should be adopted. This and other forms of therapy and

treatment are fully discussed in a forthcoming book (Cross, see Recommended reading).

'Listening posts'

This subject falls under the umbrella of craniosacral therapy and as such will be fully discussed in Chapter 10.

So far we have discussed the many individual reflected areas of the body that represent the microcosm within the macrocosm. Each has its place in analysis; some are better than others in diagnostic terms and the individual therapist will certainly have preferences of one or two against the others. Remember, however, that whichever course of training you wish to

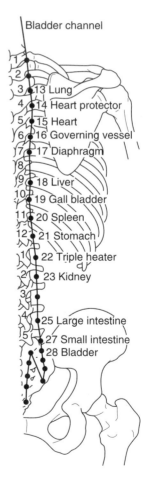

Figure 2.12 Associated Effect points

embark upon, try to choose the best and the longest course that is available. Try and be an *expert* in your chosen field. It will pay dividends in the end, not only in your capacity to heal others but also in your own self-confidence. Mention should briefly be made of the five **constitutional types** that we see in our surgeries and also explain a little of what to look out for in 'body language'. These factors can be just as important as looking at the individual 'parts' of the patient.

Constitutional types

There are several ways of differentiating the person's constitutional type. The anatomist and kinesiologist would use the body somatyping of mesomorph, ectomorph or endomorph and be able to deduce the person's capabilities, strengths and weaknesses from it. The classically trained homoeopath would use the archetyping that Hahnemann invented, namely the Miasmitic concept of dis-ease. This states that we are all born with certain hereditary weaknesses that represent a dis-ease taint or predisposition that has been handed down to us from our forebears. The dis-ease predispositions are Psora, Tuberculin, Syphilitic and Sycotic. All dis-ease is considered to stem from one of these predispositions or a combination of them. The Ayurdedic (Indian) practitioner would archetype using the **Ida** (Deep or Organic) and **Pingala** (Superficial or non-Organic) strengths and weakness; in a similar way, the TCM practitioner would classify the person's strengths and weaknesses in terms of the Yin and Yang complementary aspects of Ch'i, referred to earlier. The following simplistic archetyping of constitutional types is based upon the traditional Chinese Method of Five Elements. Generally an 'excess' body will tend to have a tight musculature, compared to a 'deficient'-type body which will have soft flesh and poor circulation. Pure archetypes are rare and patients are usually a combination and mixture of the following elemental types:

Water. Soft features. Often dark or bluish complexion. Tend to be slow, lazy and adaptable. They would have a tendency to have weak spines and also have kidney, bladder and prostate troubles. They would also have a leaning towards most types of arthritis and would have worse symptoms in the winter.

Wood. Hard, tight and strong musculature. Greenish or purplish complexion. Organized, possibly tense. Sudden rigid movement. They would have a weakness with the liver and gall bladder, would suffer migraines, headaches and also allergies. They would feel symptomatically worse in the spring.

Fire. Fine, pointed features. Wide forehead and high cheekbones. Red complexion. Sometimes nervous. Adventurous. They would suffer from circulatory troubles as well as heart and small bowel imbalance. They would dislike extremes of temperature and feel worse just before lunch time and also in midsummer.

Earth. Heavy set, often flaccid. Tendency to be overweight. Sallow complexion if not yellowy. Slow moving, calm and practical. They would have a tendency to have digestive imbalance, also immune system imbalance and also suffer from anxiety and depression. Would suffer from cold extremities and would not like wet and cold weather.

Metal. Broad shouldered, but often hollow chested and lean. White, pale complexion. Careful in movement, enjoying stillness. Rational and slightly melancholic. Would have a tendency to suffer from respiratory complaints, also skin trouble. They would feel at their worst during the early hours of the morning and in the late summer and autumn.

The following represents a brief summary of what to look for with body language, speech and emotional imbalance. Please remember that much of our physical ills are psychosomatically based. Never be afraid of asking probing questions (not necessarily at the initial consultation) regarding the patient's fears, likes and dislikes and possibly their dreams. A positive answer to some of the questions could be the golden nugget of information that you are looking for to make an adequate diagnosis.

Liver and gall bladder imbalance (Wood element). Tendency to stoop and have round shoulders, shuffle. They also speak with a 'drawl' or a 'whining' tone that can be very irritating. Emotionally they are angry, irritable and indifferent towards others. They dream of violence.

Heart, small bowel, pericardium and three heater imbalance (Fire element). Tendency to 'gabble' and chatter. Get very anxious and agitated. They are nosey and curious. They may also be giggly and very shy. Dream of laughter, being shut in and/or exposed.

Kidney and bladder imbalance (Water element). Rigid spines. Shuffle. Tend to be 'weak' people. Cowards, especially if they have dorsal scoliosis. Have extreme fear and phobias among the five types. Dream of drowning and voyages.

Lung and large bowel imbalance (Metal element). Boisterous and heavy. Very forward and will sit on the edge of their seat when interviewed. They have many fears but not as many as the Water type. They are basically shy and although 'loud' may not be able to express themselves adequately. They cry quite a lot but need to be alone to express grief and sorrow. Dream of sadness and crying, also flying, singing.

Spleen and stomach imbalance (Earth element). Have a tendency to put on weight and be indolent *or* the opposite and be very underweight. They have dark secrets and can be very fearful, anxious and depressed. Tend not to express themselves readily. Dream of food and feasting, also that body is very heavy.

The foregoing represent just a glimpse of what is possible through 'natural' diagnostic methods. Remember, though, that each is a part of the whole and that a complete picture is needed in order to find out which system or systems are in a state of energy imbalance.

Recommended reading

Academy of Traditional Chinese Medicine (1975) *An Outline of Chinese Acupuncture*. Beijing: Foreign Language Press.

Cross, J. (in preparation) *Acupressure: Clinical Applications in the Treatment of Musculo-Skeletal Conditions – 'Chinese Physiotherapy'*. Oxford: Butterworth-Heinemann.

Ellis, N. (1994) *Acupuncture in Clinical Practice*. London: Chapman and Hall.

Gerber, R. (1988) *Vibrational Medicine*. Santa Fe, NM: Bear.

Jarmey, C. and Nojay, G. (1992) *Shiatsu – The Complete Guide*. Wellingborough: Thorsons.

Lindlahr, H. (1919) *Iridiagnosis and other Diagnostic Methods*. Saffron Walden: C.W. Daniel.

Maciocia, G. (1987) *Tongue Diagnosis in Chinese Medicine*. Seattle, WA: Eastland Press.

Thompson, W. (1985) *Personalysed Diagnosis (Alternative Medicine)*. Published privately by the author.

Valentine, T. and Valentine, C. (1985) *Applied Kinesiology*. Wellingborough: Thorsons.

Vithoulkas, G. (1979) *Homoeopathy – Medicine of the New Man*. Wellingborough: Thorsons.

Part II

Healing by intention

3 Healing by intention – a research-based overview

Robert A. Charman

Introduction

For the purposes of this chapter the term 'healer' is defined as someone who practises 'healing' in the form of a deliberate act of directing an *intention-to-heal* towards another person, animal or other living system, and the term 'healee' will refer to the person who is receiving the healing intention. The intention-to-heal may be expressed as mental intention only, as in 'healing at a distance', or it may be combined with the placing of hands upon the person, or animal, to be healed. The healer may place his, or her, hands on, or over, the affected area to 'direct the healing', or pass the hands in a series of movements over and around the subject, or combine the two. Healers believe that the act of directing a voluntary intention-to-heal can have an actual effect upon the physiological, psychological or combined psycho-physiological processes, of the person or animal receiving the directed healing intention. Many healers believe in the existence of a spiritual level of being, and assume that all three aspects of bodily, mental and spiritual functioning are involved in the healing process. The nature of the response within the healee will be determined by the nature and source of the dis-ease that needs healing.

Healers also believe, and assert, that the healing outcome of their intention-to-heal, whether it has resulted, for example, in an apparent reduction, or reversal, of tumour growth, or an acceleration of wound healing, or has led to a reduction of tension and anxiety with conse-quent reduction in psychosomatic symptoms, is often substantial enough to be observed, mea-sured and recorded. They point to the consider-able body of research literature which, they feel, offers a scientific vindication of their belief that healing, as an outcome of healing intention, is a real phenomenon.

Healers believe that their *directed healing intention,* hereafter known as DHI, somehow becomes actualized into an agent of healing in its own right. It is often referred to as an 'intelli-gent agent' in that it 'knows what to do' to initi-ate, or augment, the natural healing processes in the other person, or animal, that have become relatively ineffective. Healers direct their healing intention in a spirit of love and compassion to achieve the 'highest good' of the person or animal receiving this intention. They believe that this 'highest good' may be activated at any level within the bodily, mental or spiritual dimensions of the healee according to the nature of the healing that is required.

The experience of 'receiving healing' is fre-quently described as a feeling of inner calmness and peace, often with a resultant increase in positive energy. Many who attend healers because of arthritis, for example, experience a reduction in pain, aching, stiffness and swelling during the session, and say that this relief is sustained for days, or weeks, afterwards. During the healing session the healee often experiences very definite sensations of heat, or warmth, or cold, or tingling, which may occur in any combination. These sensations are usually felt in the area under the hands of the healer and/or in the region of the body that requires healing. These sensations may be more marked if the hands of the healer are in contact, but can be just as strong if the hands are held, and moved, several inches away. They can be localized just as accurately when the healer is working behind the person, and the position of the hands cannot be seen, as when the healee can see the hands of the healer.

The healee may receive healing either knowingly, as when attending for healing, or unknowingly, as when the healer 'sends healing' at the request of a friend or relative on behalf of the healee, or the healee is given 'healing' when in an unconscious state, or an animal is brought for healing. The other circumstance in which the person 'receives healing' without knowing that they are the recipients of this healing intention is when they are taking part in a clinical trial designed to discover if the application of DHI to a person, without their knowledge, has any measurable effect upon the injury or illness parameters chosen for study as compared to matched controls.

The social context

Popular belief that some gifted people, or maybe every person in the right circumstances, can aid the desired healing in another person by DHI is widespread. In the UK there are over 20 reputable organizations that run courses leading to qualifications in healing, and there may be between 12 000 and 15 000 practitioners. Of these organizations the largest, and probably the most well known, is the National Federation of Spiritual Healers (NFSH) with over 6000 members. Courses in different systems and practices of healing, such as Chakra Energy Healing and Spiritual Healing (NFSH), are in considerable demand, and there is a course that is particularly designed for nurses and allied professionals, known as Therapeutic Touch. These three approaches to healing are discussed in separate chapters, as they are attracting an increasing number of physiotherapists who believe that this healing ability exists, and wish to offer healing as a clinical option for patients who would like to receive it. The chapter on Distant Healing reviews evidence that supports the belief that distance is no barrier to the

effect of DHI, and Chapter 8 discusses the application of healing to animals.

While belief in healers and healing is widespread, it is certainly not universal, and public opinion in the UK, as expressed in opinion polls, is very sharply divided on this subject (Clarke, 1998). Some 60% of respondents think that the possibility of one person healing another person by DHI is against all common sense and everyday experience, and that any apparent outcome can be ascribed to chance, naive suggestibility and the placebo effect. In their opinion it is impossible, and is therefore a non-existent phenomenon. On the other hand, some 40% of respondents believe that this ability definitely, or very probably, exists. If such polls reflect public opinion, then 60% of the population do not believe that healing, in this sense, exists. It is likely that the overwhelming majority of orthodox scientists across all of the scientific disciplines would strongly endorse the majority verdict on the grounds that such a claimed ability is contrary to all generally accepted scientific knowledge of how the physical world, including all living systems, actually works. For example, the consensus of opinion in the neurosciences is that mental function is a form of brain function that exists within the confines of the physical brain. The millivolt, microwatt and nanotesla to microtesla levels of electromagnetic field energies generated by any brain are far too feeble to affect anyone, or anything else, in any practical way.

A much smaller minority of scientists feel that this dismissal of the possibility that healing by DHI is a real phenomenon is far too sweeping. It ignores the strange quantum properties of the universe that underlies the ordinary world, and does not accord with carefully recorded case history experiences, or the results of laboratory and clinical investigation using accepted scientific methodology. In their opinion, this disbelief is more the expression of an *a priori* closed mind belief system than a considered judgment that has been arrived at following an impartial examination of the evidence (Benor, 1993; Dossey, 1993; Radin, 1997).

Against this background of majority disbelief within the general population and orthodox science in the claimed phenomenon of healing, and other related 'paranormal' phenomena such as telepathy, the results of a questionnaire inquiring into the personal beliefs of a cross-section of neuroscientists, neurophilosophers and other scientists who attended the Second Consciousness Conference, held at Tucson, Arizona in 1996, on the theme of 'Towards a Science of Consciousness', comes as rather a surprise (Baruss and Moore, 1998). Of the 210 participants who answered the questionnaire, 67% said that they believed that extrasensory perception is possible, 61% believed that the human consciousness is evidence for a spiritual dimension within each person, 66% said that they had experienced a transcendental or mystical experience, 82% believed that Eastern religions offered insights into consciousness, and 53% believed that consciousness transcends time. At the same time, 74% said that they believed that human consciousness cannot exist without the human brain, 59% believed that consciousness is an emergent property of the brain, and only 27% believed that personal consciousness continues after brain death. It is obvious that modern research has not resolved any of these issues concerning the relationship between mind and brain and the debate continues without resolution.

The central issue is the source and nature of consciousness. There is nothing in the known nature and processes of neurophysiology that implies an end product of emotions and conscious awareness. Correlation of localized brain area activity with particular forms of subjective experiences remains correlation. The working hypothesis of the neurosciences that neurophysiology is, somehow, mental psychology (that synaptic quanta become transmuted into *subjective qualia*) remains a useful, but unproven, hypothesis.

Two questions for answer

If healing by DHI is a genuine phenomenon, then it is possible that it may be a particular application of a more general *ability to affect* another person, animal or living system, across space without physical contact or the mutual interaction of the normal sensory systems, as in the claims for telepathy. This chapter will now confine itself to exploring the following two questions:

- *Question one.* Is there any evidence to show that a person, or persons, can affect the physiological processes, the psychological processes and/or the psycho-physiological processes of another person, animal or other living system, solely by directing a voluntary intention-to-heal, or to affect in some other desired way, that person, animal or other living system?
- *Question two.* Is there any evidence to show that a person, or persons, can affect the neuro-psychological processes, or psychological processes, of another person or persons, without having any specific intention to exert a DHI effect, or to affect in any directed way, another person or persons, but solely by their being in a particular, and unusual, state of conscious mind?

Question one

There are two main sources of possible evidence. The first source consists of individual case histories, and the second source consists of quantifiable evidence gathered from many case histories that can be converted into the comparative statistics of clinical trials.

Case histories

All medicine starts from observations and questions arising from case histories, and all medicine is based upon answers derived from case histories. The nature of the questions determines the nature of the research. The results of research determine the probable answers, and case history responses to treatment determine which of those probable answers provides the best medical answers to the original questions. Answers generate more questions leading to more research, and the cyclic process is never ending.

The literature on healing contains thousands of case histories of those who have received DHI and those who claim that they were either healed of whatever was wrong with them, or experienced considerable and unexpected improvement. The most dramatic scenarios are those cases where recovery has taken place against the gloomiest medical prognosis of imminent demise but, from the point of view of the healee, relief from the miserable pain of headache, backache or arthritis, after all orthodox therapies have apparently failed, must come a very close second.

Books written by healers such as Angelo (1994), Macmanaway and Turcan (1983), Southwood (1994) and Turner (1974), and by journalistic investigators such as Harvey (1983), Hodgkinson (1990) and Hutton (1986), are full of carefully recorded case histories implying that healers really can heal against the odds of medical prognostication. Non-believers downgrade such case histories to a more dismissive level of 'anecdotal stories' and point to suggestibility and the placebo effect or to spontaneous and coincident remission as the most likely explanation, although these explanations, of themselves, often appear more as statements of belief than explanations.

Some typical case histories are as follows:

Case history 1

A man of 65, who has smoked some 20 cigarettes a day for most of his life, but is now an ex-smoker, has lung cancer and rapidly spreading metastases which are unaffected by radiotherapy. Given a prognosis of about 8 months, he is referred by the consultant to a hospice for terminal care, is rapidly losing weight, becoming housebound, and is in a state of complete despair. At his daughter's insistence he agrees, with great scepticism, to attend a local healer centre. During the first session, lasting about 20 minutes, the healer places her hands close to either side of his chest. He feels a *warm, tingling sensation*, but nothing more, and experiences no apparent improvement in his condition. He attends weekly, finding that he feels *very relaxed* after each session, and slowly discovers that his range of activities is steadily increasing as the weeks go by. Follow-up X-rays show a steady reduction and eventual disappearance of the cancer and, some 10 years later, he remains alive and well and in sustained remission.

Case history 2

A married mother of two children has a 20-year history of acute episodes of low back pain and, in her 40s, undergoes two discectomies for intervertebral disc prolapse. After an initial 18-month period of pain relief, the pain returns with increasing severity during the next seven years. It is diagnosed as arising from postoperative meningeal membrane scarring which is untreatable. She has periods of being bedbound, and then walking in great pain with a stick, and lives with a prognosis of a likely deterioration towards a wheelchair existence. A chance meeting with a nearby neighbour who practises as a healer leads her to ask for healing. During the first session she becomes *sleepy and relaxed*, and the pain diminishes. As she receives weekly healing over the next few months the pain and disability reduce and remain within easy tolerance level and she finds that she can return to a nearly normal way of life. To her great relief she no longer has to rely on painkillers, sleeping pills and antidepressants.

Case history 3

A man in his 60s, with a 25-year history of chronic arthritis in his right hand resulting in swollen, stiff and very painful knuckles, limited movement and limited function, takes his wife, who has been diagnosed as having breast cancer, to a healer. At the end of the third session the healer turns to him and offers to treat his hand. She puts her hands on either side of his, without touching, and he feels *a lot of tingling, followed by a cold sensation that spreads throughout his hand*, with immediate relief of pain. Over the next few weeks of weekly healing the pain disappears, knuckle swelling and joint stiffness reduce, function improves, and the improvement is maintained. His wife's cancer also goes into prolonged remission.

> ### Case history 4
>
> A married woman in her mid-30s with two young children is diagnosed as suffering from primary liver cancer. She has surgery to remove the cancerous lobes, but within a few months it returns and spreads very rapidly. With a 3-month prognosis, and in the knowledge that neither chemotherapy nor radiotherapy can now offer any real hope of inhibition of the primary tumour and spread of the metastases, she attends a local cancer help centre, and is referred to a healer as part of the treatment programme. During the first session the healer slowly moves his hands over her head, and then downwards to either side of her abdomen without touching. She *feels a warmth and energy pouring in* and a sudden inner certainty that she would survive. During her weekly attendance over the next few weeks her signs and symptoms decrease, and follow-up scans confirm that her cancer has undergone rapid remission to apparent full disappearance. Ten years later she remains in full remission.

Sensations during the healing session

The reported sensations of warmth, cold, tingling and energy pouring in during the healing session, as italicized in these examples and discussed earlier, are typical, and are discussed in detail by Benor (1993, 1996). They are often mirrored as similar sensations in the hands of the healer (Turner, 1974), sometimes very powerfully and dramatically so (Weston, 1998). These sensations seem closely akin to those sensations generated by the autonomic nervous system, as in the bodily sensations that accompany being suddenly startled, surprised or shocked, or feeling intense emotional exhilaration and relief. They do not appear to be generated by any recordable changes in incoming sensory stimuli during the healing session, so their origin is probably central, possibly as a limbic system/autonomic nervous system response to a presumed DHI stimulus.

Cause and effect

It is obvious that both healers and healees are assuming a cause-and-effect relationship. They each assume that the healer, through DHI, has 'given', or 'applied', or 'channelled', a therapeutic agent called *healing* into the healee to effect the healing, whether of body, mind or spirit. Sceptics may accept a cause-and-effect relationship of expectation-triggered placebo improvement, but tend to attribute any associated remission of real physical disease to a *coincidence* of timing: in the case of cancer, to spontaneous remission, which is known to occur, or to a period of natural remission of a disorder such as chronic arthritis, or to the self-limiting signs and symptoms of a temporary condition, as in backache.

Healers may well respond by saying that if the placebo response is that powerful and effective, why was it *not* activated by the doctors and the impressive paraphernalia of orthodox diagnosis and therapy in which patients had placed their full expectation and trust in the first place? After all, the majority of people who decide to see a healer are those who feel that they have been failed by orthodox medicine and who turn to the healer in despair, and often against their own beliefs. This is just as true of pet owners who take their pets to animal healing clinics as a last resort when all veterinary skills have failed.

Clinical trials

One way to resolve this irreconcilable clash of causative interpretation is to eliminate the possibility of any expectation response, and therefore of any placebo response, by designing a clinical trial in which no one, including the subjects, knows that a healer is to direct his, or her, healing intention towards the experimental group.

Wirth and associates took this option and attempted to discover whether DHI could influence the rate of healing of a standardized skin wound. In each of these trials the research protocol, for all practical purposes, remained the same. Each healthy volunteer received a standardized, full-thickness, skin biopsy puncture wound to the skin over the left or right deltoid, and was randomly assigned to either the experimental (DHI) group or to the control group. The standard sized skin wound received standardized dressing care throughout the time of healing to completion. Attendance by both groups was daily, and the programme of

5 minutes of formal positioning of the dressed wound to receive DHI, or non DHI, commenced 30 minutes after biopsy, during which time it had been photographed and dressed. Thereafter the wound was visually inspected and photographed on given days until the end day of the trial, and the comparative rate of healing, or the number of fully healed wounds versus non-healed wounds on inspection days, was assessed by independent assessors.

Each trial was truly double blind, as neither the medical staff assessing the rate of wound healing, nor the personnel running the trial, nor the assessors, nor the subjects were told of the true nature of the trial. The latter were told that the purpose of the trial was to detect electrical fields emanating from the wound site, and that further information would be given upon trial completion. In the first trial (Wirth, 1990), the subjects thrust their arm through a hole in an opaque plastic screen behind which the healer was, or was not, present, but in subsequent trials the two were separated by a one-way mirror, which has now become the standard technique in such trials.

In discussing the outcomes of these trials it should be remembered that, as a statistical 'rule of thumb', if the differences in measurable outcome between the experimental and the control group are significant at 20:1 ($p = 0.05$), or more, against chance, then the variable under test is probably the causative factor in creating the difference in outcome between the two groups. In these trials the healers had trained in Therapeutic Touch (TT). This is rather a misnomer as these practitioners do not actually touch the healee, but place their hands in close proximity to interact with a presumed energy field around the healee (Krieger, 1979). In fact, the experimenters refer to it as 'Non contact therapeutic touch' (NCTT). In the published reports the TT treated groups were referred to as the experimental group (exp.) but this is replaced by 'TT' in this summary.

Wirth (1990). No. of subjects = 44.
TT group = 23. Control group = 21.
Inspection of the skin puncture wounds on day 8 showed that none of the subjects had healed completely, although healing in the TT group was more advanced. On day 16 this increased rapidity of healing was maintained and there was a marked difference between the two groups in the number of subjects whose skin wounds had completely healed. This latter is summarized as follows:

Day 16	Healed	Unhealed	
TT	13	10	(23)
Con.	0	21	(21)
$p = 0.01$			

The conclusion drawn from this outcome was that the most likely explanation as to why 13 (56.5%) of the TT group had healed completely within this time, as compared to none of the control group, was that the DHI of the TT practitioner was the agent that had accelerated the cellular healing processes of skin repair. The same agent was therefore responsible for the accelerated healing in the remaining 8 subjects in the TT group who were all much closer to full wound closure than the 21 subjects in the control group.

Wirth et al. (1993). No. of subjects = 24.
TT group = 12. Control group = 12.
The biopsy instrument was of a smaller diameter than in the first experiment, so assessments of healing completion, either complete or incomplete, were made on days 5 and 10.

Day 5	Healed	Unhealed	
TT	7	5	(12)
Con.	0	12	(12)
$p = 0.006$ (166.6:1)			

Day 10	Healed	Unhealed	
TT	10	2	(12)
Con.	4	8	(12)
$p = 0.041$ (24:1)			

The 2 subjects in the TT group who remained unhealed at day 10 were, again, considerably closer to full wound closure than the 8 subjects in the control group. This trial offered further confirmation of the conclusions drawn from the results of the first trial, to the effect that the DHI of a TT practitioner could stimulate a desired acceleration of cellular repair processes.

Wirth et al. *(1996).* No. of subjects = 32.
TT group = 16. Control group = 16.
By day 5 none of the wounds in either group had healed, and inspection on day 10 showed an unexpected, and statistically significant, difference between the groups that ran completely counter to the outcomes of the previous two experiments. This is summarized as follows:

Day 10	Healed	Unhealed	
TT	0	16	(16)
Con.	4	12	(16)

$p = 0.036$ (28:1)

As numbers are small, this unexpected reversal of outcome could be the result of the control group happening to include 4 exceptionally fast-healing individuals, combined with the possibility that the DHI effect of this healer was negligible. The surprise of this outcome lay in the fact that this was the same TT practitioner who had obtained apparent success as in the previous two trials. Inspection of the clinical diaries kept by all of the participants, including the healer, points to a possible, and intriguing, reason for the unexpected outcome. The diaries revealed that the healer had been suffering from severe influenzal symptoms of headaches, generalized muscle ache, temperature swings and digestive upset throughout the trial period. When the diaries of the two groups were compared, the control group diaries reported no illness of any kind but, of the TT group, 13 (81%) of the 16 subjects reported 'flu-like' symptoms of mild to medium severity. As there was no air flow contact between the healer and the TT subjects there was no possibility of viral transmission, so there was no means by which the healer could have infected any of the subjects in the TT group.

This correlation of symptoms of illness between the healer and the TT group, and the apparently reduced rate of wound healing in this group, may be chance coincidence. It does, however, agree with the convictions and anecdotal experiences of many healers to the effect that it is unwise for a healer to attempt to heal when feeling markedly unwell, as there may be symptom transfer to the healee. In a curious, and totally unexpected way, this outcome supports the belief among healers that everyone is, at some level of being, interconnected with everyone else. It also answers any charge by the sceptic that the results of the first two trials were somehow 'massaged' to 'prove' that DHI is a real phenomenon.

Wirth et al. *(1992).* In this trial the TT practitioners were asked to direct their DHI onto injured salamanders to determine whether DHI was effective when applied to another species. The objective of this trial was to assess whether healers could accelerate the rate of forelimb tissue regeneration in salamanders after surgical amputation of the forelimb at the elbow under anaesthetic. Salamanders are a naturally regenerative species following the apparently painless loss of a leg or tail when fighting or when escaping from predators. Four healers were used, both singly and in changing pairs, to test whether changing partners affected the efficacy of DHI. The comparative endpoint was the time that it took for the process of forearm and hand regeneration to reach the stage of observable differentiation into 1st finger regeneration and into 4th finger regeneration.

Number of salamanders = 154, divided into 22 tanks, with each tank containing 7 salamanders. During the trial, 11 TT tanks and 11 control tanks were singly moved and presented through an opening in front of which the healers were, or were not, sitting. The salamanders in the treated tanks received 5 minutes of DHI per day. The healers had EEG electrodes and other physiological monitors attached to them to assess whether there were any replicable physiological correlates with the 'centred' state of mind of the TT healers during the period of DHI, although any such findings were not discussed in this report.

The results demonstrated a very clear and consistent correlation of borderline to non-significant (NS) outcomes between the regeneration periods of salamanders in the TT tanks and the control tanks with those healers who disliked the trial set-up. They either found the monitoring equipment uncomfortable and distracting, or disliked treating salamanders, or felt that the whole experiment was a waste of valuable time. Conversely, one healer who normally worked with animals, who enjoyed the trial atmosphere and who felt fully confident that she could accelerate limb regeneration, consistently achieved very significant differences in regeneration times as follows:

To 1st finger differentiation.
Mean average for TT group   21.00 days
Mean average for control group   25.52 days
                                 $p = 0.01$

Less 4.52 days, or 82% less time, compared to the control group.

To 4th finger differentiation.
Mean average for TT group   27.00 days
Mean average for control group   31.82 days
                                 $p = 0.01$

Less 4.82 days, or 85% less time, compared to the control period.

When this healer was paired with another healer who also felt confident in her TT abilities, they achieved similar outcome results in acceleration of regeneration times in the TT groups of salamanders compared to the controls. One of the advantages of using animals, as in this experiment, is that there is no possibility of any placebo response affecting the outcome, and the variables can be kept to a close constant. The conclusion that the authors drew from this trial was that TT practitioners could accelerate the rate of forelimb regeneration in salamanders if they, themselves, felt fully confident that they could do so.

Discussion

The outcome of these trials would seem to support the theory that DHI, in the form of the belief system and practice of Therapeutic Touch in these particular trials, is a real therapeutic agent that can have a definite effect when 'delivered' by a healer, or by healers working together, who *feel confident* in what they are doing. The results of one trial implied, rather unexpectedly, that healers should not attempt to heal others when ill themselves. Clinical trials also demonstrate that the effectiveness of a healer dips towards non-significance in circumstances that undermine such confidence, or inhibit a desire to apply healing. This particularly applies in test conditions where it is difficult to empathize with the target subjects, such as salamanders, or the healer feels 'on trial' to obtain results. The test situation is in complete contrast to the normal healing encounter where the healer is responding to real need.

Inhibition of DHI effect

An example of the apparent inhibition of DHI effectiveness in circumstances that create a loss of self-confidence seems to be demonstrated by the outcome of the following trial:

Wirth et al. *(1994).* No. of subjects = 25. TT group = 13. Control group = 12.
The outcome assessment measures at day 5 and day 10 were identical to those used in the previous skin biopsy puncture wound trials, but the protocol was much more complicated. This was a double blind, within subject, crossover trial in which the subjects for the first 10-day trial (part A), received a skin wound over one deltoid, and then, for the second 10-day trial that immediately followed (part B), received a skin wound over the other deltoid. The same four TT practitioners, working in pairs, were used throughout both parts of the trial.

The purpose of the trial, unknown to the healers, was to assess whether the belief system of TT practitioners, which is that they must actually work within about 15 cm (6 inches) of the body surface so that they can sense and interact with the healee's energy field, would inhibit their confidence in their healing ability when they were told that subjects were either in another room elsewhere, or they were to treat through a plastic screen, or opaque smoked glass, which they believed to be inhibitory, or they were asked to treat via a video monitor or at a distance through a one-way mirror.

By day 10, the number of fully healed wounds present in the TT and the control groups for each trial was insufficient for analysis and therefore non-significant. The authors concluded that the non-significant outcome could be attributed either to genuine paired healer ineffectiveness whatever the circumstances, or to the strong dissonance that the trial created between their TT belief system and the perceived circumstances of the trial which completely inhibited any effective DHI.

Placing DHI within a wider 'intention-to-affect' context

These particular trials must now be placed within a wider context of trials designed to assess whether a voluntary *intention-to-affect*, in whatever desired way, actually does have an effect on other living systems. It seems reasonable to assume that the same mechanisms are operative whether the healer is trying to heal to the 'highest good' of the healee, or trying to influence the rate of enzyme reactions, cell division, cancer cell inhibition, germination rates of seeds, growth rates of seedlings, wound healing rates in animals, haemoglobin levels in patients, or whatever.

As mentioned earlier, it is a statistical 'rule of thumb' that if the measured difference in comparative outcome measures between the experimental group(s) and the control group(s) meets, or exceeds, a 20:1 odds against the difference being due to chance alone ($p = 0.05$), then it is considered to be statistically significant. This means that the most likely explanation for the difference may be attributed, with due caution, to the variable under test. This is not *proof* of effect, but *probability* of effect. So the greater the odds against chance occurrence, the greater the probability that this conclusion is valid.

Benor (1993) has undertaken a very comprehensive review of the vast literature on research into healing, and has divided it into controlled studies and uncontrolled studies. Benor considered the latter as fair to often very good studies whose standards did not meet the very high criteria of modern randomized clinical trials. Therefore, although their results often indicated that intention-to-affect does have an effect beyond chance, they obviously do not carry the same weight as trials meeting full scientific criteria. Benor retains the term 'healing' for all of these trials, regardless as to the intention, and points out that there has been more research into healing, in this more general sense, and more fully controlled trials on healing, than all of the other complementary therapies combined.

He found 131 trials that met modern research protocol. These include the famous series of trials carried out by Bernard Grad (1963, 1965, 1967); Grad *et al.*, 1961. He grouped and classified these trials under 10 separate headings of healing action upon enzymes, cells, fungi, yeasts, bacteria, plants, single-celled organisms, animals, electrodermal activity, human physical problems, and human subjective experiences. Each trial is summarized under its appropriate heading (summary tables in Benor, 1993, and Dossey, 1993). These 131 controlled trials can be roughly grouped into categories of different levels of statistical significance as follows:

- 56 (43%) were highly significant between $p < 0.01$ and 0.001 (100:1 < 1000:1)
- 21 (16%) were strongly significant between $p < 0.02$ and 0.05 (50:1 < 20:1)
- 12 (9%) were weakly significant between $p < 0.06$ and 0.1 (16:1 < 10:1), and therefore below the accepted $p = 0.05$ baseline, so considered as non-significant (NS)
- 42 (32%) were at the truly NS level of no detectable difference between the experimental groups and the controls.

Therefore, of the 131 trials, 77 (59%) had a statistically significant outcome, indicating that, in those experiments, an intention-to-affect had apparently had a measurable effect at a statistically significant level. Of the remainder, 12 (9%) were weakly supportive at sub-significance levels, giving 68% overall, and 42 (32%) were NS with no detectable difference between the test and control subjects. When these results are considered within the context of the numerous, but less rigorous, trials that Benor summarized under these same headings, the overall impression is that a directed intention-to-affect often has a measurable effect beyond chance expectation.

Radin (1997) refers to this outcome in his extensive review of the statistical evidence generated by nearly 100 years of trials into parapsychological phenomena. In those trials, using the tool of meta-analysis, he has found a weak, but consistent effect beyond chance outcome. Referring to Benor's findings, he feels that the odds against chance that so many of these 131 trials reached such levels of significance must be 'billions to one'. This, however, remains opinion until a formal meta-analysis is performed that can correct for differences in protocol and levels of confidence between these trials. Dossey (1993), in his review of the scientific literature on healing and intention-to-affect, points out that Braud (1989) has reviewed 149 trials, additional to those collated by Benor, in which experimenters have attempted to affect other living systems at a distance. Braud found, like Benor, that over 50% of these trials had a statistically significant outcome, supporting the hypothesis that an intention-to-affect can have an effect.

Discussion

If a directed intention-to-affect is only a subjective intention that cannot possibly have an objective effect upon another living system, as the sceptics insist, then both the experimental and control subjects, whether enzyme reaction rates, cells, animals or human beings, must be subject to the same known, and controlled, variables throughout the trials. Therefore, because they are matched and randomly assigned, any comparative outcome differences between the physically separated groups should only reach a statistically significant threshold of difference by occasional chance because, in reality, although they are physically divided for the purpose of assessment, they actually remain as one group that is subject to the same variables. In other words, of the 131 trials, instead of 77 trials (59%) showing a statistical significance in favour of a presumed DHI effect, the majority, say 120, would have shown no significant difference between the groups at all, and the rest would have shown a marginally significant difference in favour of either the experimental or control group by random chance without preference.

It is unlikely that adding clinical trial upon clinical trial of DHI, however successful the outcomes may be in favour of an assumed DHI effect, will persuade the sceptic that DHI, as an objective variable, exists because in orthodox scientific terms it just *cannot* exist. Therefore, any such persistent anomaly must have some other explanation. In other words, it is not the outcomes of DHI trials that is the real issue here, but the *claimed nature of the variable itself.* The sceptics remain convinced that those who think that DHI is the causal agent of these outcomes are making what is known as a type I experimental error of assuming something as true which is not true. Conversely, those who conclude that DHI is an agent of therapeutic effect are convinced that the sceptics are making a type II experimental error of refusing to accept something as true which is true.

Question two

The question then arises as to whether there is any sound and replicated evidence from other lines of research to indicate that one person can affect another person in a measurable and repeatable way when there is no possibility of normal sensory communication between the two. If such evidence exists, then the *a priori* grounds for rejecting DHI as a causative agent on the grounds that it *cannot* exist, because orthodox theory says that it cannot exist, are no longer valid. In this wider context DHI would be considered as the particular application of a general faculty of being able to affect something else, or someone else, by means other than the known and accepted senses and known methods of social communication.

This inquiry, therefore, must now turn to the second question as to whether there is any scientifically reliable evidence to show that one person, or particular group of persons, can affect another person, or group, by being in a *particular state of mind* without a deliberate intention to affect. Although none of the investigators use the concept directly, these trials will be considered in terms of the brain and mind of each individual acting together as an operative *brainmind system,* and a group of people will be considered as a group of *brainmind systems.* The working hypothesis will be that if transfer of information between two, or more, such *brainmind systems* in this manner can be demonstrated, then it is likely to be as a consequence of a particular mode of brainmind system functioning.

A review of the literature shows that evidence from laboratory trials using simultaneous electroencephalogram (EEG) recordings of brain wave patterns of two or more subjects in circumstances that exclude all possibility of normal sensory system communication have repeatedly demonstrated that such communication can indeed occur in certain circumstances.

Duane and Behrendt (1965). These authors decided to test popular belief that identical twins share a telepathic rapport whereby one is often aware of the circumstances of the other. They used the fact that an 8–13 Hz burst of alpha rhythm is always elicited in the brain wave pattern of a person when they close their eyelids voluntarily, as in closing their eyes on command. Fifteen pairs of identical twin volunteers were placed in separate, lighted, rooms and their brain waves were continually monitored by EEG. One, or other, of the twins was instructed to close their eyes on command to elicit the 8–12 Hz alpha burst. The EEG recording of the resulting burst of alpha rhythm in the active subject was compared with the same time EEG trace of the passive subject, whose eyes remained open, to see whether any 8–12 Hz induced alpha rhythm suddenly appeared in their EEG trace. Of the 15 pairs of identical twins tested, two pairs consistently demonstrated replicable alpha burst transfer effect. The authors made the important observation that what distinguished these two particular pairs from the other 13 pairs was that they remained calm and relaxed, whereas the latter all exhibited an appreciable level of anxiety and apprehension before and during the test. The study also included unrelated pairs of volunteers and found no evidence of induced alpha transfer effect in these cases.

Grinberg-Zylberbaum et al. *(1992).* These authors report on a series of three separate experiments designed to discover whether the EEG trace of a startle stimulation of one person, as in a sudden flash of light, or sharp sound, was simultaneously recorded as a transfer-induced effect in the EEG trace of the brainwave pattern of another person.

The particular circumstances common to each of these experiments are important, as they seem crucial to the outcome. In the first experiment, 5 successive pairs of unrelated subjects were seated side by non-touching side for about 20 minutes in a soundproof, light proof, electromagnetically shielded chamber. In complete darkness and silence they were asked to enter into a state of *empathic awareness* of each other, which the authors termed *direct communication,* and then to indicate to the experimenters when they felt that they had achieved

this state of mutual empathy. One of the pair then left and entered another shielded chamber, which was further isolated from the first chamber by an intervening electromagnetically shielded wall. Both were asked to try to maintain this empathic state while first being attached to EEG recording equipment, and then remaining in complete sensory isolation after the lights in both the chambers were switched off. The subject who remained in the original chamber was then exposed to a series of simultaneous light flashes and sound stimuli and the resulting startle effect brainwave responses were recorded as sudden blips on the EEG trace.

In each case an identical startle effect blip was recorded in the EEG record of the other, passive, subject, at each moment of active subject stimulus. The authors concluded that the startle response in the brain of the test subject induced a startle response in the brain of the non-stimulated subject as a 'transferred potential' (Figure 3.1(a)). As a guard against chance artefact, they tested pairs who entered the chambers without ever meeting and found no evidence of signal transfer between these non-empathic pairs (Figure 3.1(b)). The differences in response between the two sets of subjects is very clear and was found to be consistent.

It is important to note that while the brain of the passive subject generated a strong startle blip on the EEG record, often similar in intensity and duration to the active subject, there was **no conscious awareness in the passive subject** that this induced stimulus had occurred. This held true throughout all of the experiments, although one or two subjects did report a very vague 'something' on the edge of subliminal awareness. The two brains seemed to be the active systems that were in a state of mutual 'resonance', rather than the conscious state of the two minds. In the active 'sender', the stimulus activated a consciously received, brainmind, startle response. But the conscious processing in the receiving brainmind, even although in a state of empathic rapport, was not informed that any such stimulus had occurred.

In the second experiment, 7 pairs of volunteers underwent the same preparatory period of empathic rapport and subsequent startle test procedure, but the experimenters only recorded EEG traces from the 'passive' subjects. These were then analysed by independent observers to note where, and when, unexpected irregularities occurred. These same observers then compared their findings from the 'passive' EEG records with the EEG records of the active subjects to see whether the anomalous blip deviations matched the time of active subject stimulation. The results were just as consistent as in the first trial, so they were not the result of experimenter bias of interpretation. They received further support from those pairs who were sufficiently motivated to exchange stimulation and receiver roles with the same outcome.

In the third experiment, 4 subjects sat in one chamber and signalled when they felt that they were in empathic awareness with each other. One subject then entered the other chamber to act as passive receiver, while the remaining 3 subjects received simultaneous startle stimulation. Again the transfer effect was recorded, and this experiment confirmed the results of the previous two experiments (Figure 3.2).

In their discussion the authors made a point that is of particular importance to healers and the state of mind that may be related to the possible effectiveness of their DHI. They said that 'If the subjects *made great efforts* to communicate with each other, or used *rational strategies*, the 'transfer potential' effect could hardly be noticed. If the subjects were *sensitive*, and maintained a *fluid, natural, relaxed* attitude, the 'transfer potential' appeared with *greater clarity*' (my italics). This should be borne in mind when experimental procedures to test DHI are designed. If the healers feel under stress 'to perform', particularly when they know that the experimenters are sceptics who will exhaust every other possible explanation first if the results are positive, they are unlikely to be very successful and will merely confirm the scepticism of the investigators.

Interhemispheric EEG frequency profiles

The separate laterality of function between the left and right cerebral hemispheres, as in describing a scene (left hemisphere), and visually experiencing the scene (right hemisphere), is reflected in the very different brainwave patterns that each hemisphere generates during their operation in the busy proceedings of everyday life. When a person is relaxed, and their brain-mind system is in a non-verbalizing, quiet, and meditative mood, the EEG frequency profiles of the two hemispheres tend to fall into a rough synchrony, or coherence, that corresponds to this more unitary state of conscious experiencing. It has been found that there is a fairly consistent relationship between the observed degrees of increasing interhemispheric patterns of EEG frequency coherence, particularly with an increased voltage amplitude of low-frequency alpha waves, and reported inner states of a feeling of oneness and unity, very similar to those reported in the literature on mysticism and meditation (O'Connor and Shaw, 1978; Orme-Johnson and Haynes, 1981; Grinberg-Zylberbaum, 1982). It has also been noted (Grinberg-Zylberbaum, 1982) that when two, or more, people report that they are in a state of empathic rapport, as in the state of 'direct communication' described in the trials discussed earlier, the frequency patterns in each brain come into an increasing state of mutual frequency with the other brain or brains involved in the experiment, as if they are becoming frequency locked.

Grinberg-Zylberbaum and Ramos (1987). These authors investigated this phenomenon by asking pairs of subjects to undergo the same, side-by-side, engagement of empathic rapport as described earlier, and to remain in the same chamber with bilateral hemisphere EEG recording throughout the session. When these recordings were analysed it was found that not only was there a strong correlation between interhemispheric EEG pattern concordance within each brain as their mood of quiet, empathic rapport developed, but that their increasing awareness of each other was mirrored by an increasing synchronization of brain frequencies between their two brains. This mutual synchrony reached a maximum whenever two subjects reported that they felt that they were subjectively 'blending into a unity' with each other. It was as if this subjective unity of the two minds brought the two brains into frequency phase lock.

In this same experiment it was also found that when a third subject was unexpectedly introduced into the chamber, the EEG records from the pair clearly showed that the unwanted interruption had a destabilizing effect on the state of mutual subjective rapport, and mutual frequency of EEG recorded brainwave patterns. The pair rapidly returned to their normal separateness of bihemispheric EEG patterns as they returned to the normal state of everyday functioning as separate and individual selves.

Discussion

During a long series of experiments extending over some 15 years, Grinberg-Zylberbaum and colleagues have presented sound experimental evidence to support their contention that individual brainminds can interact directly with each other across space. What is unresolved is whether this form of communication is an intrinsic property of the *brain* as such, rather than the *mind* as such. An essential precondition appears to be the development of a subjective state of empathic rapport between the minds which, as it were, primes each brain into a *direct communication* mode. The two minds are certainly not in communication at conscious

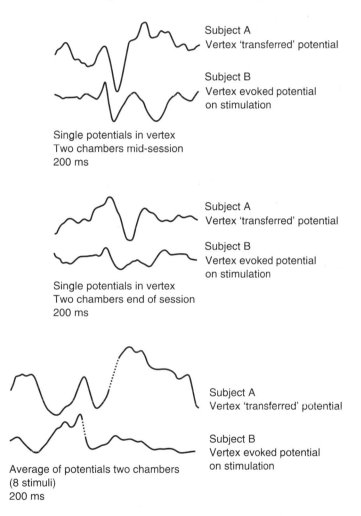

Figure 3.1(a) The three illustrations show typical examples of the EEG 'blip' trace of an evoked startle brainwave potential in an active subject (B) inducing a similar 'transferred startle potential' in the passive receiving subject (A) when each is sitting in separate, electromagnetically screened cubicles, during a period of mutual empathic rapport. These were monopolar recordings with a vertex electrode (After Grinberg-Zylberbaum, 1982)

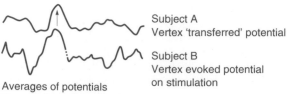

Subject A
Vertex 'transferred' potential

Subject B
Vertex evoked potential
on stimulation

Averages of potentials
Communication session in
two chambers (16 stimuli)
400 ms

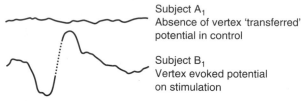

Subject A$_1$
Absence of vertex 'transferred'
potential in control

Subject B$_1$
Vertex evoked potential
on stimulation

Averages of potentials
Non-communication session in
two chambers (16 stimuli)
400 ms

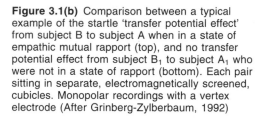

Figure 3.1(b) Comparison between a typical example of the startle 'transfer potential effect' from subject B to subject A when in a state of empathic mutual rapport (top), and no transfer potential effect from subject B$_1$ to subject A$_1$ who were not in a state of rapport (bottom). Each pair sitting in separate, electromagnetically screened, cubicles. Monopolar recordings with a vertex electrode (After Grinberg-Zylberbaum, 1992)

level as there is no transfer of any particular thought, or image, even as an induced flash of light or sudden sound. But if the state of empathic rapport is an emotional, non-verbalizing, state of communion, and if mind-to-mind communication is sustained at a non-conscious level across space, then the transfer startle response in the brain is the only objective indicator of this sustained state of mental communication.

The nature of the communicating medium does not seem to be electromagnetic, as it is not blocked by electromagnetic screening, although such screening is less effective against magnetic fields at sub-20 Hz frequencies. The 'transfer' strength also seems independent of distance, as the amplitude of the induced startle trace EEG deviation shows no apparent loss of signal strength response in the passive brain when the subjects are placed further apart.

Transferred potential from 3 subjects

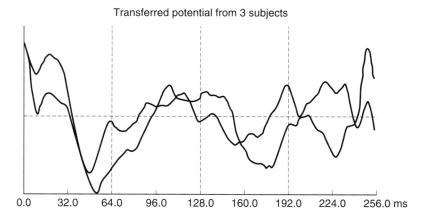

0.0   32.0   64.0   96.0   128.0   160.0   192.0   224.0   256.0 ms

Figure 3.2 Comparison between the averaged EEG records of three subjects who received a series of startle stimulations (upper trace) while sitting in one, electromagnetically screened, chamber, and the 'passive' receiving fourth member (lower trace), who was sitting in a separate, electromagnetically screened, chamber, while the whole group were in a state of empathic rapport. Monopolar recordings with a vertex electrode (After Grinberg-Zylberbaum, 1992)

A possible explanation for this may be that any loss of signal strength is compensated for by an increase in amplification by the receiving brain. Grinberg-Zylberbaum *et al.* (1994) theorize that the brain functions as a neuronal field with non-local interactions with other brain fields when in similar states.

Related research

Independent evidence to support the conclusions of this 15-year body of research by Grinberg-Zylberbaum and colleagues can be found in Cade and Coxhead (1979) who, over a similar period in London, developed an EEG unit called the 'Mind Mirror'. This could record and compare the amplitude (in microvolts) of individual frequencies across the normal frequency spectrum (from 1.5 Hz to 40 Hz) of each cerebral hemisphere at any given moment and display the two sides as an outline profile of relative amplitude, rather like the outline of a wine glass. Cade and colleagues tested dozens of ordinary members of the public, meditators, yogis and healers as they entered, and attempted to hold, different states of reported consciousness, and they found that experienced healers and meditators could 'hold' a stable EEG profile during their transcendental meditation (TM) and/or DHI states of mind (Figure 3.3), with a peak voltage amplitude of around 7–8 Hz. This ability to form, and hold, this particular profile and its related mindset was found to be closely correlated with clinical evidence of a marked ability to induce a definite healing effect in healees. Cade also found that the EEG profiles of healees tended to mirror the frequency profile of the healer during the healing session as if they had 'tuned into' the healer's DHI with a resulting 'transfer' effect of healing.

Like Grinberg-Zylberbaum and his colleagues, Cade found that the frequency profiles of meditators in TM states closely mirrored each other, and that the individual EEGs of a group of such meditators *slowly became entrained into a group synchrony of EEG beat* (Figure 3.4). Wallace (1979), in an extended series of experiments, also found that when a group of meditators entered into full TM their individual EEGs demonstrated an interhemi-spheric frequency in the alpha range, and their group EEGs tended to show brainwave entrainment. Wallace then found that the EEGs of other people, who were at a distance and *not of the same group*, showed a measurable frequency convergence towards the dominant frequency of the TM group, and that this was subjectively mirrored in a more relaxed state of mind.

This repeated finding implies that a group of people in a state of mutual TM can somehow 'bias' or 'set' the emotional level of other people in the local area towards a calmer state of mind. Such a spatially extended property of TM effect upon others seems strongly related to those demonstrated in the Grinberg-Zylberbaum experiments recording a 'transfer' startle response between two, or more, people who had voluntarily entered into a state of mutual rapport.

The 'Maharishi Effect'

The possibility that a group of people who are practising advanced TM at a level in which the meditators enter into an experiential state of 'pure consciousness' could influence, and calm, the emotional states of other people in the vicinity who are not meditating, and are unaware of the existence of the TM group, led to the idea that this effect, if real, could be used for the good of a local community or even a whole country. This possibility led to a 20-year research programme, based in the USA, to develop objective markers which could be used to measure the social influence of this presumed effect upon a local population, whole areas and countries.

The social markers chosen were the monthly official crime statistics for particular communities, broken down into robbery, assault, murder, rape, car thefts and so on. These crime statistics were then correlated with other variables, such as the weather, time of year, population age and density, economic changes, policing policies, unemployment, housing, etc., to see whether any identifiable social factor could be related to any increase, or decrease, in crime incidence, and none emerged with any consistency. These statistics of crime incidence were then subjected to a longitudinal analysis over several years to obtain overall trends, and then the crime records for particular months were compared, both before and after, with the crime records for the same month during which a sustained number of TM meditators gathered as group for a given 2–4-week period into that community.

The results were astonishing. In an extended series of over 40 trials, eventually involving several million people going about their everyday lives, it was found that there was a marked and consistent *reduction* in the crime rates during the TM 'intervention' periods compared to non-intervention periods, either within the same area or in comparison with other matched cities or urban areas (Dillbeck *et al.*, 1988). This research was extended to other countries, such as Holland and Israel, with similar, and consistent, effects. The beneficial outcomes of this TM group 'intervention' in different areas, both within the USA and abroad, became known as the 'Maharishi Effect' in honour of Maharishi Mahesh Yogi, whose original observations of the calming influence of TM practice upon other people was the starting point of the research.

He also taught the particular TM technique that was originally practised, and then introduced the even more advanced TM system known as TM-Sidhi. This is based upon the Yoga Sutris, written some 4000 years ago by Patanjali, an Indian sage, as a series of instructional verses, termed 'the stitches of unity', whereby the 'pure consciousness' of the 'unified field of consciousness' can be sustained even when engaged in everyday life ('Sidhi' means 'perfections' of experience). Maharishi originally predicted that the 'critical number' of a group of meditators practising TM should be 1% of the population to be influenced, and this became known as the '1% effect'. For TM-Sidhi, which is a much more powerful form of meditation as it can be sustained for long periods, he predicted that the 'critical number' would be the square root of 1%. For example, to affect nine million people, would require 90 000 'ordinary' TM practitioners, or 300 TM-Sidhi practitioners. This prediction was repeatedly put to the test over dozens of trials without apparent failure. The whole series of social research and experiment, extending over some 20 years, is summarized in a very

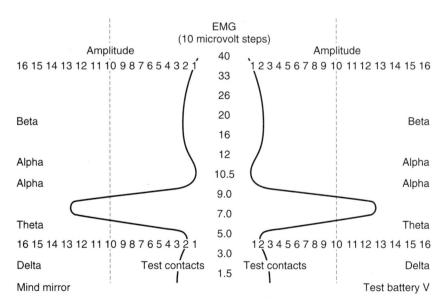

Figure 3.3 Bihemispheric, left cerebral hemisphere, right cerebral hemisphere, EEG microvoltage amplitude frequency profile that Cade, using the 'Mind Mirror' EEG unit, repeatedly found was typical of experienced healers when in the mindset of directed healing intention. He also noted that this frequency amplitude profile was sometimes evoked in the healee during a successful healing session, but not at any other time (After Cade and Coxhead, 1979)

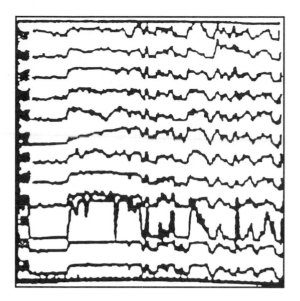

Figure 3.4 Simultaneous EEG printouts from a group of 12 people in a state of deep meditation, showing close synchronization of alpha frequency as they report that they are feeling a sense of mutual unity of group being (After Laszlo, 1996)

readable and fully-referenced book by Aron and Aron (1986).

To give one example, when some 350 meditators (1%) went to stay in a hotel on Rhode Island during the summer of 1978 the suicide rate dropped by 41.8%, the homicide rate by 40%, traffic fatalities were the lowest on record (14 instead of an expected 34), and car theft was down compared to projected numbers. After the period of TM intervention, they returned to normal levels again.

To aid this research, the Maharishi founded the Maharishi International University at Fairfield, Iowa, in 1974. The conclusion that the experimenters drew from the consistent outcomes of this extended series of social experiments, together with an extensive series of physiological measurements, especially EEG recording, with TM practitioners and volunteer subjects, was that when people are in certain states of consciousness, known as 'pure consciousness' in TM practice, they can influence other brainmind systems across space. This conclusion led to the theory of 'unified field effect'. The theory postulates that each person is an individual brainmind system that operates within an extended field that connects each to all at some non-conscious level of working. The working hypothesis arising from this research was that each brainmind has the properties of a field, and that each brainmind can be considered as an active nodal point within an extended field that embraces all brainmind systems (Orme-Johnson and Haynes, 1981; Orme-Johnson *et al.*, 1982).

Other DHI-related research

Braud and Schiltz (1991) and Schiltz (1996) have shown by a series of experiments that an intention-to-affect can stimulate, or calm, the activities of the autonomic nervous system of another person under controlled laboratory conditions when that person does not know whether the intention of the 'sender', who is elsewhere, is to increase, or decrease, tension within themselves as the 'passive' receiver.

Hunt (1995) has presented biomonitoring evidence from body surface electrodes to suggest that particular states of mind, and therefore states of brainmind systems, whether of illness, anxiety, meditation, or healing, can be correlated with bioenergy frequencies of between 100 Hz to 1200 Hz generated and emitted from the body, and that healers can induce similar frequencies in the frequency field of the healee when in close proximity.

Hand-Mediated Energetic Healing Practices

Hunt's findings lends support for the working hypothesis advanced by Slater (1996) to the effect that the practices of Therapeutic Touch and Healing Touch, in which the practitioner, having 'centred' their mind, uses his or her hands to sense and rebalance the energy fields around the patient's body, are forms of Hand-Mediated Energetic Healing Practices (HMEH). The strong and 'healthy' bioenergy field of the therapist interacting with the less healthy, and presumably weaker, bioenergy field of the patient (other belief systems invoke the life force, *Prana,* or *Chi*). The hands, in this hypothesis, are antennae that can act as sensors of field frequency and intensity. The healer acts as a tuning receiver and selective frequency transmitter back out through the hands of the healer to the healee. This rebalances the frequencies and intensities of the bioenergy field of the patient towards health and recovery.

Weston (1998) is of the same opinion. From his personal experiences as a healer, and from his involvement in research into healing, he has found that 'a charge' seems to build up over time during the healing session, which 'discharges' from his hands into the healee. Weston also supports the Maharishi Effect field hypothesis, stating that when people form a healing group, each person acts as a *human energy field* (HEF), and their united intention forms a *group energy field* (GEF) that extends outwards beyond the group boundary. He quotes several anecdotal cases of people who were passing a meeting place in which a healing meeting was in progress who suddenly felt healed of their condition, with no awareness that a healing group had been formed.

Reviews

In addition to the sources already mentioned, there are other extensive reviews of the scientific literature on healing. They include its clinical and philosophical implications together with scientific theories, often referred to as the 'New Physics' developed to try and explain these findings. Such reviews can be found in Benor (1994), Benson (1996), Bruyere (1989), Collinge (1998), Davidson (1993), Gerber (1996), Murphy (1992), Radin (1997), Slater (1996), Tiller (1997) and Woodhouse (1996). In these surveys there is often much cross-reference to parapsychology, quantum physics and energy/vibrational medicine. Clinical issues and experiments are particularly addressed by Wager (1996). New concepts of body–mind interaction that are sympathetic to this approach are explored by Capra (1996) and Pert (1997), who view the body and the mind as an interacting continuum (see also Chapter 1).

Discussion overview

This overview has been based upon examples of well-controlled trials that have been selected to demonstrate that reliable research evidence exists to support the claim that an *intention-to-heal* can have an actual healing effect upon another living system. The evidence from these

trials has been set within a wider context of 131 well-controlled laboratory and clinical trials on *intention-to-affect* (Benor, 1993). These have been grouped into bands of statistical probability that support the hypothesis that intention-to-affect can, and does, have an effect. Braud (1989) has reviewed another 147 trials with similar results. This makes some 280 well-controlled trials in total. Of these, well over 50% demonstrated an outcome supporting the hypothesis that intention-to-affect, including DHI, can have an effect. If this was not so, then only some 5% of outcomes should have supported this hypothesis by chance.

The main objection to interpreting the outcome of these trials as evidence that an intention-to-affect can have an actual effect upon another biological system is that any such intention, within the accepted laws of everyday biological functioning, remains just that, an *intention*. The subjective nature of intention cannot act as an *external* agent of effect upon another living system because subjective intention does not, of itself, possess a transferable property of effect.

It was proposed that this argument becomes invalid if there is sound evidence to show that people, as living systems, can, in fact, communicate with each other by means other than the normal sensory systems. If such evidence does exist, then the possibility that DHI can have a real effect becomes a real possibility and must be set within that wider context.

Evidence that people can communicate with each other by means other than by normal sensory contact, *when they are in a particular, and unusual, mode of functioning,* was then presented. The objective indicator used to demonstrate that such non-sensory system communication had occurred was real-time EEG recording of the brainwave activity of persons when the persons involved had no means of normal communication. One set of replicated experiments found that such *direct communication,* as the experimenters termed it, occurred when the 'sender' and 'receiver' were in the same operative mode of *empathic rapport.* Another set of replicated experiments, performed by several experimenters quite independently of one another, demonstrated that when groups of people were in the unusual mode of conscious functioning known as *transcendental meditation* (TM), their individual EEG frequency patterns tended to come into mutual synchrony as if phase locked. Other replicated experiments demonstrated that the EEG frequency patterns of people in the vicinity of TM groups tended towards a similar EEG beat, and that their behaviour became calmer and more relaxed.

A consistent finding, recognized as characteristic of this unusual mode of brainmind functioning, was that the brainwave frequencies in the left and right cerebral hemispheres of each brain tended to merge into a mutual synchrony of frequency amplitude and frequency distribution as this state of mind was entered and sustained.

An extended series of social experiments, using official crime figures as indices of change in the incidence of crime for particular months, found that the incidence of crime was consistently reduced in the target population. This consistency of effect was reached when the number of the TM group during the research period reached either 1%, or the square root of 1%, of the target population according to the mode of TM that was practised. This is the so-called 'Maharishi Effect'. Considerable anecdotal evidence was also gathered by the experimenters upon the general mood of the local population during the TM period, and it was found that they became more cheerful, more socially friendly and more optimistic.

A consistent research finding has been that this mode of non-sensory system *direct communication* is 'received' at a non-conscious level of experiencing by the 'passive' receivers, but is initiated, or 'sent', by the 'active' persons operating at an unusual level of conscious experiencing. Neither set of conscious participants in these experiments, whether of empathic rapport and 'receiver' startle blip response, TM group frequency phase locking, or TM social effect, reported any conscious awareness that such direct communication had occurred. The effect in the TM social experiments seems to be one of a subliminal 'biasing' of emotional activity in the target population towards kindness and social helpfulness, and a reduction in antisocial tendencies.

How do these findings of non-conscious level communication relate to the reported experiences of healers and healees during the DHI

transaction? The simple answer is that there are marked differences. While the mechanism of *direct communication* at non-conscious level between healer and healee may be the same, the experience rapidly 'rises upwards' and enters into the consciousness of most healees in the form of feelings and sensations that have been discussed earlier. DHI appears to be a distinctive application of *direct communication*. The difference between the two can be likened, by rather inadequate analogy, to the difference between the 'diffused light' of imageless 'empathic rapport', or 'pure consciousness', of TM compared to the 'focused beam' of the healer's active state of DHI towards the healee. The former 'illuminates' at non-conscious to subliminal level, whereas the latter activates a much more positive subliminal response that leads to conscious reception and sensory stimulus in the healee.

Some provisional conclusions

Some provisional conclusions can be drawn from this research as follows:

- *Conclusion A.* Those who conclude that the research evidence supports the working hypothesis that *intention-to-affect,* including DHI, can have a measurable effect upon another living system are **not** committing a type I error of ascribing causation to a non-existent phenomenon. The phenomenon does exist.
- *Conclusion B.* Individual people in busy, everyday life are, for all practical purposes, independent brainmind systems whose internal 'noise' effectively blocks any *direct communication* between each other for most of the time because they rarely operate in that communicative band. They cannot, therefore, 'receive' or 'transmit' in that band. This accords with each person experiencing his, or her, self as a separate and private individual who experiences rapport with others through a shared communication of ideas, emotions and relationships. Emotional distress creates even more noise in the system, which may be why the desperate desire to help others who are desperately ill, particularly other family

members, is ineffective in the DHI sense, because the emotional turbulence blocks any possibility of effective DHI to the loved one.

- *Conclusion C. Direct communication* between people, considered as individual brainmind systems, can only occur when they are in an unusual state of operation, possibly as a form of mutual entrainment. It is most consistent and effective when both brainminds are in the same state, as in empathic rapport, or in group TM. It is of uncertain and intermittent effectiveness when people are not in this mode of operation, and more likely to occur when they are calm and at rest. Direct communication is at a non-conscious level, and is most likely to be expressed, and experienced, as an optimistic and sociable change of mood within the recipient, or social group, with no awareness as to its source. It may be that individual brainmind systems can cycle in, and out of, the possibility of direct communication. If this is so, then any such communication will be received as an intermittent background influence that may, or may not, have a cumulative effect, depending upon the 'power' of the source. In the numerous cases of anecdotal, or experimental, experience of thought and image telepathy, it obviously breaks through into consciousness, but only occasionally into a conscious awareness of source. This idea of frequency cycling may offer an explanation as to why one person is affected by the hypothesised *group energy field*, but another person is not. If the brainmind system is in a state where it is receptive to entrainment, then it is more likely to occur.

- *Conclusion D.* DHI is a consciously focused application of *direct communication*. Healers first 'centre' themselves into the right operating mode of intuitive rapport. They then direct their healing intention towards the healee who, in turn, 'tunes into' this healing intention at non-conscious level, and often experiences its effect at a conscious level. Whether this direct communication from healer to healee can operate at cellular tissue level directly, as implied by the acceleration of

skin healing, and experiments upon enzyme reaction rates and cell cultures, or whether, in human or animal whole-body systems, it must work through the nervous system, via limbic, autonomic, and/or immune system directed response, is unknown.

A point that should be mentioned here, and has not been discussed in this chapter until now, is that during this DHI period, the intuitive healer often 'senses', and sometimes 'images', the inner location and cause of the healee's bodily distress and directs the healing intention to activate the healee's healing systems to heal the source of the dis-ease. This source may be at mental or spiritual level, with the psycho-somatic dysfunction acting as the outward sign and symptom of distress.

- *Conclusion E.* Healers may differ in their innate ability to enter into the operative mode of *direct communicating*. Some healers may always be more effective than others, as is true in the relative skills of every walk of life. Self-confidence, practice and experience are important factors in becoming an effective healer. Individual ability to heal may vary according to mood, inner confidence, health, rapport with the healee, or the circumstances in which the healer is supposed to 'do' the healing. This is especially so when 'under test'. If any of these variables block subjective entry into the operative mode for DHI, there will be no effect, and this may well account for the NS outcome of some 40% of the trials. Arguing from his own experience, Weston (1998) makes the point that the healer must 'generate' sufficient 'power' to be effective, and this sometimes takes up to 20 minutes to accomplish. Therefore, many trials with a NS outcome may be NS because the healer was unable achieve the critical threshold of affect for change within the target system.

- *Conclusion F.* If healers differ in their DHI effectiveness, so may healees differ in their ability to enter into *direct communication* with the healer. Some will be less receptive to healing than others, despite having the same need of healing as those in whom it has been successful. If this was shown to be so, then healees in need of healing may require some form of training so that they can more easily enter the state of mind in which they can come into direct communication with the healer.

As a working hypothesis, it is proposed that both healer and healee can be considered as relatively unstable frequency systems that can cycle into and out of 'tuning' with each other without conscious awareness. Effective healers can sustain a relatively more steady 'healing' frequency, and healees are more likely to 'tune into' the sustained frequency input.

Research into determining the nature of the healing transaction, and optimum parameters for healer–healee interaction, is badly needed. It may be, for example, that successful healers create a subliminal environment either within, or around, the healee that induces the necessary conditions for effective healing to occur.

A working hypothesis

This line of argument leads to a working hypothesis that DHI can only be effective if the healer can generate the required 'informational' healing frequency, or frequencies, with sufficient power to entrain the healee into reciprocity. In trials where the DHI, or intention-to-affect, is being directed at single cell systems, or biochemical reactions, the working hypothesis would be that such an intention will have a measurable effect only if the operator can induce a similar entrainment effect upon the desired physiological, or biochemical, processes.

Three central concepts arise from this hypothesis. One is that there is a *critical threshold of affect* within each target system that may be continuously variable about a mean. Another is that the nature of the threshold is *frequency* that is *informational* to the recipient, and that the lowest threshold of effect corresponds to a *frequency window* within the targeted system. The third is that the subjective element within the healer that needs to be 'switched on' to 'prime' and sustain the healer to healee interaction of *direct communication* is one of *empathic rapport*. Concepts of 'entrainment',

'coupling', 'resonance', 'tuning' and 'rapport' seem to be appropriate working analogies. The scientific basis for taking this approach is explored in Chapter 1.

Clinical implications

The professional relationship between the physical therapist and the person needing help, whether in intensive care, general wards, out-patients, domiciliary, private practice or the health service, is one that offers considerable potential for the use of DHI as discussed in this chapter. The various authorities quoted in this overview seem agreed that both laboratory and clinical evidence indicates that DHI can reinforce, or reawaken, the healing processes within the healee, sometimes to dramatic effect.

If this is so, then the application of DHI, whether through the sensation of touch, which seems eminently suitable in physiotherapy and lies within the practical *scope of professional practice* of chartered physiotherapists, or by non-touch intention, should enhance the natural healing systems in the patient and accelerate recovery. Applied to inpatients before, during and after medical procedures, including surgery, DHI leads to fewer complications and less emotional distress (Cox and Hayes, 1997, 1998). For patients suffering from chronic conditions, such as arthritis or bronchitis, their quality of life should be measurably improved. Those suffering from anxiety states, or depression, or are in a state of deep distress through personal circumstances, should obtain relief and regain a more positive attitude to life. All such predictions are susceptible to assessment by clinical trial. If the outcomes confirm predictions, DHI will be incorporated into evidence-based practice.

Physical therapists are people who wish to help others through their particular set of professional skills, and this includes establishing a rapport with each patient. Many therapists may well be 'healers' without even realizing it, ascribing unexpected improvement to the modality employed, instead of to themselves as unsuspecting healers who have entered into a healing rapport with the patient.

While the terms 'healer' and 'healing' have a long and honourable tradition, and are well understood, they are lay terms that some may feel are not appropriate for professional use, especially in the context of sceptical colleagues. As the working hypothesis in therapies such as acupuncture, reflextherapy, craniosacral therapy, polarity therapy and zero balancing, for example, is one of 'bioenergies' and 'bioenergy fields', therapists may feel more comfortable with the concept of 'bioenergy'. They may wish to consider the application of DHI in terms of a *bioenergy therapy* that is most likely to be effective when the therapist and the patient, or client, are in a state of mutual rapport.

Many therapists who now use this healing approach say that as their confidence develops they find that they can more easily 'slip into' the calm and 'centred' state of mind that 'releases' their DHI. This, in turn, enhances the physiological and psychological effectiveness of 'orthodox' physical therapy procedures, so that each reinforces the healing benefit of the other to the advantage of the patient.

References

Angelo, J. (1994) *Your Healing Power: A Comprehensive Guide to Channelling Your Healing Energies.* London: Piatkus.

Aron, E. and Aron, A. (1986) *The Maharishi Effect: A Revolution Through Meditation.* Walpole, NH: Stillpoint.

Baruss, I. and Moore, R.J. (1998) Beliefs about consciousness and reality of participants at 'Tucson 11'. *J. Consciousness Studies,* 5(4), 483–96.

Benor, D.J. (1993) *Healing Research,* Vol 1. Deddington: Helix.

Benor, D.J. (1994) *Healing Research,* Vol 2. Deddington: Helix.

Benor, D.J. (1996) Further comments on 'Loading' and 'Telesomatic Reactions'. *Advances,* 12(2), 71–75.

Benson, H. (1996) *Timeless Healing: The Power and Biology of Belief.* London: Simon and Schuster.

Braud, W. (1989) Using living targets in psi research. *Parapsychol. Rev.,* 20(6), 1–4.

Braud, W. and Schiltz, M. (1991) Consciousness interactions with remote biological systems: anomalous intentionality effects. *Subtle Energies,* 2, 1–57.

Bruyere, R.L. (1989, reprint 1994) *Wheels of Light.* London: Simon and Schuster.

Cade, M. and Coxhead, N. (1979, reprint 1996) *The Awakened Mind: Biofeedback and the Development of Higher States of Awareness.* Shaftesbury: Element Books.

Capra, F. (1996) *The Web of Life: A New Synthesis of Mind and Matter.* London: HarperCollins.

Clarke, N. (1998) The power of the paranormal. *Daily Mail.* 2 February, 18–19 (ICM poll of 1000 responders).

Collinge, W. (1998) *Subtle Energy: Awakening to the Unseen Forces in our Lives.* New York: Warner Books.

Cox, C. and Hayes, J. (1997) Reducing anxiety: the employment of therapeutic touch as a nursing intervention. *Comp. Ther. Nurs. Midwif.,* 3, 163–67.

Cox, C. and Hayes, J. (1998) Experiences of administering and receiving therapeutic touch in intensive care. *Comp. Ther. Nurs. Midwif.,* 4, 128–33.

Davidson, J. (1993) *Subtle Energy,* 3rd edn. Saffron Walden: C.W. Daniel.

Dillbeck, M.C., Banus, C.B., Polanzi, C. and Landrith, III (1988) Test of a field model of consciousness and social change: the transcendental meditation and TM-Sidhi program and decreased urban crime. *J. Mind Behav.,* 9(4), 457–86.

Dossey, L. (1993) *Healing Words: The Power of Prayer and the Practice of Medicine.* New York: Harper Paperbacks.

Duane, T.D. and Behrendt, T. (1965) Extrasensory encephalographic induction between identical twins. *Science,* 150, 367.

Gerber, R. (1996) *Vibrational Medicine: New Choices for Healing Ourselves.* 2nd edn. Santa Fe, NM: Bear.

Grad, B.R. (1963) A telekinetic effect on plant growth. *Int. J. Parapsych.,* 5(2), 117–34.

Grad, B.R. (1965) Some biological effects of laying-on of hands. *J. Am. Soc. Psychic. Res.,* 59, 95–127.

Grad, B.R. (1967) The laying-on of hands: implications for psychotherapy, gentling and the placebo effect. *J. Soc. Psychic. Res.,* 61(4), 286–305.

Grad, B.R., Cadoret, R.J. and Paul, G.I. (1961) The influence of an unorthodox method of treatment in the wound healing of mice. *Int. J. Parapsychol.,* 3, 5–24.

Grinberg-Zylberbaum, J. (1982) Psychophysiological correlates of communication. *Psychenergetics,* 4, 227–56.

Grinberg-Zylberbaum, J., Delaflor, M., Arellano, M.E.S., Guevara, M.A. and Perez, M. (1992) Human communication and the electrophysiological activity of the brain. *Subtle Energies,* 3(3), 25–43.

Grinberg-Zylberbaum, J., Delaflor, M., Attie, L. and Goswami, A. (1994) The Einstein–Podolsky–Rosen Paradox in the brain: the transferred potential. *Physics Essays,* 7(4), 422–28.

Grinberg-Zylberbaum, J. and Ramos, J. (1987) Patterns of interhemispheric correlation during human communication. *Int. J. Neurosci.,* 36, 41–53.

Harvey, D. (1983) *The Power to Heal: An Investigation of Healing and the Healing Experience.* London: Aquarian Press.

Hodgkinson, L. (1990) *Spiritual Healing: Everything You Want to Know.* London: Piatkus.

Hunt, V. V. (1995) *Infinite Mind: The Science of Human Vibrations.* Malibu: Malibu Publishing.

Hutton, J.B. (1986) *Healing Hands*, 2nd edn. London: W.H. Allen.

Krieger, D. (1979) *The Therapeutic Touch: How to Use Your Hands to Help or to Heal*. New York: Simon and Schuster.

Laszlo, E. (1996) *The Whispering Pond: A Personal Guide to the Emerging Vision of Science*. Shaftesbury: Element Books.

MacManaway, B. and Turcan, J. (1983) *Healing: The Energy that can Restore Health*. Wellingborough: Thorsons.

Murphy, M. (1992) *The Future of the Body: Explorations into the Further Evolution of Human Nature*. Putnam, NY: Tarcher.

O'Connor, K.P. and Shaw, J.C. (1978) Field dependence, laterality and the EEG. *Biol. Psychol.*, **6**, 93–109.

Orme-Johnson, D., Dillbeck, M.C., Wallace, R.K. and Landrith, G.S. (1982) Intersubject EEG coherence: is consciousness a field? *Int. J. Neurosci.*, **16**, 203–209.

Orme-Johnson, D. and Haynes, C.T. (1981) EEG phase coherence, pure consciousness, creativity and TM-Siddhi experiences. *Neuroscience*, **13**, 211–17.

Pert, C.B. (1997) *Molecules of Emotion: Why You Feel the Way You Feel*. London: Simon and Schuster.

Radin, D.I. (1997) *The Conscious Universe*. New York: Harper Edge.

Schiltz, M.J. (1996) Intentionality and intuition and their clinical implications: a challenge to science and medicine. *Advances*, **12**(2), 58–66.

Slater, V.E. (1996) Healing touch. In *Fundamentals of Complementary and Alternative Medicine* (Micozzi, M.C., ed.). Edinburgh: Churchill Livingstone.

Southwood, M.S. (1994) *The Healing Experience: Remarkable Cases from a Professional Healer*. London: Piatkus.

Tiller, W.A. (1997) *Science and Human Transformation: Subtle Energies, Intentionality, and Consciousness*. Stanford, CA: Pavior.

Turner, G. (1974) *A Time to Heal: The Autobiography of an Extraordinary Healer*. London: Franklyn.

Wager, S. (1996) *A Doctor's Guide to Therapeutic Touch*. New York: Perigee.

Wallace, R.K. (1979) Physiological effects of transcendental meditation. *Science*, **167**, 1751–54.

Weston, W. (1998) *How Prayer Heals: A Scientific Approach*. Charlottesville, VA: Hampton Roads.

Wirth, D.P. (1990) The effect of non contact therapeutic touch on the healing rate of full thickness dermal wounds. *Subtle Energies*, **1**(1), 1–20.

Wirth, D.P., Barrett, M.J. and Eidelman, W.S. (1994) Non contact therapeutic touch and wound re-epithelialisation: an extension of previous research. *Compl. Ther. Med.*, **2**(4), 187–92.

Wirth, D.P., Johnson, C.A., Horvath, J.S. and MacGregor, J.O.D. (1992) The effect of alternative healing therapy on the regeneration rate of salamander forelimbs. *J. Sci. Explor.*, **6**(4), 375–90.

Wirth, D.P., Richardson, J.T., Eidelman, W.S. and O'Malley, A.C. (1993) Full thickness dermal wounds treated with non-contact therapeutic touch: a replication and extension. *Compl. Ther. Med.*, **1**(3), 127–32.

Wirth, D.P., Richardson, J.T., Marinez, R.D., Eidelman, W.S. and Lopez, M.E. (1996) Non contact therapeutic touch intervention and full thickness cutaneous wounds: a replication. *Compl. Ther. Med.*, **4**(10), 237–40.

Woodhouse, M. B. (1996) *Paradigm Wars: Worldviews for a New Age*. Berkeley, CA: Frog Ltd.

4 The Chakra energy system

John R. Cross

Introduction

It is said that the human frame consists of an interpenetrating series of body forms of different vibrational frequencies, ranging from the physical to the spiritual, with the higher spiritual and mental frequency forms determining the state of the physical body. The appreciation of the existence of our invisible subtle bodies is the bedrock of our understanding of subtle body healing. The knowledge of the existence of our subtle energy bodies was taken for granted and perceived as normal by some of our ancestors. It is said that the Kuhanas, who lived in South America 1500 years ago, were all capable of *seeing* the **aura**. There are some gifted people living at present who claim to see colours, subtle shapes and various aspects of the aura and claim to be able to make an analysis of imbalance within the aura. It is the author's experience, however, that there is a greater percentage of people who can *feel* the aura and can detect anomalies in it, thus determining present or future conditions within the physical body. The subtle bodies are considered in the following text.

The Etheric body

The word 'etheric' comes from 'ether', meaning the state between energy and matter. It can be easily seen by most clairvoyants and indeed by children up to the age of 7 years, who treats its existence as quite normal. The Etheric body is, though, invisible to most of us. It ranges from 2 to 10 cm around the physical body. The breakthrough with the production of Kirlian photography assumed that it was the whole of the Etheric body that was being photographed. In a sense it was true, but the Etheric body consists of two layers – the physical-etheric and the etheric-emotional – and it is the former more dense subtle body that is seen on Kirlians. To test for the existence of our first subtle body, the following simple experiment can be tried. Hold the hands open and opposing each other about 10 cm apart. Now bring them slowly close to each other. If this is done correctly, there should be felt some degree of resistance, or buffer, between the hands.

The Etheric body is said to consist of fine tubular threadlike channels, commonly known as **nadis**, which in turn are related to the cerebrospinal and autonomic nervous system and the endocrine system. This web-like substance within the Etheric body, which is in constant motion, appears to clairvoyant vision to be sparks of bluish-white light within the light blue/grey colour of the Etheric body itself. Tansley (1972) describes the Etheric body as

> . . . consisting of fine energy threads or lines of force and light, being the archetype on which the physical body form is built. It can best be described as a field of energy that underlies every cell and atom of the physical body, permeating and interpenetrating every part of it and extending beyond to form a part of what is commonly called the aura.

The Etheric body has three main functions which are all closely related. It acts as a receiver, assimilator and transmitter of Vital Force (Life Energy, Ch'i, Ki, Prana, Odic Force, etc.) via the Chakras, which are the energy gateways between the subtle bodies and the physical. If each of the functions of reception, assimilation and transmitter of energies is maintained in a state of balance, then the physical body reflects this interchange of energies in a state of good health.

The Emotional body

This second auric body or next finer after the etheric is generally called the Emotional body (sometimes called the Astral) and is associated with feelings and, obviously, emotions. It roughly follows the outline of the physical body with heightened space above the head and sometimes hands and feet. It appears, to clairvoyants, to be coloured clouds of fine substance in continual fluid motion and extends from approximately 6 to 25 cm above the physical body. As with the other subtle bodies, it interpenetrates with its adjacent bodies. It is said that within the Emotional body a multitude of different changes are constantly taking place, even if we do not realize it, and we are continually being bombarded by external as well as internal stimuli, which in turn is said to initiate chemical changes. The changes in our emotions can prove to be most significant in eventually giving us psychosomatic conditions which eventually lead to chemical and hormonal changes within the physical body.

The Mental body

The Mental body is obviously much less dense than the previous two parts of the aura and is said to extend up to 1 m from the physical body. It deals with the assimilation of thoughts and mental processes and is considered by many to be the most important of all the auric components. The expressions 'Thought is energy' and 'Energy follows thought' come to mind when attempting to express the significance of this body. Many doctors, therapists and healers believe that a considerable percen-

tage of our ills stem from our thought patterns, in that negative thought patterns over a period of time can create chemical changes within the physical body that give unpleasant symptoms affecting the autonomic nervous system. To a clairvoyant, this very fine body appears as white/yellow shimmering light.

The other three bodies, namely the Intuitional, Monadic and Divine, do not concern us in the context of this short chapter. Furthermore, physical therapists are not likely to encounter conditions that come under their bailiwick that have an aetiology outside the proximal four bodies.

The Chakras

The Chakras are considered to be Force Centres or Whorls of energy situated from a point on the physical body and permeating through the layers of the Etheric, Emotional and Mental bodies in an ever-increasing outward fan-shaped formation. They are rotating vortices of subtle matter and are considered to be the focal points for the transmission and reception of energies. The word 'Chakra' means 'wheel'. To the clairvoyant, these energy centres can easily be seen. Each is different in form, colour and energy vibration. There are considered to be 7 Major Chakras and 21 Minor Chakras. The Minor Chakras are said to be the reflected pathways of the Majors and do not extend any further than the Etheric body outwards. They are, however, powerful acupuncture/trigger points in their own right and may be used extensively in the treatment of musculoskeletal conditions.

Anatomy of the Chakras

The Major Chakras

There are said to be seven Major Chakras: **Crown, Brow, Throat, Heart, Solar Plexus, Sacral** and **Base**. The middle five have anterior and posterior aspects on the midlines of the body, whereas the Crown and Base have only one point. As Figure 4.1 shows, there are internal energetic connections between the anterior and posterior aspects of each Chakra

Table 4.1 Relative positions of the Chakras on the physical body

Chakra	Spinal level	Ventral level
1. Crown	–	Top of the head at point Gov 20
2. Brow	Occipito-atlas junction (Gov 16)	Between the eyes (Extra point 1 – Yintang)
3. Throat	C7–D1 junction (Gov 14)	The sternal notch (Con 22)
4. Heart	D6–D7 junction (Gov 10)	Mid-sternum (Con 17)
5. Solar plexus	D12–L1 junction (Gov 6)	Below xiphoid process (Con 14)
6. Sacral	L4–L5 junction (Gov 3)	Three fingers width below umbilicus (Con 6)
7. Base	Sacro-coccyx junction (Gov 2)	Symphysis pubis (Con 2)

and vertically between the Base and the Crown. They appear as a single acupuncture point on the physical body and, as stated before, fan outwards through the Etheric, Emotional and Mental bodies. The circumference of the Chakra at the etheric-emotional level is about 5 cm, and at the emotional-mental border is approximately 20 cm. This is totally dependent on the age and health of the person. The relative positions of the Chakras on the physical body are given in Table 4.1.

Although there are strictly two points for the Base Chakra, because these two are so close together, for practical purposes, it is usually treated as one point. The abbreviations Gov and Con stand for **Governor** and **Conception**. The Governor meridian is the energy channel that flows along the posterior aspect of the body vertically up the spine, across the head and ending in the roof of the mouth. The Conception meridian flows midline on the anterior aspect of the body, from the symphysis to the lower aspect of the mouth.

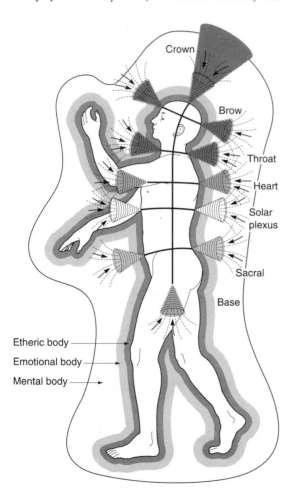

Figure 4.1 The Major Chakras

The Minor Chakras

The literature is very vague about the Minor Chakras. The existence, location and action of the Minor Chakras been occupied the author's clinical and teaching work for many years. As stated before, each of the Minor Chakras is said to be a reflected point of an associated Major Chakra. Each one is a powerful acupuncture point having several uses in acupuncture and acupressure. There are said to be 21 Minor Chakras, 10 pairs and the Spleen Chakra, which some authorities claim as being a Major Centre. They are listed below in Table 4.2 with their location and coupled Minor Chakra and Major Chakra association.

Table 4.2 The Minor Chakras with location and coupled Minor and Major Chakra association

Minor Chakra	Couple Minor Chakra	Location	Associated Major Chakra
Spleen	–	Ac. pt Sp 16	Solar Plexus/ Sacral
Foot	Hand	Sole of foot Ki 1	Crown
Hand	Foot	Middle of palm P 8	Crown
Knee	Elbow	Popliteal fossa Bl 40	Base
Elbow	Knee	Cubital fossa P 3	Base
Groin	Clavicular	Symph. pubis St 30	Brow
Clavicular	Groin	Sternal end of clavicle Ki 27	Brow
Shoulder	Navel	Tip of shoulder LI 15	Throat
Navel	Shoulder	Next to umbilicus Ki 16	Throat
Intercostal	Ear	Lateral aspect of ribs Sp 21	Heart
Ear	Intercostal	Base of ear TH 17	Heart

There are also other associations such as Key Points, Colours and Sounds that are outside the scope of this short chapter. Figure 4.2 shows the anatomical positioning of the Major and Minor Chakras. The Minor Chakras may be used in isolation or with their couples (both Minor and Major) in therapy and have been found to be particularly useful in pain relief.

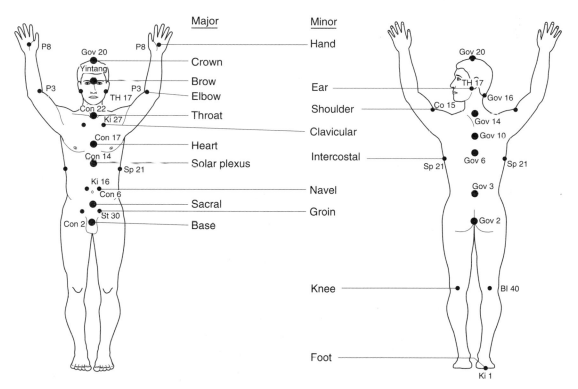

Figure 4.2 The Major and Minor Chakra energy centres

States of imbalance of the Major Chakras

An imbalance of Chakra energy may manifest itself as:

- *Congestion.* Lack of free flow of energy in any of the bodies that the Chakra passes through. This invariably causes symptoms in the physical body, although not always at the time of the congestion, but some time later.
- *Uncoordination.* This occurs between two bodies, creating a weakness which manifests itself as poor health. If the physical and the Etheric bodies are not well integrated, then debilitation and devitalization will take place. An example of this would be *impotence* which is considered to be caused by uncoordination of the Sacral and Throat centres.
- *Overstimulation.* This is where too much energy is being drawn through a particular Chakra or Chakras. This agitates the substance of the bodies involved and in so doing brings about a variety of pathological conditions. Fevers of a non-infective aetiology may be an expression of an overactive focal point of energy that is trying to disperse and flow outwards into physical expression.

'All is energy' is a phrase that is often used, and how true it is. Everything on this planet above absolute zero temperature emits a particular radiation, vibrating at a certain frequency. Even the most dormant and seemingly dead material can be considered to be alive in its molecular activity. If it is accepted that 'All is energy' is a truism, then how pointless and futile it is to suppress the symptoms of the physical body by using drugs, chemicals or electricity. Symptoms are merely the body's attempt to externally show an imbalance or its attempt to rid itself of impurities, i.e. self-healing or healing crisis. In this context, the highest and most pure forms of healing are Divine (Spiritual) Healing by laying on of hands, or by prayer and pure thought. Not everyone, though, is as gifted as those few who are catalysts or channels of healing through a Divine or Supreme Force. From this viewpoint most dis-ease can be considered as originating in the Mental and Emotional bodies and not on the Physical plane, and it is at this subtle level that both thought and therapy should be directed. In Chakra energy terms, dis-eases of the physical body may be an expression of imbalance of energy caused by the states of imbalance of the Chakras, namely Congestion, Uncoordination or Overstimulation, and it is at the Chakra level that we should apply our thoughts and therapies.

Entering the world of Chakra energies means entering the world of **true** healing of the **cause** of the patient's disease or condition. The Chakra energies can be affected at **any** level (physical, etheric and emotional) through the use of such therapies as acupuncture, acupressure, reflexology, craniosacral therapy, radionics, healing or even homoeopathy. Therefore, treatment of the individual or combination Chakras can be based upon several criteria of physical and emotional syndromes and each one is as valid as the other because each symptom that the patient has is like a golden signal to the practitioner, saying that there is something wrong somewhere and, whatever level of healing, all the other symptoms that the patient has will eventually be balanced and healed. This is a bold statement to make and not one that is made lightly, but after working with these Centres for nearly 20 years and having seen at first hand the results from dealing with this concept, it is made with the utmost conviction. The use of one or more of the following symptomatic criteria help us formulate a treatment regimen:

- An obvious imbalance of the **physical parts** of the body that are governed by a particular Chakra, e.g. a lung condition, would warrant treatment of the **Throat** Chakra.
- An obvious imbalance with the **endocrine** gland that is associated with a particular Chakra, e.g. an insulin imbalance, would be treated with the **Solar plexus** Chakra.
- An obvious or Subtle emotional state of the person that is associated with a particular Chakra, e.g. Anger or Rage, can be treated via the **Brow** Chakra.
- An obvious **skeletal** imbalance that is associated with a particular Chakra, e.g. a mid-dorsal lesion, would be treated by the **Heart** Chakra.

- An obvious **muscular** imbalance that is associated with a particular Chakra, e.g. a psoas major imbalance, can be treated with the **Base** Chakra.
- An imbalance of **Ch'i energy** felt with pulse diagnosis or by any one of the other natural diagnostic methods (see Chapter 2) that is associated with a particular chakra, e.g. a Spleen meridian Ch'i imbalance, would be treated with the **Sacral** Chakra.

Although it does not matter which type of diagnostic tool is used, there is obviously a priority in the order of importance of symptoms. They are, in order:

1. Mental and psychosomatic symptoms.
2. Ch'i imbalance.
3. Endocrine imbalance.
4. Physical or organic symptoms.
5. Skeletal imbalance.
6. Muscular symptoms.

From the above, it follows that the philosophy of the Chakra energy system may be used therapeutically with many disciplines, such as yoga (several types), meditation (several approaches), acupuncture, acupressure, reflexology, healing (hands off the body), Reiki (hands on the body), manipulative therapy, craniosacral therapy and physiotherapy. The author has, over the past 15 years, attempted to take away the mystique of these subtle energies and has attempted to make them 'therapy friendly' so they can be utilized by therapists in their everyday clinical situation, as opposed to just using them in yoga and meditation. His acupuncture doctoral thesis was written on 'The relationship of the Chakra energy system and acupuncture' (Cross, 1986).

Chakra energy associations

Each of the 7 Major Chakras are said to be associated with the following:

- a coupled Major and Minor Chakra
- one or two Acupuncture meridians
- internal organs
- acupuncture 'Key' point
- reflexes

- a colour
- a sound pitch
- an endocrine gland
- an autonomic nerve plexus
- a symbol
- muscles
- emotions and aspirations
- number of rotating vortices.

Below is a brief explanation of each of these.

The coupled Major and Minor Chakras. These have been mentioned previously. Treatment of the patient (using any of the modalities) seems to be more powerful and long-standing when the coupled Chakras are used. Also it is important before treatment of an individual Chakra commences to be able to *balance* the energies within the Chakra to its couple.

The associated meridian. This can be used when using the Chakras with acupuncture and acupressure. Stimulation of the 'source' point of the meridian, again, enhances the efficacy of the treatment. Some scholars assume that there is a direct link between the Chakra as it 'enters' the physical body and the meridians. The author believes that there has to be a system of energy that links the two. This system of energy, known as the **nadis**, also 'links' the energy of the Chakra to the associated endocrine glands and nerve plexi.

Gerber (1988) writes:

The Chakras are connected to each other and to portions of the physical-cellular structure via fine subtle energetic channels known as 'nadis'. The nadis are formed by fine threads of subtle energetic matter. They are different from the meridians, which actually have a physical counterpart in the meridian duct system. The nadis represent an extensive network of fluid-like energies which parallel the bodily nerves in their abundance. In the Eastern yogic literature, the Chakras have been metaphorically visualized as flowers. The nadis are symbolic of the petals and fine roots of the flowerlike Chakras that distribute the life-force and energy of each Chakra into the physical body. Various sources have described up to 72 000 nadis or etheric channels of energy in the subtle anatomy of human beings. These unique channels are interwoven with the physical nervous system. Because of this intricate interconnection with the nervous system, the nadis affect the nature and quality of nerve transmission within the extensive network of the brain, spinal cord and peripheral nerves.

The internal organ connection. This is a traditional link. Each of the associated organs and parts of the body are relevant in clinical practice, in that where there is an imbalance in a Chakra, it will also affect the part of the body that is associated with the Chakra.

The Key points. These are used extensively in acupuncture and acupressure. The two associated Key points are stimulated either with needle or finger pressure prior to the treatment of an individual Chakra. This is said to 'open up' the energy of the Chakra more readily. The 'Key' points were researched by the author several years ago.

Reflexes. Each of the Major and Minor Chakras has a Reflex on the foot (and hand) that can be used in treatment, hence its use in reflexology. More and more reflextherapists are using the subtle approach of 'light touch reflextherapy' which encompasses the use of the reflected Chakra points on the feet.

Colours and sound pitch. These are two interpretations of energy vibration. Each can be very effective when used in therapy. When there is shown to be an imbalance of energy within a particular Chakra, the associated colour or sound pitch can be transmitted to the Chakra either by coloured perspex or instrumentation. In some Buddhist cultures, spoken and chanted mantras are said to equate to the vibration of a particular Chakra.

The endocrine glands. These represent a powerful healing force within the Chakra energy system (Figure 4.3). The exact link between the Chakras and the endocrine glands is unknown, but mention has been made of the nadis energies. Motoyama (1988) states quite categorically that the nadis system is indeed the link. He is the first person who has attempted to quantify the

existence of the Chakras using scientific instrumentation. He has invented the AMI machine. The AMI (Apparatus for Measuring for Functional Conditions of Meridians and their Corresponding Internal Organs) is an instrument designed to measure the initial skin current, as well as the steady-state current, in response to d.c. voltage externally applied at special acupuncture points located alongside the base of the fingers and toe nails. During many years of experimentation he found that he could measure changes within the meridian system which in turn affected the Chakras *and* the accompanied endocrine glands. He found that there would be measurable hormonal changes from a particular gland. This important work is ongoing.

The autonomic nerve plexus. This is a natural extension of the above, as modern scientific medicine has shown links between the autonomic nervous system and the endocrine glands.

The symbols. The associated symbols are merely a shorthand way of showing the Chakras.

The muscles. The associated muscles have been formulated by the author as a natural progression from the research into the use of the Chakras with applied kinesiology. It has been found that when there is energy imbalance within a Chakra, the strength of the associated muscles is also affected. Once the Chakra is balanced, the muscles are automatically 'strengthened' and the strengthening can go some way towards balancing the Chakra.

The emotions and aspirations. The associated emotions and aspirations are, in the author's opinion, the most important connection of all. If the therapist can glean the patient's likes, dislikes, emotional make-up, fears and phobias, he/she can instantly tell what Chakras are balanced energetically and which ones need treatment. This was covered earlier in the chapter when it was mentioned how important the emotions are in the production of physical symptoms. There is a parallel here in the practice of classical homoeopathy. The homoeopath would repetorize the remedy by asking questions affecting the psyche to obtain the desired similimum (the single remedy that best fits the

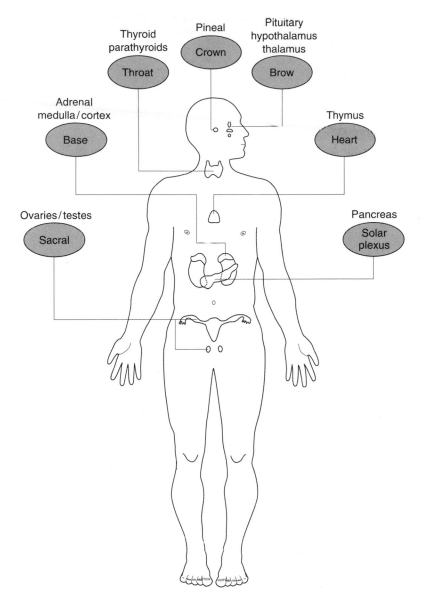

Figure 4.3 The Chakras and the endocrine glands

whole 'symptom picture' of the individual). If the patient is repetorized on the 'mental' picture, in time the whole of the symptoms, including the physical, should be improved.

The rotating vortices. These are considered by some to be factual and by others to be mythical. It is said that each of the Major Chakras has a number of rotating vortices within the etheric/ emotional part of the Chakra. Some clairvoyants can see these and other practitioners can actually feel them. There is doubt whether the knowledge of the rotating vortices is of clinical importance; however, it is significant in the fact that it shows the difference in vibration between the Chakras. For instance, it is said that there are only two rotating vortices of energy within the Base Chakra, showing its 'sluggish' vibrational frequency, but that there are 972 rotating vortices in the Crown, showing its very high frequency. It has also been said that these are merely sacred numbers with very little significance. The author once stated this at a conference of healers and was duly heckled as uttering blasphemy.

The individual Major Chakras

Chakra 1   Crown   Sahasrara

There is only one point for this Chakra and that is at acupuncture point Gov 20 which is situated on the top of the skull in the very centre between the eyebrows and base of the skull and midway laterally between an imaginary line between the front of each ear. This Chakra does not come into full functioning until a high degree of inner development has been reached. It externalizes as the pineal gland. This curious gland is active in children, but it is then thought by many to stop functioning in the physical body after the age of 7 years. The pineal gland is thought to be connected with visual perception and clairvoyancy. The Crown governs the upper brain and the right eye. It is said to be the link between a person and their spiritual plane and as such is used in many forms of yoga and meditation. It is sometimes called the thousand-petalled lotus because of the shape at its central vortex. It has, though, according to clairvoyants only 972 small rotating vortices.

Associations of the Crown Chakra

Colour	Violet
Sound pitch	B
Meridian	Triple warmer
Endocrine gland	Pineal
Organs	Upper brain (CNS) and (R) eye
Emotions	Melancholy and phobic tendencies
Muscular system	Trapezius, supraspinatus, teres major, facial muscles
Autonomic nerve plexus	None
Symbol	Lotus
Rotating vortices	972

Acupuncture Key points	TH 5 and Con 4
Anatomical position	Ac. point Gov 20

Symptomatology. Vertigo, high and low blood pressure, right-sided migraine, multiple sclerosis and other upper motor neuron conditions, delusion and melancholy. (Where there are sometimes opposite symptoms appearing with each Chakra, this shows that the energy imbalance of each Chakra may be affected in many ways. There may be a sluggishness of energy giving chronic (Yin) symptoms or a stimulation that gives acute (Yang) symptoms (Figure 4.4).

Chakra 2   Brow   Ajna

The Brow Chakra is situated spinally at the inion, which is the junction of the base of the skull and the first cervical vertebra (occipito-atlas junction). The acupuncture point there is Gov 16. Ventrally it is situated midway between the eyes. This Chakra externalizes as the pituitary gland, which is the master gland of the endocrine system. If any of the other glands are not secreting enough of their own hormone, then the pituitary will help out by secreting trophic hormone, which can often lead to imbalances and conditions such as migraine. The Brow Centre governs the lower brain (medulla downwards through the spinal cord) and (L) eye. It is extremely important when used with our various therapies for hormonal control.

Associations of the Brow Chakra

Colour	Indigo
Sound pitch	A
Meridian	Gall bladder
Endocrine gland	Pituitary
Coupled Chakra	Base
Organs	Central nervous system, (L) eye, ears, nose, eustachian tube
Emotions	Anger, rage
Acupuncture Key points	Gov 4 and Sp 6
Muscular system	Anterior and posterior neck muscles
Autonomic nerve plexus	Ciliary ganglion
Symbol	Six-pointed star

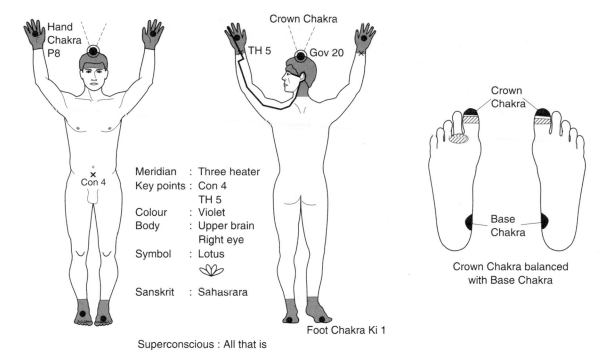

Meridian : Three heater
Key points : Con 4
            TH 5
Colour : Violet
Body : Upper brain
       Right eye
Symbol : Lotus
Sanskrit : Sahasrara

Superconscious : All that is

Crown Chakra balanced with Base Chakra

Figure 4.4 The Crown Chakra – associated with Hand and Foot Chakras. The shaded areas on the manikins represent pain relief areas when using this system of healing with acupuncture. The shaded areas on the foot reflexes are the associated areas of the reflected Chakra points.

Rotating vortices 96
Anatomical position Occipito-atlas junction and midway between eyebrows

Symptomatology. Migraine, chronic catarrh, infectious and contagious disease, deafness and altered hearing, arthritis of the cervical spine, Ménière's syndrome, stress and worry-related symptoms, vertigo, dizziness (Figure 4.5).

Chakra 3   Throat   Vishuddha

The Throat Chakra is situated at the junction of the 7th cervical and the 1st dorsal vertebrae (C7–D1) at the base of the neck. The acupuncture point there is Gov 14. Anteriorly, it is at Con 22 which is in the sternal notch. This is a powerful Chakra and very active, relating to the higher creative faculties. It is said to be the lowest Chakra of the upper part of man (heaven). It manifests on the endocrine level as the thyroid and parathyroid glands. It tends to be the first line of defence when the body is fighting bacteria and viruses, and indeed viruses that are still active can cause a great deal of imbalance at this centre, e.g. glandular fever or dormant asthma. It is said to be in a state of imbalance in people who are reclusive or introvert and who cannot easily express themselves. Damage to this Chakra can be caused by emotional shock such as grief or other such turmoil.

Associations of the Throat Chakra

Colour	Blue
Sound pitch	G
Meridians	Lung and colon
Endocrine glands	Thyroid and parathyroid
Coupled Chakra	Sacral
Organs	Lungs, bronchi, vocal apparatus, alimentary canal
Emotions	Shyness, paranoia, introvertness
Acupuncture Key points	Con 6 and Li 5

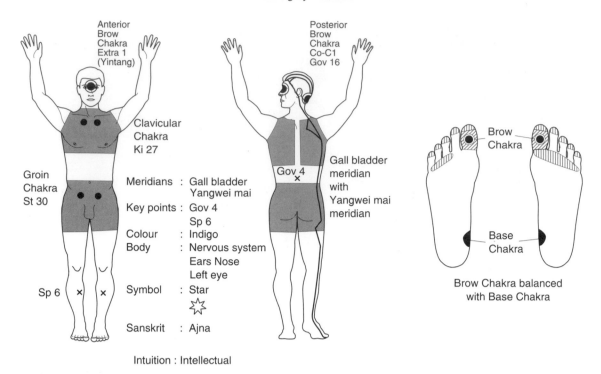

Figure 4.5 The Brow Chakra – associated with Clavicular and Groin Chakras. The shaded areas on the manikins represent pain relief areas when using this system of healing with acupuncture. The shaded areas on the foot reflexes are the associated areas of the reflected Chakra points.

Muscular system	Latissimus dorsi, pectorals, triceps, forearm muscles
Autonomic nerve plexus	Superior cervical ganglia
Symbol	Crescent
Rotating vortices	16
Anatomical position	C7–D1 and sternal notch

Symptomatology. Migraine, chronic and acute sore throats, tonsillitis, shyness and introvertness, asthma, loss of taste, chronic and acute bronchitis, colitis and irritable bowel syndrome, sexual imbalances, ileocaecal valve syndrome, chronic skin lesions such as eczema and alopecia (Figure 4.6).

Chakra 4   Heart   Anahata

The Heart Chakra is situated at the centre of the dorsal spine in between the shoulder blades at the junction of D6 and D7. The acupuncture point there is Gov 10. Anteriorly, it is at Con 17 which is halfway down the sternum. The glandular counterpart of this Chakra is the thymus which is involved in the autoimmune response of the body. When this Chakra is overactive it can produce the amoral, irresponsible individual. Energy flooding uncontrolled can have devastating results and affects the personality of the person, especially with affairs of the heart. Overstimulation can produce the idyllic state of sheer bliss, as when falling in love, which can give an almost out-of-this-world feeling. Weeping comes easily and also getting upset over trifles. Executives and tycoons can suffer from heart trouble as a consequence of everyday stress and strain. Doctors and therapists in the caring professions who cannot detach themselves from their patients are in a similar plight (therapists please note!).

Associations of the Heart Chakra

Colour	Green
Sound pitch	F

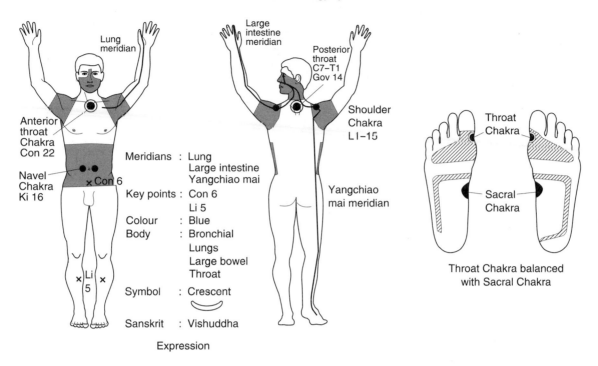

Figure 4.6 The Throat Chakra – associated with Shoulder and Navel Chakras. The shaded areas on the manikins represent pain relief areas when using this system of healing with acupuncture. The shaded areas on the foot reflexes are the associated areas of the reflected Chakra points.

Meridians	Heart and small intestine
Endocrine gland	Thymus
Coupled Chakra	Solar plexus
Organs	Heart, blood, circulation, vagus nerve
Emotions	Tearful, anxious, giggly, detached
Acupuncture Key points	Ht 1 and Gov 7
Muscular system	Erector spinae
Autonomic nerve plexus	Inferior cervical ganglion
Symbol	Cross
Rotating vortices	12
Anatomical position	D6–D7 junction and anteriorly at mid-sternum

Symptomatology. Tumours and growths, cysts, fibroids, heart conditions ranging from heart failure to mitral stenosis, ischaemic heart disease, nausea, palpitations, varicosities, tearfulness, anxiety, vertigo, insular and introvert, angina (Figure 4.7).

Chakra 5   Solar plexus   Manipura

The Solar plexus Chakra is situated at the junction of the dorsal spine and the lumbar spine at D12–L1. The acupuncture point there is Gov 6. Anteriorly, it is situated just below the xiphoid sternum. The glandular counterpart is the pancreas, where insulin is secreted in order to adjust sugar metabolism. This Chakra represents a vast clearing house of energies found below the diaphragm. In most people it is over-stimulated, resulting in nervous disorders, stomach, liver and gall bladder disease as well as diabetes. Dysfunction of this Chakra is considered to be one of the most potent causes of cancer. It is always important to balance the energies of the Solar plexus Chakra to that of the Heart Chakra while treating the patient, as the emotional symptomatology and aetiology are similar and connected. The experienced practitioner spends more time balancing and treating this Chakra than any other. It is the Earth Centre and as such the rest of the bodies

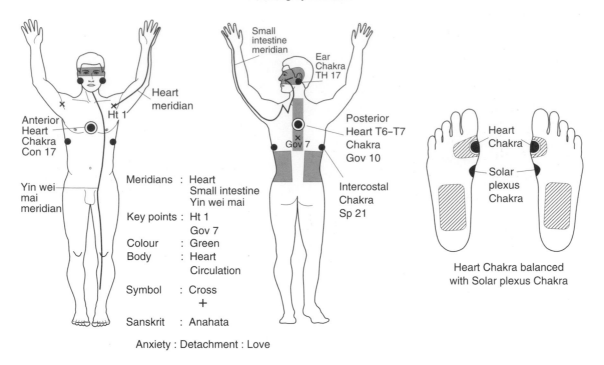

Figure 4.7 The Heart Chakra – associated with Ear and Intercostal Chakras. The shaded areas on the manikins represent pain relief areas when using this system of healing with acupuncture. The shaded areas on the foot reflexes are the associated areas of the reflected Chakra points.

are dependent upon its stability, which in the vast majority of humankind is simply not the case.

Associations of the Solar plexus Chakra

Colour	Yellow
Sound pitch	E
Meridians	Liver and stomach
Endocrine gland	Pancreas
Coupled Chakra	Heart
Organs	Stomach, liver, gall bladder, pancreas, spleen
Emotions	Depression, anxiety, phobias
Acupuncture Key points	Con 17 and TH 4
Muscular system	Abdominals and quadriceps
Autonomic nerve system	Coeliac plexus and coeliac ganglion
Symbol	Circle
Rotating vortices	10

Anatomical position D12–L1 junction and below the xiphoid sternum

Symptomatology. Skin conditions such as acne and eczema, stomach ulcers, cancerous growths, worry and depression, hepatitis, gall bladder colic, glandular fever, autoimmune system infections, allergies of *any* kind, chronic fatigue syndrome, hay fever (Figure 4.8).

Chakra 6   Sacral   Svadhisthana

The Sacral Chakra is situated at the junction of L4 and L5 near the base of the lumbar spine. The acupuncture there is Gov 3. Anteriorly, it is situated about 3 cm below the umbilicus at a point Con 6 which is also known as the Hara. This Chakra is said to be important in the reproductive system and as such it is used extensively in the treatment of conditions associated with that system. It is also called the Chakra of water balance and is closely tied in with fluid balance of the body, including urine and semen. It is coupled with the Throat Chakra and this couple is used to treat such conditions

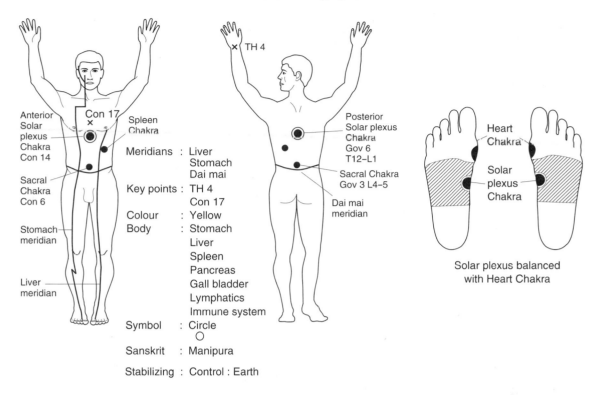

Figure 4.8 The Solar plexus Chakra – associated with Sacral and Spleen Chakras. The shaded areas on the manikins represent pain relief areas when using this system of healing with acupuncture. The shaded areas on the foot reflexes are the associated areas of the reflected Chakra points.

such as chronic sore throats and impotence, as well as pelvic disorders.

Associations of the Sacral Chakra

Colour	Orange
Sound pitch	D
Meridians	Spleen and pericardium
Endocrine gland	Gonads
Coupled Chakra	Throat
Organs	Reproductive system, fluid balance
Emotions	Jealousy, envy
Acupuncture Key points	Gov 12 and P3
Muscular system	Hamstrings, anterior tibials
Autonomic nerve system	Inferior mesenteric ganglion
Symbol	Triangle

Rotating vortices 6
Anatomical positions L4–5L junction and anteriorly CV6 (Hara)

Symptomatology. Low vitality, intestinal and gastric conditions, irritable bowel, chronic tiredness, impotence, libido high or low, chronic sore throats, imbalance with heating mechanism including chilblains, menstrual and menapausal conditions, oedema, swollen ankles, rheumatoid factor conditions (Figure 4.9).

Chakra 7 Base Muladhara

The Base Chakra is said to be responsible for anchoring the body upon the physical plane and providing a channel for the will to express itself. It is said to be dormant in the mass of humanity, but its activity is on the increase due to the stress of modern living. It is situated at the sacrococcyx junction at Gov 2 and is associated with the adrenal medulla which is concerned with the production of adrenaline.

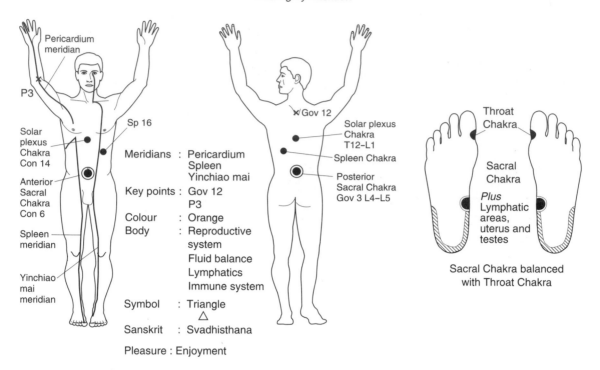

Figure 4.9 The Sacral Chakra – associated with Solar plexus and Spleen Chakras. The shaded areas on the manikins represent pain relief areas when using this system of healing with acupuncture. The shaded areas on the foot reflexes are the associated areas of the reflected Chakra points.

This centre is used for the treatment of *any chronic* condition which is miasmatic or heritable. It is also used in any condition to do with the spinal column and the kidneys.

Associations of the Base Chakra

Colour	Red
Sound pitch	C
Meridians	Kidney and bladder
Coupled Chakras	Crown and Brow
Organs	Spinal column, kidneys, lower limbs
Emotions	Insecurity, insanity
Acupuncture Key points	Con 22 and Li 8
Muscular system	Psoas major/iliacus, soleus, gastrocnemius
Autonomic nerve plexus	Pelvic plexus
Symbol	Square
Rotating vortices	4
Anatomical position	Sacrococcyx junction

Symptomatology. Low vitality, osteoarthritis, ankylosing spondylitis, lethargy, stiff joints, nephritis, cystitis, prostatitis, kidney calculii, gravitational ulcers, growing pains, Scheuermann's disease and other 'bone'-related conditions, also depression and insanity (Figure 4.10).

Treatment of conditions

As the reader is by now aware, the Chakra energy system is a vast topic that covers many facets of healing. As has been stated before, this philosophy of subtle energy healing can be used by several modalities of therapy, each being as pertinent as another. Although this system can be used extensively in the treatment of acute conditions, it is in its approach to the treatment of chronic conditions that it excels. This is because the therapist is truly treating the *cause* of the condition and not just palliating the symptoms.

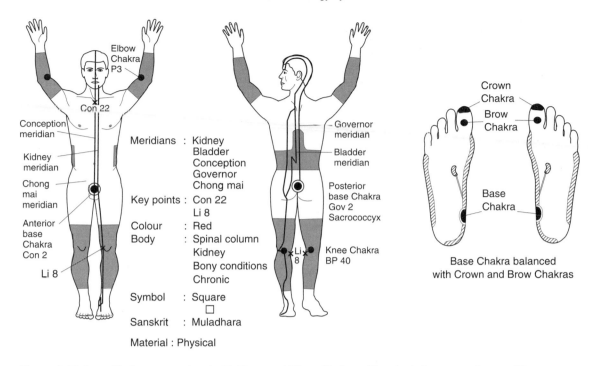

Figure 4.10 Base Chakra – associated with Knee and Elbow Chakras. The shaded areas on the manikins represent pain relief areas when using this system of healing with acupuncture. The shaded areas on the foot reflexes are the associated areas of the reflected Chakra points.

The author is at present preparing a book, *Healing with the Chakra Energy System*, which will include the approaches of acupuncture, acupressure, reflexology and craniosacral therapy, as well as briefly mentioning treatment by colour, sound, yoga and meditation.

References

Cross, J. (1986) The relationship of the Chakra energy system and acupuncture. *Doctoral thesis*. Copyright held by the British College of Acupuncture.

Gerber, R. (1988) *Vibrational Medicine*. Santa Fe, NM: Bear.

Motoyama, H. (1988) *Theories of the Chakras: Bridge to Higher Consciousness*. Wheaton, IL: Theosophical Publishing House.

Tansley, D.V. (1972) *Radionics and the Subtle Anatomy of Man*. Saffron Walden: C W Daniel.

Recommended reading

Brennan, B.A. (1987) *Hands of Light*. New York: Bantam Books.

Ellis, N. (1994) *Acupuncture in Clinical Practice*. London: Chapman and Hall.

Gimbel, T. (1980) *Healing through Colour*. Saffron Walden: C W Daniel.

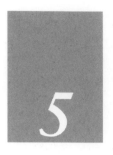

5 Spiritual healing

Bernadette Dunne

Introduction

Manifestations of the 'divine' can be as readily glimpsed in the equations of quantum physics as they can be seen in the symbols of orthodox religion. What is evident are the varying expressions of an ultimate truth. Simplicity and diversity coexist at the most fundamental level of reality. On a social level, humanity has evolved through a multitude of different cultures, and yet certain characteristics of humanity are common to all. Spiritual healing is one of the most ancient and holistic approaches to wellbeing. The expressions of spiritual healing are as diverse as the cultures and personalities from which they spring: North American Indian healers encouraged a holistic relationship with their environment, and practised in the name of the Great Spirit. In contrast, Lawrence LeShan, an American clinical and research psychologist, became known as 'the man who scientifically trained himself to become a healer'.

'Healing' derives from the Anglo-Saxon word '*haelen*' – to be or become whole. It is a return to wholeness through recognition of what is deepest within us. Following such a path involves commitment, and may lead to the attenuation, or occasionally, complete healing of physical symptoms. Conversely, a person's journey into wholeness may be facilitated not by 'cure,' but by learning to cope with physical difficulties.

Historical perspective

It must have been with a great sigh of relief that healers in Britain greeted the repeal of the Witchcraft Act in 1951. Prejudice and fear had made them liable to prosecution. Western understanding of the 'witch doctors' of aboriginal peoples has been similarly misinformed. They were, after all, one of the earliest groups of healers. Witch doctors were often chosen for the wisdom that comes with age, and functioned as a powerful, positive force within their group.

The healing ministry of Jesus and the early Christian church has been the predominant influence in Western spiritual healing. The characteristic laying on of hands, associated with many healers, has continuity however, not only with the early church, but with ancient practice in China, Egypt and Greece.

The self-healing techniques of the Indian Ayurvedas were well established when the pyramids were built. Ayurveda ('Ayus' life, 'Veda' knowledge or science) is the body of classical Indian medicine which is based upon the texts of the ancient yogis or 'Rishis'. The main tenet of their writings is that mind creates a flow of life within the body. Their philosophy has many of the hallmarks of contemporary consciousness studies. Vedic wisdom states: 'The universe's wisdom extends from smaller than the smallest to larger than the largest.' (Chopra, 1989)

A unifying field, supporting and inviting diversity, is suggested in quantum physics at the level of the Planck scale. Here the photon, or smallest, indivisible unit of light can be observed as either wave or particle. At the level of human consciousness, aberration from the true nature of a person's being, where simplicity is paramount, but where potential is unlimited, can be the cause of disease. Ayurvedic techniques, which restore the balance of consciousness, can be the means of resolving disease. All have their basis in meditation.

Disease can be overcome in two ways: by an awareness of the purity and power of consciousness, in the light of which the symptoms of illness become less important, or by focusing the power of consciousness directly on the problem.

Ayurveda engages the whole person and encourages commitment to enhancing the body's natural ability to heal itself. Herbal medicine, self-purification techniques and meditation are means by which this can be attained.

By the mid-nineteenth century, Western healers were beginning to see the manifestations of disease in the context of the whole person. Phineas Quimby, a clairvoyant healer from the USA, gave full support to the belief that many diseases were psychosomatic in nature. Christian Science under the guidance of Mary Baker Eddy, went on to develop these ideas: that spirit is the only enduring reality, and that, in some instances, a breakdown in physical health is a reflection of a problem at a deeper level.

One of the better known British healers, Harry Edwards, said: 'Healing has to get into the mind.' He encouraged and empowered people to cooperate in the healing process by helping them to address the cause of the problem. His holistic approach included massage, exercise and movement. Regarding arthritis, he said:

> The purpose of the healing is to build upon what movement there is. The movement must be gently yet purposefully encouraged, seeking 'just that little more'. (In Hammond, 1973)

Edwards believed that he was only a channel for healing 'by a non-human agency'. He did not believe in Karma, but he did believe in life after death and in the ability of spirit 'guides' to assist in the healing.

The co-founder, in 1955, of The National Federation of Spiritual Healers, Gordon Turner, believed that he was more than a channel for the healing power of God. He also emphasized an awakening of healing power within the person themselves:

> I think we have gone along the wrong lines in our research in healing. I think we have tended too much to be concerned with the physical changes which take place in our patients. . . . The power passing through the healer . . . and in asking 'where does the power come from?' I don't think it comes from anywhere, it's *here* the whole time. (In Hammond, 1973)

Healing for Turner was a process which occurred relative to the level of consciousness achieved. Through a change in consciousness brought about by meditation, the healer seeks attunement with his higher self, and through this with the divine. He simultaneously seeks attunement with the other person: 'One essence becomes totally intermingled with another essence.' This is a level to which healers aspire. It is at this level of focus that spontaneous healings are said to occur.

Turner was responsible for the introduction of healers into the hospital environment. He envisaged two specific roles for healers: the non-professional healing counsellor, and the paid professional, i.e. nurse healer, doctor healer. He would certainly have welcomed the physiotherapist healer.

It was Ronald Beasley, a British healer contemporary with Harry Edwards and Gordon Turner, who emphasized the karmic nature of healing:

> The person may have a big program of personality development to carry out within his consciousness; some of this is painful. Often what people think of as pain is evolution working through the consciousness. It isn't illness you have got to help, it's the person! (In Hammond, 1973)

This is a sentiment echoed by many involved in healing. Helen Schucman writes: 'Think never of the body. Healing is the thought of unity. Forget all things that seem to separate.' (In Carlson and Shield, 1989)

Beasley, like Turner, was convinced of the importance of thorough training. He organized courses for healers, lecturing on subjects from anatomy to psychotherapy. He expected from the healer 'dedication, discipline and a complete belief in his ability'.

Lawrence Leshan also expected rigorous mental discipline from his students. His workshops included exercises to heighten the powers of concentration, encourage a deeper understanding of the concepts of time and space, and facilitate the changes in consciousness necessary for healing to take place (Hammond, 1973).

Some healers are clairvoyant or clairaudient. Some teachers of healing recommend a course in anatomy and physiology, while others are wary of treating physical symptoms as they feel that this may divert them from treating the cause of the illness. Some healers are assisted by spirit guides or doctors, and some adhere to a particular religious belief. All these factors are incidental. The essence of healing, and this would appear to be upheld by all healers, is a desire for wholeness on the part of the healer and for all with whom they come into contact. The Buddhist promise takes this one step further: 'I vow to attain enlightenment in order to save all sentient beings from suffering.'

Healing concepts

Belief and commitment

Belief is of central importance in spiritual healing. Its presence can be demonstrated overtly, on the part of the recipient, or more subtly, for example when another expresses faith on their behalf. The belief of the healer is also relevant here. In Jesus' healing ministry, as recorded, He frequently looked for a sign of commitment and trust, either from the recipient, or from those interceding for them:

Bartimaeus was persistent in his demands that Jesus should help him, and Jesus responded accordingly:

'Rabbi I want to see'!
'Go,' said Jesus, 'your faith has healed you!'
(*Mark, Chapter 10, verses 51–52*)

The centurion was rewarded for his belief that Jesus could heal his servant from a distance: 'Go, it will be done just as you believed it would.'

(*Matthew, Chapter 8, verse 13*)

When Paul and Barnabus were preaching at Lystra, Paul responded to the silent faith of a man in the crowd: 'Paul looked directly at him, saw that he had faith to be healed and called out 'Stand up on your feet!'
(*Acts of the Apostles, Chapter 14, verses 9–10*)

The effect of intercessory prayer on patients in a coronary care unit was studied in a double-blind trial in the USA in 1988 (see Chapter 7). The patients were unaware of prayers offered on their behalf and yet a significant impact on their recovery was demonstrated. (One could question whether or not the potential 'faith', or open-mindedness of those conducting the experiment, might have influenced the outcome.)

Animals do not consciously express faith in healing, but they are very responsive, and many successes have been reported with absent healing in animals. Perhaps one of the most important factors regarding belief is lack of resistance. Human beings have the freedom to choose wholeness. Animals follow this path instinctively, and the healer intercedes on their behalf.

Human choice is often a series of commitments made over a period of time. Healing therefore may occur gradually, building upon the person's own desire for wholeness.

Time and 'intension'

The Ayurvedic Rishis mastered the art of truly 'being' in the present moment. They spent prolonged periods of time in meditation, and their 'intension' or intense focus of consciousness was relatively pure. Their ability to heal could be instantaneous.

Alexis Carrel, a scientist who studied the effects of prayer at Lourdes, commented on such a quantum leap in healing:

In a few seconds, a few minutes, at the most a few hours . . . pathological symptoms disappear . . . the miracle is characterized chiefly by an extreme acceleration of the processes of organic repair. (In Horstman, 1964)

Carrel was recognized by his fellow scientists as an impartial observer. He was also known as a man of prayer, a healer in his own right, who interceded for the suffering.

For the most part, healing takes part over a longer period of time. The actual passing of time can have a beneficial effect. Likewise, time spent with another can be the means by which the infinite is glimpsed. Bruyere has said: 'The healer establishes a sacred space or Temenos . . . in which energy may be generated.' (In Carlson and Shield, 1989)

Worthiness

The source of healing must be approached with humility and respect. To many healers, this source is a God of love, to be approached with childlike simplicity: likewise the gift of healing. Historically, the relationship of the healer to this gift has been interpreted in different ways.

Rolling Thunder, born a Cherokee Indian, believed that self-purification was a prerequisite for healing through the power of the Great Spirit. His demonstrations of spontaneous ritual during healing were highly intuitive, and responded to each individual's specific needs.

Rasputin could be said to have had many characteristics which were at variance with his undoubted ability to heal: his moral faux pas were more than peccadilloes. A lot of his work was accomplished, however, at a distance. This is considered by many practitioners to be healing in one of its purest forms.

For the author, it is reassuring to know that healing is not dependent upon human effort and moral purity. From the Christian standpoint, it is the grace of God which is active in the healer. St Paul speaks of a 'thorn' in his flesh, which he is simply unable to overcome. He is assured by Christ: 'My grace is sufficient for you, for my power is made perfect in weakness.' (*2 Corinthians, Chapter 12, verse 9*)

Thorns, weaknesses, character flaws have a valuable role to play. They may help to soften the ego and awaken the healer to a reality which is infinitely grander than they would otherwise believe.

Touch

The concept of touch in healing appears relative to the healer and the culture that they represent. At certain times Jesus would touch a specific part of the body, for example the eyes. He made a definite point of touching lepers. In Harry Edwards' healing ministry it is evident not only that he touched people, but that he handled them with some authority. Our current Western practice of laying on of hands has become complicated. Fears of litigation are inhibiting some groups from placing hands directly on the body.

A human energy field or 'aura', extending beyond the body, is upheld by many ancient teachings, including Hindu vedic texts, and the more recent Jewish Kabbalah (sixth century BC). This energy field is thought to precede and give life to the physical body. In Western practice, the concept of 'treating the aura', by placing one's hands at a slight distance from the body, has occasioned considerable debate. If the aura does extend beyond the body as a field, then such a practice can be upheld.

The term 'layer,' when referring to the aura, can be misleading, as it leads to a belief that each layer is placed on top of the one below. The term 'body' is more appropriate, each auric body, considered as a vibrational field, suffusing the physical body and extending further outwards than one of a lower vibration. The implicate order of physicist David Bohm is relevant here. The implicate order pervades and gives meaning to the explicate order or observable universe, just as the existence of a vortex depends upon the water that surrounds it. The implicate order exists in every particle of observable phenomena; likewise every part of a hologram reflects the image of the whole.

It follows, then, that in healing, with whichever part of 'the body' one comes into contact, one is, in effect, treating the whole being.

Personal experience

The event which triggered the author's involvement in healing was a sudden return to England from Canada several years ago. A very special cat had to be left behind. Distance was not experienced, however, as a barrier to communication; it rather heightened the awareness that love and consciousness cannot be constrained by the bounds of time and space. Spiritual healing is a point of contact or 'communion' where this universal flow of love or energy can be shared.

The author has subsequently been involved in animal healing and with a local spiritual healing group. The ethos of the group is to offer healing in as simple a way as possible. After all, according to Bruce Shield, 'The shortest distance between two points is an intention'.

People request healing for chronic illnesses, stress-related problems and life-threatening conditions. It is important for people to talk freely if they choose. It is rare that someone will seek help for a physical problem without divulging a source of stress in their life. The physical problem is sometimes the validation that the person may feel they need in order to ask for healing.

After communicating in this way, the process of attunement begins. The author has found it very useful to have a symbol of attunement. This can be a thought or image used exclusively for the purpose. Concentration on the symbol can bring about the meditative state almost immediately. Some physical contact takes place at this time, either holding the person's hands or with hands placed on their shoulders. The breathing patterns of both people will often synchronize. From the point of view of attunement, nothing else is needed. For distant healing, the person or animal does not even have to be in the same room. Contact, however, is a 'sacrament' of the divine: it can help to incarnate the infinite. It can also help people to feel at ease.

James Oschman (see Chapter 1) refers to the capacity of the human brain in the meditative state to condense and magnify the earth's Schumann waves. This high-intensity, low-frequency output can be transmitted very effectively through the hands of the healer. (The right hand has a positive, and the left a negative polarity.) Contact with Chakra points has definite value (see Chapter 4). During healing, most

people become very relaxed and many will report feeling a sensation of warmth where the hands are placed.

Although there is an obvious element of ritual, the healer remains as open as possible to guidance throughout healing. Energy is focused on the other person's highest good. Attention to physical symptoms is relative to this. People will usually return for healing several times, and will often need reassurance that they are most welcome to do so.

Relevance to physiotherapy

Many hospitals and GP practices now employ healers as part of their team of complementary therapists (there is a growing GP healer network in Britain). Nurses practise Therapeutic Touch (see Chapter 8); it has become a recognized facet of their professional input, especially in the USA. Physiotherapists, likewise, may bring another dimension to patient contact through spiritual healing or other healing techniques.

The author's approach can be described as discreet, with the intention of incorporating healing into actual patient contact. To approach the other person with attention and respect is surely central to everyone's practice. For the author, it is the connection from which 'instant' attunement is possible. Attunement is not time-dependent. If the orientation of the healer is appropriate, the focus of 'intension' can be almost instantaneous. In the clinical setting, this is invaluable.

There are many instances, however, when it is necessary to spend more time with people, for example oncology patients and those receiving palliative care. The ITU presents a similar challenge, as the stress to which patients are subjected is phenomenal. The case here for a period of systematic healing, with aura and Chakra work, is clear. There is also an obvious need on the part of the relatives involved.

Lifestyle and anxiety-related illnesses, such as myalgic encephalitis and hyperventilation syndrome, would also benefit from a holistic approach which included spiritual healing.

Chronic pain presents another significant patient group. The aim would be to empower the person either to cope with or overcome their illness. The attenuation, or healing, of physical symptoms would be a welcome manifestation of a positive change in the whole person.

The treatment, by healing, of a localized problem could be either incorporated into our existing 'hands-on' contact, or formalized as a specific healing therapy for many patients. Such a problem, however, may be a symptom of a deeper concern, and will begin to resolve only when attention is paid to underlying issues.

Joel Goldsmith encourages the healer to focus on the ultimate:

> The Spiritual healer, anchored in spiritual wisdom, remains relaxed in God and lets the Spirit flow. . . . When you are swimming, let the water carry your body, and when you are giving a treatment, let the Spirit, let the Truth carry the treatment! (Goldsmith, 1960)

Physiotherapists are involved in many situations which provide the opportunity for more than physical treatment. Each person that presents to us has a considerable capacity for self-healing, and physiotherapists have the expertise to help them achieve their physical potential. Spiritual healing has at heart the infinite potential of each person. A perspective such as this brings challenge and depth to our physiotherapy practice.

References

Carlson, R. and Shield, B. (1989) *Healers on Healing*. Los Angeles, CA: Tarcher.

Chopra, D. (1989) *Quantum Healing. Exploring the Frontiers of Mind/Body Medicine*. London: Bantam.

Goldsmith, J.S. (1960) *The Art of Spiritual Healing*. London: Allen and Unwin.

Hammond, S. (1973) *We Are All Healers*. London: Turnstone.

Holy Bible, New International Version (1973) London: Hodder and Stoughton.

Horstman, L. (1964) *An Introduction to Spiritual Healing*. London: Rider.

Recommended reading

Laszlo, E. (1996) *The Whispering Pond. A Personal Guide to the Emerging Vision of Science*. Shaftesbury: Element.

6 Therapeutic Touch

Ann Childs

Introduction

This therapeutic modality is a contemporary interpretation of ancient and traditional healing practices, yet remains free of any religious doctrines. It is an innate, natural human potential that can be learned and practised by anyone who has the intention to help and heal. In 1992, the Nurse Healers Professional Association (NHPA) defined Therapeutic Touch (TT) as 'a consciously directed process of energy exchange during which the practitioner uses the hands as a focus to facilitate healing'. Interestingly, TT incorporates *a non-touch* technique, by accessing the body's external energy fields rather than the physical skin. There are times when the physical body is touched, yet the intention is still to maintain energy contact. TT is practised over the patient's clothing.

Historical context

Tracing the ancient traditions of *laying on of hands healing and touch* within the context of religion and culture gives some insight into our today's present sensitivity of the subject, combined with the developing scientific bias (Brennan, 1993; Richardson, 1995).

In the 1960s and 1970s, to counteract the mystique surrounding psychic/spiritual healing, Drs Grad, Miller, Smith and Vogel collaborated with established healers, Worral, Hill and Estebany, to run a series of experiments (Gerber, 1988). They were pioneers in the use of creative and exacting research methods and the detection and measurement of the effects of the human energy field (HEF). These effects included alterations of the surface tension and hydrogen bonding in healer-treated water compared to a non-treated control sample and the effects of the electrical and magnetic properties of the HEF on the alteration of growth rate in plants, wound repair in animals and changes in enzyme reaction rates. Many of these experiments are summarized by White and Krippner (1977) and Gerber (1988).

In 1971, Dr Dolores Krieger, Professor of Nursing at New York University, who later coined the term 'Therapeutic Touch', joined the well-known healers Oskar Estebany and Dora Kunz as a fellow researcher to study the biological effects of healing. Krieger looked specifically at the resultant increased blood haemoglobin levels of TT-treated patients compared with controls (Krieger *et al.*, 1979). Having validated a reliable biochemical yardstick to measure haemoglobin levels following TT, Krieger was taught by Kunz to use her hands for healing, the effect of which improved with practice. Krieger's students are also able to increase their hand sensitivity to TT perception, with practice, and obtain therapeutic results (Paes de Silva, 1996).

After further research, Krieger felt strongly motivated to teach Master's Degree nursing students in a programme called 'Frontiers of Nursing'. However, owing to the cynical associations of any form of psychic/spiritual healing with the health care professionals, Krieger decided, as mentioned above, to rename the technique Therapeutic Touch, as a less threatening and more innocuous term accepted by the nursing and medical staff. TT continues to be taught in over 80 universities in the USA as part of their nursing degree programme, and in the schools of nursing of more than 70 other countries, continuing to be used in many mainstream hospitals (Bronstein, 1996).

Conceptual framework

Therapeutic Touch is imbued with an array of metaphysical ideas. In order to give some understanding of TT, Krieger drew out of Eastern philosophy a supportive framework on which to base the concepts of energy interaction between therapist and patient. During the past 20 years quantum physics, the wave-particle phenomenon, areas of more sensitive physics research, and new paradigms of interconnectedness and interrelationships between energy and matter, have begun to give explanations as to the function and interactions of the human energy field (Brennan, 1993; Laszlo, 1996). The concept of quantum physics is used by energy medicine practitioners to explain the phenomena of TT (Vaughan, 1995). These new concepts in physics, together with a deeper understanding of Eastern philosophy concerning the nature of matter, clarify the significance of the limitations of a purely structural approach.

The components of the Human Energy Field (HEF) can simply be described as the etheric, emotional, mental and intuitional fields, the latter related to our source of belonging in the universe. Awareness of this Universal Energy Field (UEF) and our connectedness to it underlies the principle of energy flowing from the UEF through the therapist to another person without draining the therapist. Hover-Kramer (1990) continues this line of thought with the phrase 'Through our own health and healing we access our capacity for compassion and genuine giving, knowing there is enough love in the UEF for each of us'.

Somehow as human beings we are constantly putting concepts of mind, spirit and identity into locatable categories. This tendency to locate and compartmentalize could be interfering with our understanding of energy concepts. Peck (1990) talks of the

> . . . boundaries of an individual being more of a permeable membrane. Just as our conscious mind is continually partially permeable to our unconscious mind, so is our unconscious permeable to the mind without. [Collective consciousness? or interconnectiveness?]

During the same time that Krieger was developing TT at New York University, another Professor of Nursing, Martha Rogers, was developing the conceptual framework of the Science of Unitary Human Beings. This is based upon the concepts of energy fields, open systems, pattern and pandimensionality (a nonlinear domain without spatial and temporal attributes) (Johnson Lutjens, 1991). Rogerian science talks of energy process and the human energy field's relationship with the environment, rather than the Krieger concept of energy transference between two people. To explore this further, Biley (1995) explores these concepts and their clinical implication in depth.

An important factor underpinning TT, is the *intention* to help or heal, expressing a deep inner desire to augment the process of healing, to the best of our knowledge and skill. There is an experience of connectedness with the patient through unconditional love and, paradoxically, a position of detachment as to the outcome. The intention relates more to the balancing or repatterning of the patient's energy fields, hence placing them in an optimum position to mobilize their own healing energy more effectively, rather than having a specified outcome in mind, e.g. increased range of movement of a localized joint.

Quinn (1982), a leading exponent of Rogerian thinking, describes TT as 'an attempt to focus on the well-being of the patient in an act of unconditional love and compassion'. Krieger speaks of a 'healing meditation' (Krieger *et al.*, 1979). The debate continues.

During a study to measure physiological parameters of the healer–healee interactions, significant findings were revealed regarding brainwave activity. An unusual amount of rapid rhythmical beta electroencephalogram (EEG) activity was recorded during TT. This would correspond to approximately 20–30 Hz associated with a bihemispheric state of active attention. The frontalis electromyogram motor unit activity (EMG) subsided, indicating that the rapid beta frequency was not an artefact of muscle action. The electro-oculograms (EOG) showed slight divergence and no movement, another indication of deep concentration.

During TT the patients displayed *high-amplitude alpha wave activity*, approximately *7–12 Hz*, both with eyes open and closed. This frequency is associated with a passive, meditation state in which the self is stilled, the body relaxed yet the mind remains alert. Physiological indices indicated they were indeed relaxed (Krieger *et al.*, 1979).

Considering the work of Cade and Coxhead (1979), in which both the healer and healee enter into a rough synchrony of bihemispheric high-amplitude alpha frequencies of approximately 8–10 Hz, there may be different mechanisms of healing, characterized by the different frequency output of the healer and the *transference* or *induction* of similar frequencies in the healee. A working hypothesis could be considered where the belief system of the healer regarded themselves as an *open tuning channel* to a greater universal energy source and in essence, used as a *conduit* to the healee, involving the meditative state of high-amplitude alpha frequencies. An alternative hypothesis could be considered where the healer is directing their own energy fields as a *generating source of energy*, with active attention characterized by fast beta activity, not as a passive conduit. Thus, to date, research offers tantalizing glimpses of healer–healee interactions of which a fairly constant feature is a change from separate left and right hemispheric EEG patterns to a *common bihemispheric beat frequency* which seems to correlate with an intention to heal and a readiness to receive healing.

The author's experience of TT is reflected in this quotation by Carl Rogers, the instigator and developer of Person Centred Counselling who requires the core conditions of the therapeutic relationship to be unconditional acceptance, honesty and empathic understanding. He observes that

> When I am closest to my inner, intuitive self, somehow in touch with the unknown in me, when perhaps I am in a slightly altered state of consciousness in the relationship, then whatever I seem to do seems to be full of healing. Then simply my presence is releasing and helpful. There is nothing I can do to force this experience. . . . At these moments it seems that my inner spirit has reached out and touched the inner spirit of the other. Our relationship transcends itself and becomes a part of something larger. Profound growth and healing and energy are present. (In Thorne, 1991)

Technique

The following is a brief description of the 5-step procedure involved; however, in reality the experienced practitioner will merge the sequence, giving opportunity for creativity and intuition. The recipient may be standing or seated but usually lying supine and prone to access anterior and posterior aspects.

Centring. This is a shift of the practitioner's external awareness to an internal focus in order to achieve a sense of calm and being grounded. It is essential preparation for all energy work and is maintained throughout the process. Thought of as a meditative state, it enables the practitioner to find within him/herself an inner reference of stability.

Assessment. Moving the hands some 5–15 cm (2–6 in) above the physical body, until the whole surface has been covered, assesses the energy field (*scanning*). Note is made of subtle energy cues in the energy field pattern such as differences in temperature, pressure, changes in rhythm and flow and localized tingling or electric and magnetic-type feelings using the natural sensitivity of the hands. There is a sense of *listening and tuning in* to the person.

Clearing. The hands are swept longitudinally over the body from head to toe, with the intention of facilitating a symmetrical, rhythmical flow of energy to areas of the field that the practitioner perceives to be sluggish, congested or static. This phase often brings about a deep relaxation response.

Balancing or repatterning. The hands are used to redirect the areas of accumulated tension or energy to depleted areas, thus helping to re-establish the perceived energy flow. Energy imbalances which were felt in the original assessment are addressed by conscious direction using intention, visualization and appropriate hand movements to assist the recipient to repattern their own energy fields, via interaction with the practitioner's own energy fields. This may be discerned as loosening and clearing congestion, cooling a warm area, or to calming and soothing an overactive location.

Evaluation. Reassessment by scanning, using sensory cues, demonstrates to the practitioner a perceived improvement, synchronicity and bilateral symmetry in the patient's energy flow. Completion of repatterning is often experienced intuitively, together with clues such as the patient sighing or changing the breathing pattern. After having *centred and tuned in* to the patient, the practitioner has both a sense of cognitively and energetically *disconnecting* to finish. This is postulated to maintain the integrity of the practitioner's own energy field once TT has completed.

Clinical effectiveness

Spence and Olsen (1997) reviewed quantitative work from the last decade (1985–95) and found evidence to support the practice of TT for the reduction of pain or anxiety.

Pain relief

Keller and Bzdek (1986) found that TT reduced the pain of tension headaches in a significant number of subjects (90%), to a significant degree (70%). The effect was enhanced over 4 hours following the intervention, reducing the need for medication. The control group was subjected to a placebo intervention which did reduce the headache pain, but the effect did not occur as often, was not as great and did not last as long as the effects of TT.

The pilot study of Vaughan (1995) investigated the health status and health perception of patients attending a small GP outpatient clinic. There were no exclusion criteria based on diagnosis. One of the indicators included pain experienced as part of their overall health problem. The subjects showed significant improvement in the perception of pain relief after the first session and a continuation of the pain relief 1 week later, compared to both the control and placebo groups. During the following week, particularly with traumatic injury, a warm glow was felt inside the body around the site of injury reported by the experimental subjects but not the control or placebo group.

In a study by Peck (1997), pain and distress were significantly decreased in subjects with chronic arthritis, after the first application of TT, and further decreased after subsequent treatments. A second group of patients were taught progressive muscle relaxation techniques. They exceeded the pain-relieving effects of the TT group. Both groups showed a statistical, clinical improvement of arthritic pain relief and reduction of stress, followed by an improvement in daily functional activities. Peck discusses the requirement of client involvement, motivation and cognitive understanding using the muscle relaxation techniques, compared with the ease of TT with clients unable to cooperate with treatment. However, a practitioner must be available for every treatment.

Biley (1996) explored the psychological concept of body image and traditional biomedical treatment of phantom limb pain compared with a human field image perspective treated by TT. It would appear that loss of a body part may result in an alteration of an individual's three-dimensional body image, while the human energy field remains, although perhaps in some kind of altered form. Before an amputation there should be a congruency between the body image and the human energy field image. After an amputation, it is suggested that there develops an 'image incongruency' or 'integrated awareness dissonance' giving the phantom limb sensation as part of the modification of the total body image. Biley discusses several qualitative case studies relating to phantom limb pain and the use of TT, termed by Biley as *positive human field image patterning*. The results described a significant impact on pain, altered sensation and altered body image.

Anxiety

Cox and Hayes (1998) initiated a qualitative exploratory design describing the experiences of two critically ill patients who received TT on an intensive care unit. The case studies indicated an increase in relaxation, a sense of comfort and peace and an ability to understand more about themselves which contributed to their psychological well-being.

Hover-Kramer (1990) found significant reduction in anxiety after TT as compared with casual touch in hospitalized children.

An investigation by Olson *et al.* (1992) was designed and implemented in the 2 months following Hurricane Hugo in the West Indies, to study and help a large group of individuals with post-traumatic event anxiety. In the first two sessions, TT was administered and the third session became a control session in which the same procedures were followed, with the exception that no TT was done. Both physiological and psychological outcome measurements were used. Mean anxiety scores after receiving TT were reduced by more than half, compared with the pre-TT scores. The control group showed no decrease in anxiety scores.

Hughes *et al.* (1996) undertook a qualitative study of adolescent patients with mental health problems, looking at their perception and experience of TT. They reported being less agitated, happier, more energetic, more in control of feelings and more able to express feelings appropriately. Behaviour changes were brought about by the ability to translate the new awareness into self-perception and new coping skills (e.g. being able to calm themselves). Through the course of treatments the adolescents perceived an improved relationship with the nurses, manifested by improved communication and trust. After the study, both the subjects and other observing therapists wanted the treatments to continue.

Literature reviews

Daley (1997) undertook a comparative analysis of five trials conducted on the efficacy of TT for wound healing. Of these five rigorously controlled trials, two indicated statistically significant accelerated rates of dermal healing,

one had the opposite effect, in that the controls healed more quickly than the TT-treated group (see Chapter 3) and the other two showed no clear effect. Despite the fact that the five studies reviewed did not demonstrate a consistent replicate TT effect, Daley recommends Wirth *et al.* (1994) for their seminal research efforts. The design features utilized in these experiments are considered by many, both within orthodox and complementary healing circles, to be some of the most scientifically rigorous, methodologically sophisticated experimental protocols ever utilized in the field of healing. The original concept and approach of using TT through a barrier, at a distance, and without the subject's knowledge, eliminates suggestion, expectation and the placebo effect.

From the studies it may be seen that, given the clinical nature of TT, there are inherent drawbacks in attempting to demonstrate experimentally what is essentially a clinical phenomenon. The use of subject cross-over experimental protocol where the subjects acted as their own controls is an excellent methodological design feature, but from a clinical perspective potential problems are created from a carryover treatment effect.

A brief mention of the study by Rosa *et al.* (1998) would be pertinent at this point as an illustration of a seemingly good experimental design to test TT's basic premise that a practitioner is able to perceive another person's energy field. Within the experiment there appeared to be a strong bias of scepticism, high stress factors to perform and emphasis on test procedure rather than a clinical ambience, intent to heal or development of rapport, all of which reduce intuitive sensitivity. These essential factors for TT are reflected in the poor outcomes. Again this calls for a more sensitive and creative, yet at the same time exacting, stringent approach in the design of research methodology.

Rosa *et al.* (1998) conducted an extensive literature analysis from 1972 to 1997 identifying 853 abstracts. Only one study, Quinn (1982) demonstrated independent confirmation of any previous positive studies. They emphasize the increasing need to replicate and confirm previous positive studies, together with an evaluation of the many shortfalls implicated in the experimental designs.

Hughes *et al.* (1996) refer to the fact that present knowledge remains based more in theory and practical experience than rigorous scientific research. Spence and Olsen (1997) clearly state there is an incongruity between the research statement, conceptual framework and the findings. TT is not well differentiated from other related concepts nor is it clearly distinguished from other *intentional* or *energetic healing* modalities. The search for a more apt name and clearer concept is ongoing. It would seem that both qualitative and quantitative explorations are of equal importance, both of which are needed within the same study.

Further implications discussed by Spence and Olsen (1997) include using multiple therapists in a single study to minimize the therapist effect and more accurate assessment tools to measure the multiple levels of qualitative responses. TT practitioners other than the researcher should perform the intervention, while a non-TT practitioner should perform the mimic TT.

Quinn's pilot study looked for the psycho-neuroimmunological effects of TT in both the practitioner and recently bereaved recipients (Quinn and Strelkauskas, 1993). The magnitude of the changes and the consistency of the pattern of diminution in the T8 suppresser cells across both recipients and practitioners were unequivocal. There was a significant increase in positive affect (mood) and decrease in negative affect in both practitioners and recipients (68% in Affect Balance Index). From this investigation an entirely new area of study has emerged which could relate to an altered state of consciousness occurring in TT. This corresponds to the perceived time distortion (difference between actual and estimated time taken) and its direction, i.e. under- or overestimation, experienced by both practitioners and recipients.

Hughes *et al.* (1996) succinctly speak of 'those who conduct research in TT struggle with the problem of destroying the very thing they seek to study, through stringent controls and delimitations'. For example, significant benefits have been shown to result from more than one treatment, lack of time constraints, accountability of intent and building rapport. Equally it has become apparent that to prevent the assumed TT occurring in a control/placebo mimic situation is exhausting, stressful and difficult to maintain for the therapist (Vaughan, 1995).

To conclude, if successful TT requires the well-being of the therapist, any stress to the therapist could have a detrimental effect on the treatment outcome, including research programmes.

Compatibility with other therapies

Therapeutic Touch is an ideal therapy to integrate and enhance other modalities, whether this is bodywork, mind-based or energy-orientated therapy, traditional medication or surgery. As TT supports the body's own inherent healing system, it may be used as a therapy in its own right but within the context and as part of the total medical health care system.

Some therapists find that combining an Aura-Soma pomander enhances the effectiveness.

Physiotherapy application

Therapeutic Touch is almost exclusively based in the nursing profession. The vast majority of research arises directly from nurse practice and is mostly confined to nursing journals. The following explores thoughts and experiences the author has encountered within physiotherapy practice.

In order for the therapeutic intervention to be successful, TT need not involve verbal communication, cognitive understanding or specific patient responses. Thus it gives access to people with learning difficulties, those with profound physical disabilities, babies, children, animals, movement disorders – the possibilities are endless. Conversely, the same factors require greater ethical consideration when seeking informed consent.

The technique may be applied at the beginning of a therapy session to reduce anxiety and promote relaxation, thus enhancing the effectiveness of the other modalities. To ameliorate local symptoms, especially pain and inflammation, TT can be integrated with massage, soft tissue work, joint mobilization and reflextherapy. Probably for greatest effect, TT can be used as the concluding modality, especially when working on several locations of the body to bring about an overall amalgamation, integration and balance of both body awareness and the energy fields.

The use of TT within mental health has only recently been explored, probably because physical touch, let alone complementary therapy, has been so largely ignored. The study by Hughes *et al.* (1996) explores the sensitive issues around negative experiences of touch, feelings of safety, changing therapeutic relationships and communication with the therapist/nurse, the body/mind connection, behaviour changes, somatic and relaxation responses. This study encompasses some of the many beautiful and creative responses that the body/mind experiences during TT. Although subjective, these astute observations have a ring of truth, depth and relevance to both the therapist and patient.

Case histories

Case history: Jill

Jill had an extensive lower limb and hip amputation 20 years previously, was independently mobile with a full hip and leg prosthesis and had been receiving treatment for low back and hip pain, muscle imbalance, postural control and stamina. Previous treatments with positive outcomes included massage, soft tissue and joint mobilizations, applied kinesiology and Chakra energy balancing. On this occasion the therapist used TT to support the energy balancing to the entire body with special reference to phantom limb discomfort and hip pain. Surprisingly, both the therapist and Jill reported that the etheric field of the amputated limb could be felt by both of them in the empty space. After the energy field had balanced, Jill was quite overcome with joy at the new found sense of feeling her 'amputated leg' with normal proprioception, dimensions, etc, as she had remembered it 20 years ago, rather than the contorted, smaller phantom limb she had become accustomed to. However, once the prosthesis was in place, Jill found it extremely difficult to balance upright and walk, because her gait pattern had changed so dramatically owing to the altered limb perception.

Later at home, ecstasy changed to grief as she re-experienced fully the loss and denial of the feelings associated with her leg and overall self-image. Being the exceptional person she is, Jill competently worked through the feelings on her own (a contact phone number was available). After 3 days the kinaesthetic sense of the phantom limb had returned to its original state, but without the discomfort, hence Jill's gait and postural balance were functional again with reduced pain and discomfort. In hindsight, Jill appreciated and learnt much from the one experience of TT. Her regret was that she 'did not have TT early on in her rehabilitation'.

Case history: Colleague

While away on holiday, a colleague badly sprained her ankle and was unable to bear weight. TT was given as a first aid measure, resulting in decreased pain and oedema, enabling partial weight-bearing with a stick. Five days later, after she had returned home, the ankle was X-rayed and found to have a displaced tibial fracture with a well-forming callus. The fracture was reduced under anaesthetic and maintained in plaster of Paris, while TT was continued afterwards. The ankle regained full pain-free function. This illustrates how the delay in appropriate orthodox medicine can have a detrimental effect on patient care. However, this case also demonstrates the pain-relieving properties and accelerated rate of tissue repair properties of TT. A poetic example of the need for complementary therapy and orthodox medicine to work alongside each other!

Case history: Mary

Mary was admitted onto the mental health ward requiring close observation. She had seriously injured herself after jumping from the second floor, whilst in a psychotic state. This resulted in severe compression fractures at several sites in her ankle and foot, including the calcaneus. Although advised to be non-weight-bearing, Mary was non-compliant. Owing to her mental health section, Mary was not allowed to leave the ward and was on 'close observation'. The feeling of restriction from the plaster of Paris was reinforcing her overall mobility restraint. The pain was exacerbating her mental condition and overall anxiety. TT was used as the main treatment modality to reduce both her general level of anxiety and, locally, over the plaster of Paris to effectively reduce pain. This was repeated twice daily for approximately 20 minutes and then the time interval slowly extended. On the few occasions when the physiotherapist did not use TT, Mary reported no reduction in pain relief. Shoulder and neck massage was reported as helpful, but in Mary's opinion not as effective in her anxiety management as TT. When TT was not given for more than 4 days Mary's behaviour deteriorated, resulting in renewed aggressive incidents. Throughout her orthopaedic rehabilitation Mary failed to comply with, or attend, conventional physiotherapy sessions; however, she would return to the mental health physiotherapy department and ask for TT. After TT, Mary would happily comply with soft tissue mobilization and exercises.

Case history: Linda

Linda has many behavioural and mental health problems stemming from childhood abuse. Alongside her general mistrust of touch and of building relationships is an impassable phobia regarding anything touching her feet. Contact on the floor is impossible unless she is wearing trainers. From energy, mental and physical points of view, hands-on therapies would help her lower limbs, but this would be totally unacceptable to Linda. TT is acceptable because of the non-touch and unthreatening nature of the technique. During the first session, Linda felt warmth and tingling in her legs. This resulted in a greater acceptance and connection with her own body image and awareness. Interestingly, Linda reports feeling more 'grounded', her legs are perceived as heavy and more 'in touch' with the floor and there is more focus and clarity in her thinking. After several sessions her increased level of trust enables the therapist directly to massage her legs and she is now secure enough to be without trainers! During high levels of anxiety, irrationality and agitation, TT remains the therapy of choice to help bring her sufficiently into the here and now to enable her to work with both touch and cognitive therapies, empowering the management of her own therapeutic process.

Training

The British Association of Therapeutic Touch (BATT) was launched in 1994 to register and accredit TT practitioners: BATT, 33 Grange Thorpe Drive, Burnage, Manchester M19 2LR, UK.

Many advanced courses in specific complementary therapies work with energy fields using non-physical touch. These tend to be known by the associated therapy, e.g. Chakra balancing and reflextherapy rather than TT.

References

Biley, F. (1995) Providing a conceptual framework for practice. In *The Theory and Practice of Therapeutic Touch*. (Sayre-Adams, J., Wright, S., Biley, F. and Richardson, M., eds). London: Churchill Livingstone.

Biley, F. (1996) Rogerian science, phantoms and therapeutic touch: exploring potentials. *Nurs. Sci. Quart.*, **9**(4), 165–69.

Brennan, B. (1993) *Light Emerging*. New York: Bantam New Age Books.

Bronstein, M. (1996) Healing hands. *Canad. Nurse*, **92**(1), 32–36.

Cade, C.M. and Coxhead, N. (1979, reprint 1996) *The Awakened Mind; Biofeedback and the Development of Higher States of Consciousness*. Shaftesbury: Element Books.

Cox, C. and Hayes, J. (1998) Experiences of administering and receiving therapeutic touch in intensive care. *Comp. Thera. Nurs. Midwif.*, **4**, 128–33.

Daley, B. (1997) Therapeutic touch, nursing practice and contemporary cutaneous wound healing research. *J. Adv. Nurs.*, **25**(6), 1123–32.

Gerber, R. (1988) Psychic healing. In *Vibrational Medicine* (Gerber, R., ed.). Santa Fe, NM: Bear.

Hover-Kramer, D. (1990) Implications for the science of human caring. *Imprint*, **3**, 81–82.

Hughes, P.P., Meiz-Grochowski, R. and Duncan Harris, C.N. (1996) Therapeutic touch with adolescent psychiatric patients. *J. Holistic Nurs.*, **14**(1), 6–23.

Johnson Lutjens, L. R. (1991) *Martha Rogers, The Science of Unitary Human Beings*. London: Sage.

Keller, E. and Bzdek, V. (1986) Effects of therapeutic touch on tension headache. *Nurs. Res.*, **35**(2), 101–105.

Krieger, D., Peper. E. and Ancolis, S. (1979) Physiological indices of therapeutic touch. *Am. J. Nurs.*, **14**, 660–62.

Olson, M., Sneed, N., Bonnadonna, R., Ratcliff, J. and Dias, J. (1992) Therapeutic touch and post-Hurricane Hugo stress. *J. Holistic Nurs.*, **10**(2), 120–36.

Paes de Silva, M.J. (1996) Teaching therapeutic touch: a report of an experience. *Revista Latino – Americana de Enfermagem*, **4**, 91–100.

Peck, S.M. (1990) *The Road Less Travelled*. London: Arrow.

Peck, S. (1997) The effectiveness of therapeutic touch for decreasing pain in elders with degenerative arthritis. *J. Holistic Nurs.*, 15(2), 176–98.

Quinn, J. F. (1982) An investigation of the effects of TT done without physical contact on the state of anxiety of hospitalised cardiovascular patients. *Dissertation*, New York University.

Quinn, J.F., Strelkauskas, A.J. (1993) Psychoimmuniologic effects of therapeutic touch on practitioners and recently bereaved participants: a pilot study. *Adv. Nurs. Sci.*, 15(4), 13–26.

Rosa, L., Rosa, E., Sarner, L. and Barrett, S. (1998) A close look at therapeutic touch. *J. Am. Med. Assoc.*, 279(13), 1005–10.

Sayre-Adams, J., Wright, S., Biley, F. and Richardson, M. (eds) (1995) Ancient beginnings in religion. In *The Theory and Practice of Therapeutic Touch*. Edinburgh: Churchill Livingstone.

Spence, J. and Olsen, M. (1997) Quantative research on therapeutic touch. *Scand. J. Caring Sci.*, 11(3), 183–90.

Thorne, B. (1991) Carl Rogers in person-centred counselling. In *Therapeutic and Spiritual Dimensions* (Dryden, W., series ed.). London: Whurr.

Vaughan, S. (1995) The gentle touch. *J. Clin. Nurs.*, 4, 359–68.

White, J. and Krippner, S. (1977) Millner's methods of detecting and measuring healing energies. In *Future Science* (White, J. and Krippner, S., eds). Garden City, NY: Anchor Books.

Wirth, D.P., Barrett, M.J. and Eidelman, W.S. (1994) Non-contact therapeutic touch and wound reepithelialization: an extension of previous research. *Complement. Ther. Med.*, 2, 187–92.

Distant healing

John D. Chacksfield

Introduction

Distant or *absent* healing, also called *psi healing*, refers to the process by which a healer can affect the mind and body of the person receiving healing without needing to be present in the same location. This chapter will focus on this idea and the forms it can take. Distant healing is discussed in the light of the author's own experience and some of the scientific and anecdotal evidence available. Finally the value of the technique for the clinician is discussed and recommendations made as to techniques for implementation.

A difficult concept

The idea that healing can be effected from a distance without contact with the patient is difficult for many to grasp. It seems illogical and unbelievable to most of us who are acquainted with the core of Western science and contemporary thought. Some dismiss the idea completely and are unwilling to even test it. Some fall on superstition and see healing by touch, let alone distant healing, as an evil power at work. Both of these ideas are, in reality, unscientific. The true scientist retains an open mind to all phenomena and uses reason to test and examine cause and effect. It is in this spirit of true scientific enquiry that we recommend this chapter be read. As with many things which were once misunderstood and are now regarded as common fact, it is likely that new scientific theories will be developed to explain phenomena such as distant healing.

The phenomenon of distant healing

A long history

Before science can act, an idea must be formed. Before an idea is formed, an observation must be made. This chapter is written from the perspective that distant healing has been seen to work, despite the fact that it has not yet been fully explained. Observations of the results are far from recent. Like many medical discoveries, which existed long before they were found, distant healing has been accepted within human societies and civilizations since time immemorial. Many examples exist within Frazier's (1922) classic, *The Golden Bough*. From examples in ancient Greek and Egyptian records, to instances within Native American and African tribal lore or biblical anecdotes, Buddhist texts and ancient Hindu writings, there can be found the mention of the concept of healing by distance. Many of these cultures still practise their traditional healing techniques. Kelly (1995) explores some of these and suggests that much can be learned by occupational therapists through observation of how these healers operate.

In the West, 'traditional healing' has long been practised within the complementary therapies as well as within religious groups. Absent healing is included. For example, Christians have believed strongly in the 'power of prayer' to heal the sick for centuries. Pagan religions, such as Druidism and Wicca, carry out elaborate healing rituals to effect cures at a distance. Healers within Spiritualist and other religious groups carry out absent healing in a systematic and often structured form. It is in Spiritualism, in particular, where distant healing began to be made more systematized, particularly through the work of famous healers, such as Harry Edwards, and healing organizations such as the National Federation of Spiritual Healers. Others include the Healer Practitioner Association International (affiliated to the Institute of Complementary Medicine) and the White Eagle Lodge which focuses much of its work on distant healing. Edwards (1974) even goes so far as to say that

As Absent Healing and its implications become more fully appreciated and understood, so in future years this form of healing will assume ascendancy over other methods, and be a major factor for the prevention of disease.

In Edwards (1974), the chapter on 'Absent healing', although wordy, is probably one of the most comprehensive written on this subject from a healer's own experience. His main assertion is that healing involves the transmission of energy.

Although basic, these investigators and practitioners of distant healing have formed the basis for the much more scientific investigation of *psi healing* within the field of parapsychology.

Associated areas of enquiry

A number of concepts also relate to distant healing. 'Mind over matter', or the belief that the mind can influence the physical body or other material, is not new. The concept of 'psychosomatic illness' is also gaining ground in acceptability. Ideas such as telepathy are beginning to be explained by physicists. Furthermore, the importance of the magnetic field, which surrounds the human body and other living matter (bioenergetics), has become a developing area for scientific enquiry. Many therapists recognize the value of biofeedback, or the

systematic training, through electronic feedback, of one's own mind to relax, operate specific muscle groups and control impulsive behaviour. Some of this can take place through visualization of mental images that promote relaxation or represent their goal, e.g. imagining a muscle in a relaxed state. Visualization and guided imagery are techniques often used in the treatment of illnesses such as cancer (Burke and Sikora, 1992).

A further developing field of investigation is the science of consciousness. In 1994, a conference was held to explore the scientific possibility of 'non-local mind' (Freeman, 1994). This, probably the first of its kind, was held at London University's Institute of Psychiatry and involved some of the world's leading scientists, including Professor Sir Roger Penrose, Rouse Ball Professor of Mathematics at Oxford University and Dr Rupert Sheldrake, former Research Fellow of the Royal Society. All of these areas are beginning to widen the possibilities for us to further develop our understanding of the universe.

Distant healing in the modern world

Most practitioners of healing energy therapy, spiritual healing, Reiki or Therapeutic Touch, have, as part of their training, some input on methods of distant healing. Other people see healing in connection with their particular religion and integrate distant healing with prayer. What is clear is that healing is a universal concept. Scientists too are starting to investigate the ability of the human mind to influence living systems from a distance, including 'psi healing'. A number of people have begun to gather evidence of its effectiveness.

Daniel Benor, a doctor and healer, has collected 155 examples of the effectiveness of healing, including distant healing (Benor, 1993). Although Benor's review may need to be more rigorous (Solfvin, 1997), it presents an interesting collection of experiments. Distant healing experiments include some on seeds and bacteria as well as humans. Seeds and bacteria that received distant healing were found to grow much faster than those that did not. In human beings, Benor includes examples of distant healing, such as that of Miller (1982) who studied its effectiveness in lowering blood pressure.

Within the field of psycho-kinesis (PK), or the study of the influence of mind over matter, considerable evidence has been gathered which demonstrates the power of the mind to affect the human body. Studies involving attempts to influence living systems (direct mental influence on living systems, or DMILS) so far seem to produce stronger results than those involving non-living systems such as electronic equipment. They are also more directly relevant to one of the main practical questions of parapsychology: Is there a psychic component to alternative healing practices? Thus DMILS work will continue to be an important component to parapsychology research. Further information on DMILS research is available on the Internet via the University of Edinburgh's 'Koestler Parapsychology Unit' and the Dutch DMILS on-line experiment. These Internet sites are listed at the end of this chapter.

Eysenck and Sargent (1993), two acclaimed psychologists, reviewed some of this kind of research. They make particular reference to a large body of evidence gathered by American scientist William Braud and his co-workers. In one example, Braud carried out experiments to examine the effects of PK on changes in blood cells, where a person used PK to prevent the natural disintegration of blood cells. These experiments demonstrated significant results. Schmeidler (1990, cited in Eysenck and Sargent, 1993) reviewed six significant studies attesting to the ability of the mind to affect small organisms, such as Salmonella and *Escherichia coli* bacteria and yeast. Distant healing on rats infected with a blood disease (Snel and van der Sidje, 1991) was given by a healer who looked only at their photographs. The healer (who lived 20 miles away) was asked to strengthen the 'defences' of the rats. Compared to the control rats that were not given healing, the treated group demonstrated a significantly lower proportion of infected red blood cells.

Another developing scientific field is that of consciousness studies, which has included healing as part of a wider discussion on consciousness. For example, Lansky (1997), a computer scientist, discusses 'energy-based systems of medicine', such as in Chinese medicine, and the influence of consciousness on this energy system. She cites examples of distance healing within this discussion and presents a mathematical model to explain her ideas.

Prayer

The healing power of prayer has been observed in clinical trials by Dr Larry Dossey (Dossey, 1993), who carried out experiments on 400 heart patients. He found that 200 of these, randomly selected, were found to have fewer deaths and three times fewer complications than the group not prayed for. Another double-blind study of intercessionary prayer (IP) on coronary care patients (Byrd, 1988) investigated 393 patients which were randomly allocated to the IP group ($n = 192$) or a control group ($n = 201$), with no difference between the groups on pre-experimental measures. The IP group only, received IP by participating Christians praying daily for rapid recovery and prevention of complications and death. These 'intercessors' were all located outside the hospital and knew only the first name, diagnosis and general condition of each patient. Each patient was assigned to between three and seven intercessors. Data on each patient was collected systematically and included presence of a range of diagnostic symptoms and therapeutic events. On follow-up, the IP group had a significantly lower severity score ($p = 0.01$) and required less therapeutic intervention.

Although this experiment may have needed more explanation of bias due to extra-experimental factors, it still represents one of the most significant evidence of the effectiveness of healing by prayer.

Two recent studies provide further support for the efficacy of group prayer, offered for patients known only by their first name, in reducing the incidence of adverse outcomes following admission to coronary care units. The MANTRA Study Project, was an informed consent, 150-patient, five-arm pilot study at the Duke Clinical Research Institute on the therapeutic effects of different complementary therapies (CT). It found an overall reduction in the incidence of adverse outcomes in the CT group of 30 per cent compared to the standard therapy control group. The prayed for group showed a 50 per cent to 100 per cent reduction of adverse outcomes

(Horrigan, 1999). A major 1500 patient MANTRA trial is now in progress. In another trial at St Lukes Hospital, Kansas City, patients were secretly enrolled into either a prayed for group or a control group, with neither patients or medical staff being aware of the study, thus eliminating any placebo effect (Harris *et al.*, 1999). Hospitalization time was the same for both groups, but it was found that the 466 patients in the prayed for group had less adverse outcomes than the 524 patients in the control group.

An informed consent study (Sicher *et al.*, 1998) of 40 patients suffering from advanced AIDS found a significant reduction in the incidence and severity of AIDS related illnesses, hospitalizations, inpatient time and visits to doctors, in the randomly allocated prayed for group of 20 subjects compared to the 20 subject control group during the six month trial period. Changes in positive mood and outlook also reached statistical significance in the prayed for group. Taken together, these trials indicate that distant healing, offered in the form of group prayer in these instances, has a beneficial effect beyond chance outcome.

Spiritual healing and health care

Spiritual healing, generally, has also come to be accepted as a recognized treatment available on the British National Health Service. At first, it was recognized particularly in cancer treatment (Burke and Sikora, 1992), and has since spread more widely. It is advocated by many health professionals, who now also train as healers and use it as part of their work, notably nurses, physiotherapists and a growing number of doctors. One of the largest sub-organizations of the Confederation Healing Organisations (CHO) recently reported that 15% of its trainees were nurses and 25% were nurses or other health workers (Booth, 1994). An increasing number of these also carry out distant healing.

The mechanism of distant healing

Distant healing, specifically, is best investigated through one's own careful experimentation, following well-tried methods and ideally under the guidance of an experienced instructor. It is recommended that anyone setting out to do this should first read about it, then follow a specific plan and, ideally, record their results in a notebook. It would also be advantageous to learn more from one of the recognized healing organizations and to meet other absent healers. According to Edwards (1974), healing is a natural talent which many people have, and which only needs development and the opportunity for expression.

Systematic distant healing

Preparation

The most important precursor to performing distant healing is the state of mind. This requires a *relaxed mind* and *positive attitude*. Also important are the ability to focus the attention and to mentally visualize images. It is therefore essential that the healer is *not* operating under the influence of alcohol or other drugs, is not feeling anxious, and is of a stable mind at the time of the healing.

Relaxed mind and body

The healer must develop the ability to approach a distant healing session in a calm, relaxed (but not sleepy) manner. An effective way to relax is to use a technique such as reverse breathing, meditation or progressive muscular relaxation. 'Reverse breathing', for example, involves first observing the breath as it happens, then changing the pattern so that the outbreath is emphasized, allowing the inbreath to happen naturally as the diaphragm 'springs back into place'. A short period of this kind of breathing can usually bring fast and effective relaxation.

Positive attitude

The healer must also create the right attitude. This requires the thinking to be positive, happy and balanced. The easiest way to enter this state of mind is to read a poem, say a prayer, listen to music or look at a picture – any of which is likely to trigger these feelings. Another way is through *affirmation*. Affirmation involves repeating an appropriate phrase in one's mind or out loud, until the desired state is achieved. The following are examples of affirmations.

- I am peace, I radiate peace.
- I am happiness, I radiate happiness.
- I feel positive, I feel great!

Laughter is another great mood-lifter, and can be stimulated by thinking about a humorous story, happening or simply making oneself laugh – this can feel so ridiculous that you end up laughing anyway!

It is also useful to generate in oneself positive feelings towards the subject of the healing, and a wish to transmit one's own positive mood. Healing works best when entered into unconditionally, or without a feeling that one wishes to be acknowledged or rewarded for the effort of doing so. These kinds of feelings can block one's ability to focus on the 'healee'.

Once the healer is in the right frame of mind, or relaxed and positive, the healing can begin.

Other preparations

A number of other preparations are necessary. It will help the process if the healer sets up a peaceful atmosphere, perhaps by taking the telephone off the hook, lighting a candle and playing some peaceful, gentle music to cover any background noise and create the right mood. It is important for the healer to be alone, unless they are deliberately working with a group of healers who are all focused on the task of sending out healing together.

Next it is useful to have the details of the person or people who require healing written down in front of the healer, with a photograph, although this is not absolutely necessary. Many distant healers keep a record book with the date of entry, name, location, diagnosis and space for brief progress notes – if reported.

The distant healing technique

Distant healing involves mental imagery and the projection of healing energy to a sick person. This generally involves creating a mental picture of the patient, mentally requesting they be healed, and imagining healing energy flowing to them (using an image such as light from the sun or bright white light). Finally the patient is visualized as whole and free of illness. This procedure is then repeated at regular intervals for a greater or lesser period, depending on the severity of the illness. Different approaches to distant healing exist, which advocate specific images, techniques and ways to structure the healing session. Some of these, which are considered 'tried and tested', are presented below.

Different distant healing techniques

The Harry Edwards' technique

Harry Edwards was a great advocate of distant healing and collected several million letters testifying to its effectiveness, between 1948 and 1974 (Edwards, 1974). Edwards, through years of practice as a healer, came to believe distant healing to be 'an advanced spiritual science', more evolved than contact healing, and more than simply 'faith'. He describes it as a 'thought process' based on a planned act, having both intention and direction. This then allows for universal healing forces to flow through the healer to the patient. Edwards' method follows three stages:

1. *The seeking of attunement.* This involves the important preparation stages outlined above, so that the healer is in a positive frame of mind and receptive to the healing energies. His mind is free from distraction. If the healer believes in God, then this can aid their attunement (many say a prayer before beginning healing), although it is not absolutely necessary to do this.
2. *Making a 'mental contact' with the patient.* The healer thinks about the patient, trying to picture them and their predicament – if they do not know what the patient looks like, then they should simply try to create a representative picture. They then mentally request that they be healed, that the pain or problem be removed. This process should be purposeful and directed, not casual and complacent or under stressful concentration or in an emotional state.

3. *Ending the healing episode.* After the healer has made their mental request, they then allow this train of thought to stop before progressing on to the next patient or ending their session. Lengthy intercession will not add to the efficacy of the healing. Some healers end with a prayer. Again this is not absolutely necessary.

At the end of the session the healer should then let their mind relax, imagining they are strolling through a peaceful, sunlit wood or a garden, or similar beautiful scene. They should take their time and stop when ready.

Edwards emphasizes that healing is a gift to be developed, and practised, together with attempting to live a healthy, peaceful lifestyle. This will help the healing ability to grow.

A similar method is advocated in the *Training Manual for Probationer Healers*, produced by the Healer Practitioner Association International. They suggest that to stage 2 (above), the healer 'may wish to visualize a state of well-being in the people that the healing is being directed to'. This idea is also part of the White Eagle Lodge method of healing, which suggests visualizing the person who needs healing perfect within the light of the sun, or a six-pointed star (which is a symbol used by this organization as a focus for healing).

Distant healing and use of colour

Some approaches to distant healing involve a greater use of the ability to visualize the healing happening (e.g. during stage 2 of the Harry Edward's technique). As part of this, the healer might picture bright colours around the patient. Some healers say that specific colours can help particular illnesses or conditions to be healed more effectively, such as green for mental distress, or yellow for neurological problems. Distant healers at the White Eagle Lodge make use of colour, mentally directed by a group of healers under the guidance of an experienced leader. They also advocate the direction of healing colours to particular areas of the body, including Chakras, which are considered to be aspects of the human 'energy body' by many Eastern medical systems (see Chapter 4).

There is a growing body of research about the effect of colour on physical systems. A recent article in the *New Scientist* (1998), for example, presents remarkable evidence of changes in plant growth rate under different coloured light. Many advocates of distant healing using colour strongly support its effectiveness. However, there seems to be no clear research evidence in the area as yet.

Group healing

A common approach to healing is to operate in a group, it being felt that the patient can have a more powerful healing. Healing with a group can also help learning and help the healer to be motivated to maintain a regular distant healing session.

Contraindications

There are generally no contraindications for distant healing as a treatment. Most healers recommend training and the use of a structured system. Some distant healers who use colour in healing say that inappropriate use of particular colours can be harmful and therefore training is essential. Credible healing organizations also work under a specific Code of Conduct, which emphasizes things like not exploiting patients, always cooperating with doctors, not diagnosing illnesses and not using drugs or alcohol. Healers tend not to promise a cure, either. The general principle of most distant healing is that the healer is a channel for healing energy and that it is not for them to take credit for any cure. In this spirit of humility, genuine distant healers will not accept money for their work, quite apart from any difficulty proving that their efforts led to a cure.

Conclusion

Distant healing is clearly one aspect of a wide range of complementary therapies which are gaining increasing recognition within modern society. It is important to remember that distant healing, like most therapies, can be described as art as well as science. As with any art, there will be those more 'gifted' in its operation and the fact that it will improve with practice. Furthermore, certain practitioners will find themselves more suited to, and effective with, healing certain illnesses or conditions than others. This art side should not be given any less importance than the scientific study of the subject. With the scientific method, the collection of evidence and observations, which describe the phenomenon of distant healing, is equally important. Contemporary examples and a growing body of well-conducted research are beginning to expand and rewrite modern scientific assumptions. Personal experiences and observations are reforming individual assumptions and opinions about the effectiveness of phenomena like distant healing.

Finally, distant healing is something worth trying out. Many practitioners of other healing arts find they can combine these with distant healing easily and sometimes with an enhanced effect.

This chapter has described just some of the ideas surrounding distant, or absent, healing. Further reading is recommended, as well as seeking information through some of the main healing organizations.

Internet sites

- Colorado Health Net: Section on Prayer and Mental Healing:
  http://www.coloradohealthnet.org/holistic/mind/mind_3j.htm
- The Koestler Parapsychology Unit:
  http://moebius.psy.ed.ac.uk/index.html
- The Dutch DMILS experiment:
  http://www.psy.uva.nl/resedu/pn/EXPMNTS/DMILS/dmils.html
- National Federation of Spiritual Healers Distant Healing Page:
  http://www.nfsh.org.uk/NFSH/distant healing.stm

References

Benor, D.J. (1993) *Healing Research*, Vol. I: *Research in Healing*. Oxford: Helix.

Booth, R. (1994) Keeping in touch. *Nurs. Times*, 90(44), 29–31.

Burke, C. and Sikora, K. (1992) Cancer – the dual approach. *Nurs. Times*, 88(38), 62–66.

Byrd, R.C. (1988) Positive therapeutic effects of intercessory prayer in a coronary care unit population. *South. Med. J.*, 81(7), 826–29.

Dossey, L. (1993) *Healing Words: The Power of Prayer and the Practice of Medicine*. New York: HarperCollins.

Edwards, H. (1974) *A Guide to the Understanding and Practice of Spiritual Healing*. Shere, UK: Healer Publishing.

Eysenck, H.J. and Sargent, C. (1993) *Explaining the Unexplained: Mysteries of the Paranormal*. London: BCA.

Frazier, J.G. (1922) *The Golden Bough: A Study in Magic and Religion*. London: Macmillan.

Freeman, A. (1994) Conference report: The science of consciousness: non-locality of mind. *J. Consciousness Studies*, 1(2), 283–84.

Harris, W.S., Gowda, M., Kolb, J.W., Strychacz Vacek, J.L., Jones, P.G., Forker, A., O'Keefe, J.H. and McCallister, B.D. (1999) A randomized controlled trial of the effects of remote, intercessory prayer on outcomes in patients admitted to the coronary care unit. *Arch. of Int. Med.*, 159(19), 2273–78.

Horrigan, B. (1999) The MANTRA Study Project. An interview with Michael W. Krucoff MD. *Alt. Ther.*, 5(3), 75–82.

Kelly, L. (1995) What occupational therapists can learn from traditional healers. *Br. J. Occupational Ther.*, 58(3), 111–14.

Lansky, A.L. (1997) Consciousness as an active force. Paper presented at the 'Towards a Science of Consciousness' Conference, 1996. Available on-line: *http://www.renresearch.com/consciousness.html*.

Miller, R.N. (1982) Study of remote mental healing. *Med. Hypotheses*, 8, 481–90.

New Scientist (1998) Rainbow growing. 24 October.

Sicher, F., Targ, E., Moore, D. and Smith, H.S. (1998) A randomized double-blind study of the effect of distant healing in a population with advanced AIDS. *Western J. Med.*, 169(6), 356–63.

Snel, F.W.J.J. and van der Sijde, P.C. (1991) The effect of retro-active distance healing on *Babesia rodhani* (rodent malaria) in rats. *Eur. J. Parapsychol.*, 7, 123.

Solfvin, J. (1997) Book review: *Healing Research: Holistic Energy Medicine and Spirituality*, Vol. 2, by Daniel Benor. *Eur. J. Parapsychol.*, 13, 130.

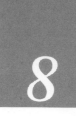

Healing touch therapies for animals

Lorraine Cookson

Introduction

Physiotherapy for animals was first recognized back in 1939. At that time, Sir Charles Strong, a leading physiotherapist, was employed by Lord Mountbatten to treat his polo ponies, after having received veterinary permission to do so. Soon afterwards Sir Charles decided to form a recognized group of practitioners, and over the next 20 years the practitioners struggled on, while trying to follow the rules of professional conduct of the Society of Chartered Physiotherapists (CSP). It was later during the 1980s that Mary Bromiley, a prominent figure at that time, gathered support and discussions were held between the physiotherapists, the CSP and the Royal College of Veterinary Surgeons. Government legislation affecting veterinary practice, insurance and physiotherapy modalities applicable to the treatment of animals were considered. As a result the Association of Chartered Physiotherapists in Animal Therapy (ACPAT) was established on 9 March 1985, and it was agreed that all members were to abide by the Veterinary Surgeons Act 1966 which states:

> The Veterinary Surgeons Act 1966 provides that with certain specific exception only veterinary surgeons may carry out acts of veterinary surgery on animals. Veterinary surgery is so defined by the act as to include the making of a diagnosis and the carrying out of tests for diagnostic purposes. Of the

exceptions created by the Veterinary Surgery (Exemptions) Order 1962, one permits the treatment of an animal by physiotherapy, provided the veterinarian who has examined the animal has prescribed treatment of an animal by physiotherapy.

It is absolutely essential that all members operate within the guidelines set by both professional bodies. Standards of knowledge, communication, assessment and documentation together with those of safety have been produced for members.

Personal note

Having worked for the Health Service since 1980, mainly in orthopaedics and orthopaedic outpatients, and having attended many lectures as a category B member of ACPAT, the author was eventually given the opportunity to work alongside local equine practitioners, veterinary surgeons and horse trainers. Since then she has been able to subscribe as a category A member and has steadily adapted her physiotherapy skills to the physical and emotional problems encountered by animals. It is since working with animals, however, that her attitude to medical practice has changed. Over the last two years the author has considered many different approaches, as it has become obvious that animal owners are becoming increasingly aware of complementary therapy. As a conventionally trained analyst and practitioner, any therapy that has not been proven, and lies outside orthodox practice, has always seemed a little far-fetched. However, she, like many others, is now beginning to realize the value of complementary therapies.

Background

Many therapies that have evolved from ancient Asian healing traditions help the body to respond in a way that helps it to heal. These therapies have proved themselves to be effective over many years and have been beneficial in the treatment of animals. Various treatments have been described in early veterinary texts; however, many feel that with modern approaches such as nuclear medicine, laser surgery and a broad spectrum of antibiotics for use in animal care, we have surely progressed. On the other hand, some are of the opinion that by following the philosophies of these therapies, that is, of manipulating the body and balancing the energy within, these therapies can still help alongside modern medicine, and it might be that where conventional methods fail, some ailments may in fact respond well to alternatives such as acupuncture, herbology, massage, chiropractic, aromatherapy and homoeopathy.

In the past when asked to treat an animal, particularly the horse, mobilization, stretching, massage, stimulation by low-level lasers, other electrical and magnetic sources, ultrasound, rehabilitative exercises, hydrotherapy and the application of heat and cold have been the techniques of choice. Despite being trained to look at the body of the animal as a whole, focus is often aimed at a specific joint or series of joints, given the limited time. It is, however, very necessary not to overlook the psychology of the animal, and that of the owner as well, if one is to be successful in one's approach. Books written by experienced animal trainers and those who follow the philosophy of natural horsemanship give valuable insight into the behaviour of horses and their handlers. The work of Linda Tellington-Jones, a Canadian horsewoman, has captured the minds of many.

TTeamwork or TTeam – the acronym for Tellington-Jones Equine Awareness Method –

is seen as a successful method of training and healing horses, based on classical horsemanship and the work of Dr Moshe Feldenkrais, an Israeli physicist, who believed that by the use of non-habitual movements, one could reprogramme the nervous system thereby relieving pain and discomfort and allowing the body to become more aware of its actions and sensations, and that this increased awareness would lead to improvements in flexibility, balance, coordination and posturing.

Endorsed by equine experts and vets worldwide, it is not difficult to see how TTeamwork can be adapted in the treatment and rehabilitation of neuromuscular conditions in animals. Those who have practised the work have realized its potential as a holistic approach to training, healing and communicating with animals, with much of the work resembling that which others would consider to be along the lines of acupressure, Shiatsu and Reiki. The first step is to go over the animal's entire body in a mindful way to determine whether and where there is tension or pain. If this is detected, a system of touches is then used to relieve any tension and anxiety, to increase circulation and influence the patterns of nerve impulses that are transmitted to the brain. It is believed that by opening up new neural pathways to the brain, the sensation of pain can be overridden, and at the same time the animal's awareness of itself is influenced.

The TTouches are simply a series of circles and strokes performed at different pressures and speeds according to what is required. Surprisingly the TTouches are very light in nature, but appear to work well where ordinary massage might fail. Often a single session can have a long-lasting effect and, particularly in horses, posture and performance is seen to improve. Not only does the animal become more focused, if the TTouches are practised with therapeutic intent, while remaining open-minded, the practitioner becomes relaxed around the animal, becomes more aware of what they feel and often enters an almost meditative state. Breathing deeply in time with the movement of the circles enables the TTouch to be given almost effortlessly. It is while in this state that one seems very able to pay attention to what it is one is feeling and how the animal is responding.

The techniques are 'less invasive' than massage and mobilization. There are those who would see this only as the 'laying on of hands', yet Tellington-Jones theorizes that 'one is making a cell to cell connection and a oneness with the animal', and that by doing this one is able to alter the individual cell's memory of pain. This is true in clinical practice, although science has yet to prove how this works. As a result of the TTouch, pain is relieved and excess muscle tone and spasm is reduced, often leading to an effortless increase in the range of pain-free movement. If one combines the TTouch bodywork with the series of 'ground exercises' devised by Tellington-Jones, one is able to further encourage normal movement within the affected parts, which further improves balance, coordination and posturing. This has the effect of teaching the animal obedience, self-control and patience. Examples of the ground exercises referred to are (a) working the horse, in hand, within a set configuration of wooden poles on the ground, and (b) leading the horse between obstacles such as, barrels, plastic sheets and ropes, once the horse is responding to subtle signals or spoken commands.

The 'power of touch' has probably been underestimated by many. It has been suggested that the skin is the largest producer of hormones and immune cells in the body, so when stimulated by touch there will be increased levels of vitalizing hormones and immune cells available to sustain health. The local increase in circulation is well recognized and also the action of the receptors in the skin conveying messages to the brain to stimulate the release of the body's own endorphins. The way in which we touch, and what we feel during touching, can tell us a lot about an individual. Animals are very aware, and when touched they know when we are tense or calm; and where words would fail in the training of animals, touch can be used instead to demonstrate what is required. It is recognized that where there has been touch deprivation in the early stages of life there have been inhibitions in the emotional and physical growth of a child, and equally in the animal world this need for physical contact continues through adulthood. Apart from the mechanical and physiological effects on specific tissues and their associated organs, which serve to unlock physical tensions in the body, touch has the ability to comfort, share empathy and help relax and unwind the mind, so touch works on a psychological as well as a physical level.

A loving touch can soothe away mental stress and help settle the emotions. As with humans, animals suffer from stress, which is detrimental to health and can lower the body's natural defences and limit its ability to fight disease. By using a system of touches it is possible to reach the mind/body complex. Many emotions and memories can, in fact, be released as the body relaxes, so demonstrating the psychosomatic link. In dealing with animals and their handlers there is often a noticeable change in the behaviour and attitude of both when this happens. In many cases the muscular tensions may be the result of repressed emotions and not of injury. Where the problem lies with poor self-image and self-esteem, there are often problems of habitual bad posturing leading to chronic tension in the body. However, by stimulating the nervous system and specific centres in the brain, by applying TTouch techniques to various parts of the body, it is believed that these problems can be alleviated. This is as true for human beings as it is for animals.

Through a desire to understand how TTeam and TTouch can often have such amazing results on the animals, and their owners, some physiotherapists have developed an interest in other forms of bodywork for animals. Based on the philosophies of Traditional Chinese Medicine (TCM), the ancient healing art of Reiki, which is considered by many as a means of relieving stress, would seem to complement TTeam and TTouch therapy. A large volume of scientific literature on Therapeutic Touch (see Chapter 6), which is thought to be similar to Reiki, can be found in most medical libraries. Reiki can be seen as a bioenergetic system for relief of stress and is very easy to use. The word 'Reiki' means 'vital life force energy', i.e. the energy that connects us and every other living thing. In the context of TCM, Reiki seems a way to synchronize and energize vital meridians and acupuncture points in the body, thereby assisting the body in its own level of healing and wellness. This healing energy is greatly beneficial to all life forms. In practice it can be seen as a consistent way of relieving stress and associated tension and hypertension. Working on the mind/body complex it can be used to help control anxiety and anticipation often associated with illness and disease. As with other forms of bodywork it has a calming effect on the body, and since adapting the Reiki technique used for humans as a therapy for animals, the author has found it of considerable benefit, especially in the treatment of horses.

Horses are 'fight/flight' animals and soon become anxious, stressed and confused. When reacting reflexly their cardiorespiratory rate is easily increased. By using a combination of hand positions on major parts of the body, it is believed that one can channel the vital energy to balance the emotional issues easing the worry and fears, so promoting calmness, and as a result muscular tension in the body is reduced. Breathing slows and deepens and heart rate is reduced as relaxation ensues. As with TTouch, the use of the hand contact alone will stimulate proprioceptive transmission, which will bring an awareness to the area being addressed at that time, and consequently this will increase overall body awareness and help in the grounding of the animal. Experience shows that the horse appears to resort less readily to the instinctive behaviour of 'fight and flight' once this has been triggered.

Practitioners often report on the sensations that they feel while performing Reiki and other forms of bodywork. These can vary from tingling in their fingers, to heat, icy cold or pulsing, and their skill is in their ability to pay attention to and focus in a relaxed state on what it is they actually feel 'at that moment', and then how to respond to it and use it as a healing therapy. As a recipient one can experience strange sensations, ranging from a pulsing in other parts of the body to those being touched, and even a movement of the table on which one is laying. As to what it is the animal feels it certainly seems to promote a sense of well-being as the animal becomes more relaxed throughout its body, and animals do seem to let you know when they have had enough. Those who practice TTouch report similar experiences.

There are times when veterinary and physiotherapy diagnoses have failed to explain the reason for the 'not quite sound' movement of the horse, for its stumbling, biting, resistance to working and bucking, for example, and that these problems are now being considered by many as being the result of mental pain and stress caused by the environment. After treatment with Reiki and TTouch some of these problems can be alleviated and a new level of trust seems to develop between horse and handler. Such hands-on therapy can also help in identifying problem areas. Following intuition and being non-judgemental, it is often surprising how the practitioner can be drawn to certain areas and how often the horse presents the appropriate area for touch. It would seem that the horse can sense the person and the intention clearly, whether one senses what is really happening or not, or whether one believes in the rebalancing of energies, or the existence of 'cellular memory'. In her book *The Tellington TTouch*, Tellington-Jones comments on how, in the past, a person having less than an hour's TTouch instruction achieved satisfying results, and that one doesn't have to be a specialist to be successful. By keeping an open mind and developing an awareness of self and feeling, the therapist can make a difference. Having experienced this state of heightened awareness, and allowing intuitive thought and action to develop, many can appreciate the value of this work in evaluating and treating the symptoms and source of ill-health.

Case histories

Case history 1

Ted is a big, strong-willed horse. He is 10 years old and stands at 17.1 hh. Prior to sustaining a broken neck Ted was a grade 'B' show jumper. He broke his neck while scrambling to his feet, after having caught his front legs in his turnout rug. The vet had advised euthanasia, but as there was no neurological damage the owners wanted to give him a second chance. Subsequently he was given a long period of box rest and expensive medication. Five years later, he has continued to make steady progress, though has not been easy to handle. The author was asked to examine Ted after he had started bucking so violently that he would almost fall over. At the same time it was becoming increasingly difficult to groom him without him biting or kicking out. On examination, Ted displayed extreme high-headedness and a gross imbalance of the neck muscles. He appeared to be overdeveloped on the right and contracted to the left. He had a corresponding hollow in his back, had several old jumping wounds, and there was X-ray evidence of arthritic changes in the joints of the forelimbs. His tail was clamped extremely tightly. On palpation, his skin was tight and the tissues stiff and he resented even the lightest pressure on his back and through his shoulders. As Ted violently reacted, a full objective examination was impossible. Here was an animal in fight/flight mode, acting on instinct and in great need of help. Once he was contained in the stable, it was possible to approach the problems using random TTouch circles and strokes all over his body, gradually working towards the problem areas. The author was conscious of being mindful and breathing into each circle and followed her intuition as to where she touched next. Within minutes Ted was becoming more focused and less reactive to the pressure of the hands, his eye had noticeably softened and he had begun to take a deeper breath. It would seem that as he became aware of different parts of his body that he was developing more self-control. After only 10 minutes of TTouch, Ted began to lower his head. It was surprising how quickly the author was able to touch his ears and the top of his neck. It was as though Ted was actually asking to be touched here. His apparent discomfort or his expectation of discomfort in these areas had been changed. By the use of a flat hand exploration down his neck the author was able to ascertain the degree of tension in the tissues. She was then able to ask Ted to stretch around after a carrot, which he did despite the obvious physical limitation of the contractures in his muscles to the left. His owner was pleased to see an increase in his range of movement and the apparent ease in which it was performed. The owner was given a few simple active exercises for the horse, which were to be done until the next visit. Although the author felt that considerable progress had been made, she was totally unprepared for the message that awaited on the fax at home. Apparently, 20 minutes after leaving, Ted had been led like a lamb from his stable to the field, and for the first time in five years had been seen to get down and roll completely over on both sides. His owner was ecstatic. Ted has since had two more sessions of TTouch and TTeamwork and each time there has been a noticeable change in his behaviour and physical ability. His balance and coordination have dramatically improved as he has developed a greater sense of body awareness and has become less reactive.

> **Case history 2**
>
> Sam is a 16-year-old gelding. He suffers from arthritis of the stifle joints of the hindlimbs, and despite having been given injection therapy his pain and stiffness were still apparent when first examined. He was intermittently lame behind and had difficulty in engaging his hindquarters when asked to move on a circle. He resented even gentle passive mobilization. The stifle area on a horse is often a very sensitive area and Sam was very quick to react. Touching him in the conventional way was unacceptable, and it was only after a few sessions of TTeamwork, using both the TTouches and ground exercises, that improvement started to occur. The range of flexion in the stifle, and consequently the hocks, increased though he never looked totally relaxed in his work. He would hold tension in his mouth, begin to hold his breath, and sweat easily. Having established the degree of tension in Sam's back muscles after a period of work, the author practised the hand positions of Reiki healing. After only a few minutes of holding her hands with healing intent across his lower back, and focusing on him with soft eyes, she began to feel just how icy cold he was in that area. A few centimetres towards his head the temperature felt normal. Although it is difficult to accept the concept of channelling energy by such simple means, nevertheless it did seem to have a far-reaching effect on Sam. When horses relax they often begin to lick and chew, breathe more deeply and also sigh and yawn. These are responses of the parasympathetic nervous system, which counteracts the responses of the sympathetic nervous system in preparing an animal for flight or fight. This had been triggered in Sam. Once he was in this relaxed state he seemed to cope with the work asked of him. Further sessions of TTouch prior to and immediately after work have helped him since.

Discussion

It is recognized that any medicine must follow a plan of treatment. In conventional medicine a prescribed route is followed based on scientific study and diagnosis. In complementary medicine the route is not so strictly prescribed and is based more on intuitive clinical observation. Generally it would seem to defy scientific reasoning, yet provided that the practitioners of complementary medicine have specialized knowledge and skills there seems no reason why it cannot be used for animal disease and injury. It is seen to complement that which has been started by the veterinarian and indeed there are many vets, both in the UK and abroad, who have seen its value and have included it in their practice. Modern veterinary medicine may be successful at easing symptoms, but it doesn't always encourage healing.

Physiotherapists recognize that when cells function they create and use energy. When cells are damaged they display abnormal activity, yet this can be corrected by stimulating the healing process by applying various frequencies of energy to the injured parts, e.g. in the form of laser, electromagnetic fields and ultrasound. Seen in this way many believe that physiotherapy may represent the link between modern medicine and the ancient healing therapies. This man-made energy, however, is not suited to all injuries, so in our desire to improve circulation, lymphatic drainage and function, we begin to provide other energy stimuli such as massage and manipulation. In its simplest form, when a part is touched, circulation is increased, bringing healing substances to the area, and at the same time the skin signals to the brain, so stimulating endorphin release.

Yet, in conclusion, it is often the most sensitive hands offering the lightest of touch which seem to address not only the physical problems, but those problems of attitude and emotional pain and stress. Relief of these symptoms encourages relaxation, and allows the body to let go of its habitual holding patterns and limitations. These therapies would appear to energize the body and the mind to heal itself.

Recommended reading

ACP (1994) *Association of Chartered Physiotherapists in Animal Therapy Handbook*. London: ACP.

Kasselle, M. and Hannay, P. (1995) *Touching Horses*. London: J.A. Allen.

Physiotherapy Frontline (1997) Animal therapy: how it all began. *Physio. Frontline*, 3(7).

Snader, M.L., Willoughby, S.L., Khalsa, D.K., Denega, C. and Basko, I.J. (1993) *Healing Your Horse*. New York: Howell Book House.

Tellington-Jones, L. and Bruns, U. (1988) *The Tellington-Jones Equine Awareness Method*. New York: Breakthrough Publications.

Tellington-Jones, L. and Taylor, S. (1992) *The Tellington TTouch*. New York: Viking Penguin/Cloudcraft Books.

Wyche, S. (1996) *The Horse Owner's Guide to Holistic Medicine*. Marlborough: The Crowood Press.

Bodywork therapies

9 Acupuncture and related therapies

Lynn Pearce

Introduction

Acupuncture, and the related therapies of electroacupuncture, acupressure and moxibustion, are complementary therapy techniques which can and have been readily integrated into physiotherapy practice (Alltree, 1993).

Acupuncture

As a technique, acupuncture simply involves the insertion of a needle into/through the skin (Latin *acus*, a needle; *punctura*, a prick/perforation). As a part of Traditional Chinese Medicine (TCM) it has its origins in ancient China (Kaptchuk, 1983; Ropp, 1990). Historically, 9 types of needle were depicted (see Figure 9.1). While the material of today's modern needle is generally different (stainless steel, copper, zinc, gold and silver), there remains a high degree of correlation in terms of shape and usage with the needles of old (Figures 9.2 and 9.3).

The demand for sterile needles, and the emergence of the pre-sterilized disposable needle, has altered the technical method of practice for many acupuncturists. However, TCM principles still underpin many of the approaches found in diagnosis and treatment. Acupuncture needles can be inserted through the skin, into:

- TCM acupuncture points (anatomically located points throughout the body, which lie along specific lines of energy, called meridians or channels)

- trigger points (areas of reflex hyperactivity within muscles)
- points based on 'same segment' neuro-anatomical innervation
- local points of pain (called 'ah shi' points).

Electroacupuncture

This can be defined in two ways:

- direct application of an electric current to acupuncture needles whilst *in situ*
- stimulation of the skin related to an acupuncture point (this would include TNS, H-wave, electroacupuncture pens).

Acupressure

This involves direct pressure, usually with thumb, finger or elbow, on the skin, over an acupuncture point. The obvious extension of this as a technique is Shiatsu (see Chapter 15).

Moxibustion

Moxibustion involves the burning of 'moxa' which is a substance derived from the *Artemesia vulgaris* plant (also known as mugwort or Chinese wormwood). The leaves are dried and can be used in a number of ways to provide a deep heating effect:

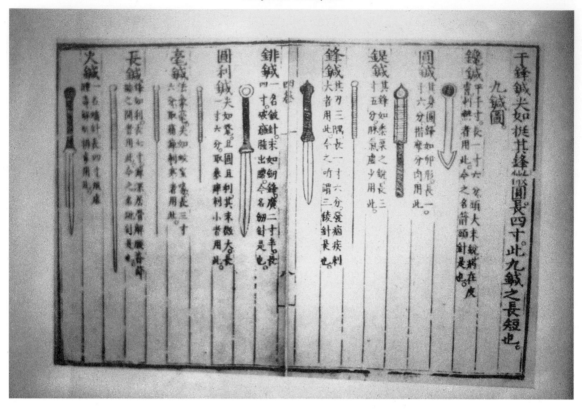

Figure 9.1 Traditional needles used in acupuncture © Lynn Pearce 2000

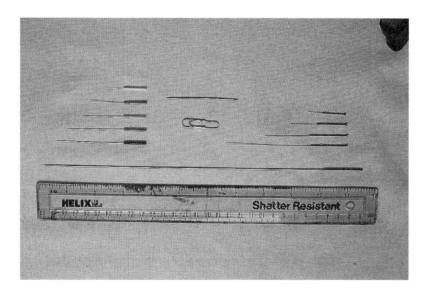

Figure 9.2 Modern acupuncture needles © Lynn Pearce 2000

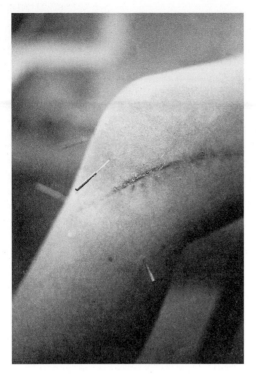

Figure 9.3 Modern acupuncture needles in position around a knee © Lynn Pearce 2000

- as a 'punk' – moxa punk is loose moxa, can be shaped by the practitioner into cones or small balls for use directly on the skin, on acupuncture needles or within a moxa frame
- as a stick/roll, resembling a large cigar (Figure 9.4) – can be held over acupuncture points or congested areas within surface tissue.

Background

Although the Western practice of acupuncture may differ widely from the TCM approach, the indisputable fact remains that it is towards the China of 5000 years ago that we must look for the origins of acupuncture and moxibustion. Needles of stone and bone have been found in China dating from 3000 BC (Ropp, 1990). Throughout the past 5000 years there has been an ebb and flow of acceptance of acupuncture, both in China itself and across the continents to Europe and America up to the present day.

One influence in the introduction of acupuncture and its related techniques to Europe stems from the Dutch East India Company of the seventeenth century. This company employed physicians who, on their travels, were exposed to Japanese practitioners of acupuncture. One notable doctor, Willem ten Rhijne, interpreted the acupuncture charts he was shown, as representations of vascular and neuroanatomical

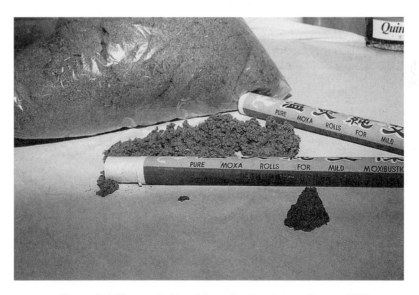

Figure 9.4 Moxa rolls for mild moxibustion © Lynn Pearce 2000

structures known to him at that time. In reality, the charts showed the meridian or channel pathways – a network of invisible vessels central to TCM practice, through which flowed 'Qi' (pronounced 'chee'), or the energy of life. It was from these roots that physicians in the West began to question and develop the type of acupuncture more commonly found today within Western medicine.

A boost to present-day interest in acupuncture practice came from President Nixon's visit to China in 1970, made possible after the Cultural Revolution in China of the late 1960s. Here, he and his team witnessed surgery under acupuncture analgesia. Subsequently, interest and scientific research has grown rapidly across Europe and America. Acupuncture, in becoming part of the 'integrated medical scene' of the late twentieth and early twenty-first centuries, lends itself well to the present sociological climate of active investigation into complementary therapies.

How acupuncture works

Two modes of action can be considered for acupuncture, as described below.

The Western scientific model

There are known physiological processes explaining the mechanism of acupuncture when used to treat pain (Stux and Pomeranz, 1997; White, 1998). Neurochemical pathways are recruited, blocked, and the release of endogenous opiates has an effect on pain transmission and inhibition. Other systems within the body can also be affected, such as the cardiovascular system. Reflex normalization is another potential explanation for specific techniques, like trigger point acupuncture (Baldry, 1993).

The Traditional Chinese Medicine model

Acupuncture, and the related techniques of moxibustion and acupressure, are components of a much larger system of medicine, just as manual therapy and drug therapy are parts of

the wider system of Western medicine. In TCM terms, ill-health is seen as the result of a poor circulation of energy (Qi) throughout the body. Normally, Qi is carried within a defined yet invisible network of meridians or channels, collectively termed the Jing Luo. There are twelve main meridians named after the major body organs with which they have a connection. The meridial system is visualized as a network of vessels (Luo translates to 'net') and there are Extra meridians, and further combinations of points, creating layers of channels throughout the body (Figure 9.5(a–c)). Along these meridians are positioned acupuncture points. These are precisely located areas where the Qi can be influenced, be it with an acupuncture needle, acupressure, electrotherapy, etc.

Another of the key principles upon which TCM is based is that of Yin and Yang. The Ancient Chinese philosophy of Taoism attempted in the fourth and fifth centuries BC to explain, through observation, the existence of mankind within the world. The way of life of man is a reflection of the way of life of the universe, the macrocosm should be represented in the microcosm and vice versa, with harmony between the two – a state of flux but balance. Not so much a religion, but more a way of guidance as to how man should live in harmony with the world/universe/heaven, one of the basic principles of Taoist thought relates to Yin and Yang. Everything in life can be broken down into two 'opposites', yet at the same time, these opposites cannot exist without the other. A positive electrical charge is meaningless without its opposite of a negative charge. A superior structure in anatomy is only superior because there is an inferior structure to which it relates (*Essentials of Chinese Acupuncture*, 1980; Maciocia, 1989).

The original Chinese characters for Yin and Yang show the path of the sun over a hill or mountain, and the TCM explanation of Yin encompasses all that relates to the 'shady side of the hill' (e.g. darkness, night, passivity, potential). Yang qualities were explained in terms relating to the 'sunny side of the hill' (e.g. light, day, activity, movement).

It is possible to make an extensive list of opposites relating to anything in life, but to maintain a focus on physical therapy and the

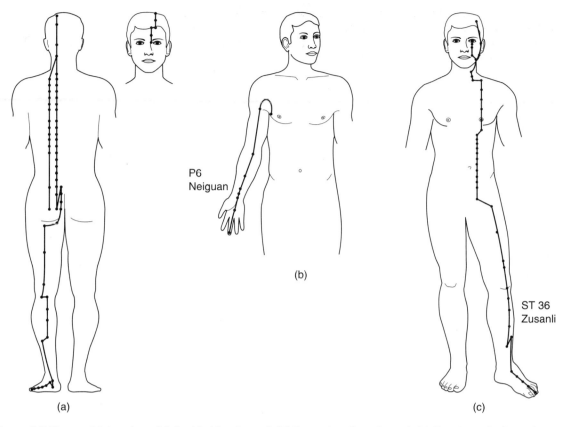

Figure 9.5 The meridial system: (a) the bladder channel; (b) the pericardium channel; (c) the stomach channel

treatment of the human body the list in Table 9.1 may prove more useful. This is by no means exhaustive, but gives an idea as to how the body may be viewed.

Table 9.1 Some Yin and Yang opposites

Yin	Yang
Front – ventral	Back – dorsal
Inferior	Superior
Caudal	Cephalic
Cold	Hot
Internal	External
Medial	Lateral
Dull, deep pain	Sharp, surface pain
Passive	Active
Chronic	Acute

TCM diagnostic methods

Traditional Chinese Medicine diagnostic methods are based on observation and the linking together of a collection of signs and symptoms (see Chapter 2). Work, home life, environment, relationships, emotional tension and the behaviour of the condition for which a patient is seeking treatment, all form part of a Chinese diagnosis. In addition to direct questioning, the TCM diagnosis places emphasis on observation of the patient themselves, and of their tongue, which reflects the state of the inner organs. The tongue body and shape reflect the state of some of the inner organs, the Blood and the Qi; the coating on the tongue reflects the state of the body's fluids and Qi. The position and type of change indicate the nature and area of disharmony within the body.

Palpation of the Chinese pulses. Three distinct areas over both radial arteries at the wrist give an impression of the strength of the 12 major organs of the body, and how they relate to one another in terms of function. This is a highly skilled yet subjective technique.

Eight principles

The observations a practitioner collates from his or her patient can be grouped into one of 4 groups, defining the condition for which the patient was seeking treatment. Within each of these groups are 2 'opposites': 4 groups containing 2 subjects each = 8 principles. The 4 groups are:

Yin/Yang   Full/Empty
Hot/Cold   Internal/External

An 8-principle diagnosis will indicate the nature of a condition (e.g. an ankle sprain would be Hot, Full, Yang and External).

Five elements

The Chinese developed an elaborate way of linking the 5 earthly elements of Wood, Fire, Earth, Metal and Water, as they believed the health of an individual was inextricably linked with the cycle of the elements, seasons and way of life of the natural world. The 5-element theory comes into its own diagnostically when the Correspondences are added. The Correspondences relate to a number of other influences which can be charted onto a 5-element diagram. These Correspondences are all factors which have a connection with each other, be it clinically, environmentally or emotionally.

The 5-element cycle can consequently help fit these elements into the overall clinical picture. This can be represented more easily in diagrammatic form (Figure 9.6):

Wood gives rise to fire, from which ash gives rise to earth, from whose depths is mined metal, whose polished surface may attract dew (water) which causes wood to grow and thus to complete the cycle. (Tsou-yen, *c.* 350–270 BC)

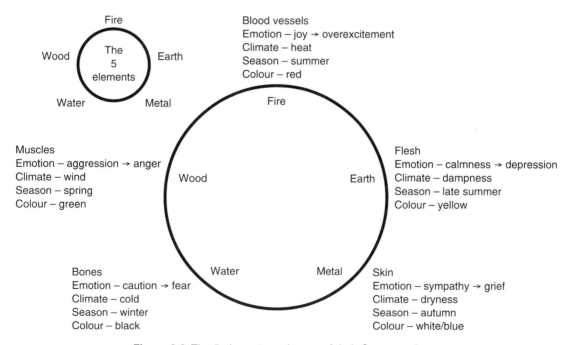

Figure 9.6 The 5 elements and some of their Correspondences

A TCM diagnosis encompasses many aspects of a patient's condition. The language used to describe this results in the statement of a pattern of disharmony.

Acupuncture points and meridians – do they exist?

Some practitioners state that acupuncture points do not exist at all (Mann, 1998) and hold steadfastly to a system of practice based on Western observation. It has been shown that acupuncture points are often related to small nerve bundles (Stux and Pomeranz, 1997), and some studies have highlighted the sympathetic nervous system, with points having a lower electrical impedance than surrounding tissue (Bensoussan, 1991; Chen Kuo-Gen, 1996).

In terms of what the meridian system is encoding, it has been suggested that the structural and functional existence of an organ within the body results in an emission of an electromagnetic field. With embryological development, the internal organs will have an electrical outlet onto the skin, via pathways which have been shown to exist through the use of an electrodermal screening system (EDSS) (Chen Kuo-Gen, 1996). This type of investigation provides evidence for pathways throughout the body which have increased electrical conductivity when compared to surrounding tissue. These have shown spread of radioactive tracers along their route (Darras *et al.*, 1992; Chen Kuo-Gen, 1996). These pathways mirror the meridian network as described in TCM. If the organ's function is disturbed, the electromagnetic field and electrical conductivity around the area will alter. This will, naturally, through the laws of physics, affect other organs within the system. This could be one explanation as to why complex patterns of disharmony can be allowed to exist, with their origins related to the disturbance of one aspect of the body's function. It could be said, therefore, that the meridian system is reflecting the electrical/electromagnetic state of the body.

Clinical applications of acupuncture

Through its complex evolution as part of a larger medical system in TCM, acupuncture can be used to help treat virtually any condition. If all disease, in TCM, is based on poor flow of Qi, then restoration of that flow is paramount, and acupuncture can be one way of achieving it. The Western medical model, however, veers towards the acceptance of acupuncture in practice, within fields which can be readily researched from a biochemical, bioneurological point of view.

The prime area for this is acupuncture analgesia. Through investigation into the physiological changes (Stux and Pomeranz, 1997, and others) produced in the body with acupuncture, its use can be justified further within most aspects of Western medicine – respiratory conditions (notably asthma), cardiovascular conditions (e.g. hypertension), digestive disorders, mental illness, addiction and particularly musculoskeletal disorders. Primarily these effects relate to stimulation of the opiodergic system which is recruited when acupuncture is used (White, 1998).

Acupuncture and nausea – anti-emetic properties

Traditional Chinese Medicine practitioners have long used a particular acupuncture point for the treatment of nausea and motion sickness, this being Pericardium 6 (Chinese name Neiguan) (see Figure 9.5(b)). A second commonly used point, often suggested for non-specific nausea, is Stomach 36 (Chinese name Zusanli) (see Figure 9.5(c)).

Use of these points has drawn increasing interest from the Western medical world, with particular reference to post-operative nausea, chemotherapy-induced nausea, morning sickness in pregnancy and travel sickness. A number of anti-emetic drugs have side-effects which acupuncture does not. Consequently, acupuncture may offer a safer and more pleasant alternative than drug therapy for the relief of some types of nausea.

Neiguan has been shown to have an anti-emetic effect in a number of well-designed studies (McMillan, 1994). 'Sea bands', commercially available wrist bands with a pressure button positioned over Neiguan, are based on the principle of acupressure.

Some effects associated with acupuncture

The following are some of the more common effects which can be associated with acupuncture:

- *Drowsiness.* Acupuncture can make individuals feel very relaxed, to the point of 'serene', and this can be associated with drowsiness. This should be taken into account when planning treatments, especially if a patient has to drive a long distance.
- *Skin reaction.* Erythema – around the needle. Beware patients who have metal allergies, as they may not tolerate any length of time for retention of needles. Itchiness – local histamine release. Bleeding – on removal of the needle.
- *Relaxation in muscle tone.*
- *Increased capillary action.*
- *Raised neurochemical reactions within the nervous system.*
- *Temporary aggravation in symptoms.* Much like many manual therapy techniques, it is not unusual for patients to have an increase in their symptoms. This is perfectly normal and patients should be reassured/forewarned.
- *Stress response.* Dry mouth; light headedness.

Deqi

Acupuncture sensation, or deqi (pronounced 'der chee'), is the sensation a patient should experience from and around the needle area. Sensations have been variously described as feelings of: distension; aching; heaviness; soreness; cramping; tingling; warmth.

The numb aspect of needle sensation is thought to be produced by stimulation of large diameter A beta fibres, whereas the heavy feeling is from stimulation of large diameter A delta fibres. Some studies quote that outcome of acupuncture treatment is likely to be better if there is a regular sensation of deqi during the treatment (Takeda and Wessell, 1994).

Complications and adverse effects

1. Acupuncture

Poor technique may be indicated in many of these adverse effects.

Death

From sudden cardiorespiratory insult (pneumothorax, and others – see below).

Trauma

Cardiovascular:
  endocarditis
  cardiac tamponade
  bleeding – beware patients on anticoagulants or haemophiliac patients.
Pneumothorax.
Haemothorax – These are rare, and often associated with specific congenital abnormalities.

Cross-infection of patient and therapist through needlestick injury

HIV.
Hepatitis.
Septicaemia.

(The National Blood Transfusion Service will accept patients as blood donors, after acupuncture, as long as they can produce a certificate, signed by the acupuncturist. The certificate, available through the acupuncturist's professional body, shows that they are a Registered Practitioner.)

Needle-related adverse effects

Retained needle:
  stuck
  broken
  bent.

Other

Fainting/syncope.
Fitting.

2. Moxa

Burning.

3. Auricular

Perichondritis.

4. Electroacupunture

Shock.

Treatment for the onset of such adverse effects are as for any other situation in which they occur.

Cautions

Strong reactors

Individuals who experience the deep relaxation that acupuncture can produce, after only a short time of treatment, are likely to be strong reactors. These patients also occasionally report the acupuncture sensation travelling away from the needle, apparently in the directions as depicted by meridian charts.

Weak patients

Anyone who has had long-standing ME, or is generally of a 'weak constitution', will not be able to tolerate prolonged spells of needling. Treatment times should be kept relatively short and the number of needles kept to a minimum.

Diabetics

Care needs to be taken from the point of view of the poor circulation which diabetics often have. Also, some acupuncture points appear to raise the blood sugar level, so strong treatment should be avoided. Impaired sensation must also be considered.

Patients on anticoagulants

Do not use deep needling. Assess the risk, in terms of how much anticoagulation the patient is on.

Withdrawal of drug therapy

If a patient is responding to acupuncture for their condition, the acupuncture practitioner and GP/Consultant should work together to reduce the therapeutic dosage of relevant drugs.

Certain points

Care must be taken with needling of certain points over the thorax, where there is a risk of pneumothorax. Oblique needling should be used.

Contraindications

Patient

Do not:

- treat an unwilling patient – needle phobic
- treat a patient who cannot understand you, or understand what the treatment with acupuncture entails, or a patient who cannot cooperate (e.g. mentally disabled)
- treat a patient who is very weak/hungry because of alteration in blood chemistry.

Pain

Do not:

- treat pain of unknown medical origin. If in any doubt, or needing further investigation, consult with the patient's physician (e.g. grumbling appendicitis, bony pain from metastatic disease). *Be sure of what you are treating.*

Orthopaedic

Do not:

- treat locally any area which may be relying on muscle tone to provide stability (e.g. in cases of spinal trauma, spinal malignancy or infection).

Pregnancy

Do not:

- treat a pregnant woman in the first trimester of pregnancy with strong-acting acupuncture points because of potential miscarriage. Certain conditions may be treated by some practitioners, but with great care and knowledge.

Paediatric

Do not:

- treat into fontanelles of children
- treat, with acupuncture, small children who cannot remain still. Acupressure may be more appropriate.

Dermatology

Do not:

- treat directly into moles/lumps of unknown origin.

Vascular

Do not:

- treat haemophiliac patients (danger of intra-articular bleed which may go unnoticed if deep points are used)
- treat some patients on anticoagulant therapy (see Cautions, above).

Certain points

Do not treat the forbidden points:

- nipple
- umbilicus (with acupuncture – can use moxa).

Contraindications to techniques

Moxa

Do not:

- treat directly on the face
- treat near any orifice, or the eyes
- treat over major blood vessels – popliteal artery/neck
- treat over the anterior chest wall/nipple area
- treat over areas of reduced temperature sensation – beware diabetic patients for this reason
- treat over area where there is impaired circulation.

Electroacupuncture

Do not use with:

- pacemakers – demand pacemakers can be inhibited by electroacupuncture.

Auricular acupuncture

Do not:

- leave small press needles *in situ* in patients who have diabetes, rheumatic valve disease, are on immunosuppressants or steroids – increased risk of infection.

Acupuncture and pain

An increasing knowledge base of proposed neurochemical and neuroanatomical pathways involved in the transmission, inhibition and appreciation of pain has provided a foundation from which to research the effects of acupuncture within this field.

The general consensus for acupuncture's mode of action is that acupuncture analgesia is created by an opiodergic mechanism (Stux and Pomeranz, 1997, and others). Cholecystokinin octapeptide (CCK-8), and naxolone, both opioid antagonists, reverse acupuncture-obtained analgesia, so confirming the role of the opioid-driven system (Cheng and Pomeranz, 1980).

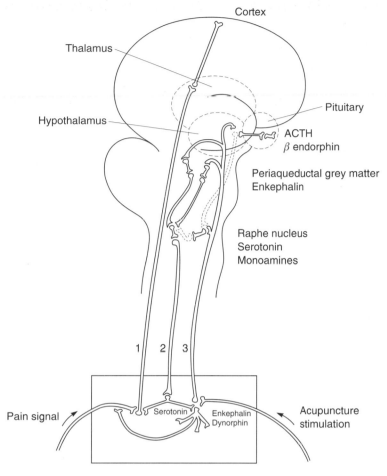

Figure 9.7 How acupuncture analgesia is achieved: 1, spinothalamic tract – ascending; 2, descending dorsolateral tract; 3, anterolateral tract – ascending

In summary, the central nervous system response to acupuncture stimulation is a multi-site release of opioid-like endorphins and related neurohormones. These either inhibit or modify transmission of the pain signal at the cord, brainstem or cortical levels. Figure 9.7 shows an overview of the key aspects of pain transmission and how acupuncture analgesia is achieved at varying sites within the nervous system.

Segmental acupuncture

A segment in neuroanatomy, for example L4, consists of a dermatome, myotome, viscerotome or sclerotome which are linked through embryo-logical development. Through this shared inner-vation, a part of the segment sending or receiving an abnormal neurological message will potentially see that message mirrored in other same segment elements (Figure 9.8). Thus, a cutaneous abnormality may in time result in an abnormal visceral function and so on through the group.

The level of neurological activity remains pri-marily a spinal one, with different elements of the segmental stimuli, inhibiting or exciting other elements. The aim of segmental acupunc-ture and related therapies like acupressure is to renormalize the aberrant segment by stimulation of a particular nerve fibre type. By stimulating fast-conducting A delta and A beta fibres, the

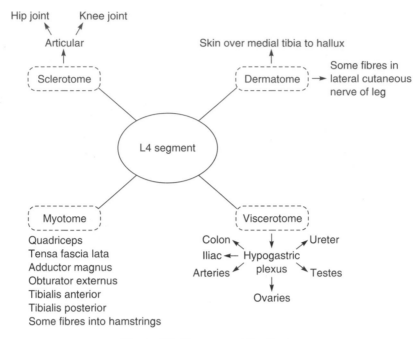

Figure 9.8 The segmental pathway

smaller A delta and c fibres are blocked at the spinal cord. This will result in reduced pain transmission, and a reduction in associated muscle spasm. In turn, this may result in a cessation of abnormal cell stimulus.

Trigger point acupuncture

Primarily used for the treatment of musculoskeletal pain, this technique is widely used by manual therapists. Based on the research put forwards by J. Kellgren in the 1930s, the referral pattern of pain from the soft tissue structures of muscle and fascia has been charted and investigated. Much work has been added by Travell and Bigelow (1946) and Travell and Simons (1983), and the neurophysiological basis of trigger point acupuncture is now well established.

A trigger point is defined as a 'focus of neural hyperactivity' (Baldry, 1993), generally found in muscle, which refers pain to adjacent or distant structures. Treatment directed at the trigger point, will affect the referred pain pattern (see Case history 1, later).

Trigger points are primarily tender areas within the muscle, but there is also often a close association in the surrounding area, with palpable fibrous bands or nodules (myofascial bands). Direct needling into these points is an extremely beneficial treatment – relieving pain and regaining muscle viability in the associated musculature. This can be particularly useful for manual therapists wishing to progress to more direct techniques.

Auricular acupuncture

Acupuncture to the auricle (ear) is a microsystem approach to acupuncture. In 1955, Paul Nogier, a French doctor, was intrigued after coming across a lady practitioner in Lyons who used to cauterize a certain point on the ear to help cure sciatica (Nogier and Nogier, 1985). He developed a system, after careful observation, which resulted in a working hypothesis of the ear as a 'microsystem' of the body. He felt the effect of treatment was through a scientific reflex system. There are references to the technique of auricular acupuncture in ancient Chinese texts, but general credit is given to Nogier for the development of the auriculotherapy of today.

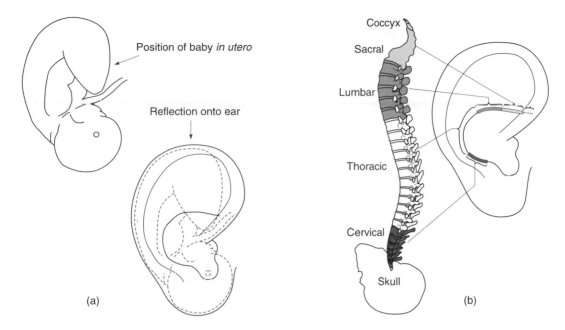

Figure 9.9 (a) The connection between the shape of the ear and a fetus; (b) connections of the ear with the spine

Nogier's 'man in the ear' shows a connection between the shape of the auricle, and a fetus (Figure 9.9(a)). These auricular charts are often slightly different from one text to another, and serve only as a guide to point location (Figure 9.9(b)), much like the acupuncture charts of the meridians or channels.

In 1984, R. Dale explored further the system of 'microacupuncture', and concluded that the body functions by a set of 'organ-to-cutaneous and cutaneous-to-organ' reflexes. As an example, a problem at the fifth lumbar vertebra will result in a reflex disturbance elsewhere in the body, not just through same segment innervation. Acupuncture to the point in the ear which corresponds with the fifth lumbar, will create a reverse reflex, cutaneous-to-organ, which may result in sedation of the hyperactivity.

Auricular acupuncture is the most commonly used technique when treating with acupuncture for withdrawal of substances such as drug addiction and smoking – considered as an addiction in biochemical terms. Combined with electroacupuncture, it works on the principle that the release of endogenous opioids provides the 'chemical fix' craved by these patients. There

have been a number of studies on this subject (Ken and Yongqiang, 1991), and although the evidence remains inconclusive, like many findings with acupuncture, there are often successful reported effects by patients.

Electroacupuncture

Electroacupuncture primarily refers to the application of an electrical current directly through an acupuncture needle while it is inserted into tissue. The use of electrical stimulation over an acupuncture point, be it with transcutaneous nerve stimulation (TENS), interferential, H-wave or commercially available hand-held 'pen' stimulators, can be considered an extension of this technique. Electroacupuncture machines are designed to apply a variation of currents, with variable amplitudes and frequencies. There is often a choice of waveform.

Frequencies and neurotransmitter release

Certain neurotransmitters are released in greater volume in response to certain frequencies of stimulation. Han and Sun (1990) found the two most useful frequencies for stimulation were 2 Hz as a constant, with bursts of 15 Hz. Other references cite higher frequencies to increase recruitment of the serotonergic system (Bensoussan, 1991; Hobbs, 1994). Low frequency (1–4 Hz) stimulates the c and smaller A delta fibres, so recruiting the endorphin network. The analgesia obtained from low-frequency use is first obtained through the chemical release of met-enkephalin and then enkephalin, both of which have a slower and more lasting effect than the beta endorphin. The low-frequency currents also activate the descending inhibitory pathways involved in pain transmission and blockage.

It has been found that the segmental release of dynorphin and enkephalin is most effective if the frequency of electroacupuncture is kept between 1 and 3 Hz (Han and Sun, 1990). High-frequency stimulation (50–100 Hz), or higher, stimulates large A beta fibres and will give a short-term analgesia.

Electroacupuncture, when used in the treatment of addictions, is most effective in aiding withdrawal, with frequency ranges from 75 to 300 Hz for narcotics and sedatives, 1 to 2 kHz for amphetamines, and 5 to 10 Hz for nicotine (Bensoussan, 1991).

Transcutaneous nerve stimulation

TENS is a familiar treatment technique to physiotherapists and is often used to treat chronic pain. Use of TENS directly over acupuncture points can enhance the overall effectiveness of the technique. Machines used in current practice now give the therapist and patient the choice of a much larger range of electrical stimulation – recruiting the low-frequency range of 2–4 Hz which appears to be the most useful for utilizing the pain-relieving mechanisms of acupuncture, as well as the more traditionally used higher frequencies.

There are four currents in use with TENS in today's clinical environment:

- Conventional TENS – high frequency (100 Hz)/low intensity (*analgesia obtained by recruiting spinal segmental effects*).

- Acupuncture-like TENS – low frequency (1–4 Hz)/high intensity (*analgesia obtained by recruiting spinal and descending inhibitory control mechanisms*).
- Burst train TENS – baseline low frequency (1–4 Hz) (*analgesia obtained by recruitment of segmental and central mechanisms*).
- Brief intense TENS – high frequency (100–150 Hz), high intensity (*analgesia obtained as per local anaesthetic – short duration, segmental effect*).

TENS provides the patient with an extension of their treatment, and some control and inclusion in their own rehabilitation. It allows a therapist to maintain/improve on their patient's pain relief in between actual treatment sessions. Using it in conjunction with theories of acupuncture is one approach.

Laser

Low-level laser can also be used over acupuncture points, although its method of action is still far from understood. From the perspective of pain relief, there is considerable contention as to its mode of action.

It does not stimulate the serotonergic systems, involved in acupuncture analgesia, and it does not stimulate the A delta fibres, involved in segmental control of pain with acupuncture (Pontinen, 1992). It may be more appropriate to consider the pain-relieving properties of low-level laser as being those which go hand in hand with the healing response which is stimulated with its use.

Acupressure

Put simply, this technique involves the use of finger, thumb, whole hand or elbow pressure over acupuncture points. The most obvious extension of this as a technique is Shiatsu (see Chapter 15). As a specific technique, acupressure can thus best be described within the confines of Shiatsu.

Moxibustion

Moxa is a substance derived from the *Artemesia vulgaris* plant (see chapter Introduction). This principle behind the use of moxa has more of a place within the TCM framework of practice, as it is said to supply Qi to an area, or deficiency. It is worth remembering that, in TCM, acupuncture *moves* obstructed Qi, moxa *supplies* and moves Qi.

As a method of applying heat to an area, moxa produces all the effects of any application of heat as used within physical therapy.

It is perhaps not a very convenient method of use, particularly within hospital departments, with its characteristic sweet smell (much like cannabis – which usually raises a few eyebrows!), while the smoke it produces can become hazardous (smokeless rolls of moxa are available, but they take a long time to reach a therapeutic heat level, and patients do not find the heat as penetrating as pure moxa).

Fire alarm systems have to be considered, and practitioners can become affected by it (it can cause sore throats and headaches if used in abundance).

Patients do, however, comment that it has a penetrating warmth, and find it very comforting.

Cupping

Cupping is very much a manual technique, creating a movement of blood and tissue fluids in the area underneath it, once it has been applied to the skin. The principle of application is that a vacuum is created within the cup which is placed over the skin where there is deemed to be congestion, or directly over an acupuncture point. As the vacuum develops, the skin and soft tissue underlying it are drawn up into the cup. The capillaries passively dilate and superficial engorgement occurs. Suction cups on interferential machines often create a similar mechanical effect.

Patients must be warned that this technique will leave quite noticeable marks on their skin for some days, but this is perfectly natural with the kind of technique being used.

Case histories

Case history 1

Miss H, a personnel director in a large company, presented with a second episode of severe left-sided neck and scapular pain. She felt this episode was related to an increased administrative load and long working hours over the last two weeks. She is right handed. She had previously had a workplace assessment which had highlighted aspects such as desk height, and where possible these had been corrected. These measures had helped resolve the first episode of pain, along with soft tissue massage and manual stretching techniques. Cervical spine movement was restricted in *right* rotation, *right* side flexion, with increased muscular pull on the *left* in forward flexion. Limiting structures were primarily the *left* upper trapezius, but also levator scapulae, scaleni and splenius capitus – all on the left. There was a large and palpable trigger point, as shown in Figure 9.10(a), and when palpated this referred pain up into the left side of the neck and across the superior aspect of the scapula.

Following a few minutes of soft tissue massage, which highlighted the centre of the trigger point, acupuncture was used in the points, as shown in Figure 9.10(b). Needles were inserted superficially and left for 5 minutes. After this time, a deeper insertion was sought, into the trigger point itself, and again needles were left for 5 minutes after being rotated to elicit a twitch response. This was followed by manual stretch and contract/relax techniques to upper trapezius. The first treatment resulted in a 60% reduction in pain. Range of movement increased by 70%.

At her second visit, Miss H stated that she had no problems with movement and restriction, but was still aware of the 'very local area' of the trigger point. She had slept very well the same night of her treatment, and felt much better in herself. Acupuncture was repeated, again with 5 minutes of superficial insertion. During the second 5 minutes, of deeper insertion, an electric current of 2 Hz was also applied to the needle, provoking muscle twitch. Again manual stretching was performed, and the patient was instructed in exercise to maintain/increase the stretch now gained in the muscle. Follow-up appointment was 2 weeks after this second appointment. At her third appointment, Miss H stated she had not really been aware of pain, but when she palpated the trigger point area she realized there was still 'a knot' and some discomfort. Her cervical spine ROM was normal. Acupuncture was repeated, directly into the remaining palpable fibrous band at the trigger point site, and this time electric current was applied immediately. This was left for 10 minutes. Soft tissue massage was used after the acupuncture this time, and the whole area around the left scapula and left side of cervical spine was loosened. *All* associated musculature in the area was stretched. Miss H was discharged with stretching exercises (the seven-way stretch particularly relevant to anyone using a VDU or working in administration). She had no pain, and full ROM at discharge.

Case history 2

A 52-year-old woman, Mrs C, presented with *left* sciatica of 6 months' duration. Pain emanated from L5/S1 on the left and radiated posteriorly to mid-calf. Onset had been after an overreaching injury sustained while playing tennis. The injury occurred while Mrs C was on holiday in the USA, and in the period immediately post-injury Mrs C had received osteopathic treatment. When she presented for physiotherapy in the UK, the injury had improved to the point

that her spinal mobility was good, but constant referred pain caused her to mark herself 6 out of 10 on a 0–10 pain scale. Soft tissue massage showed palpable congestion along the course of the bladder channel and the gall bladder channel. Direct palpation of L5/S1 facet joint was minimally tender. After patient consent, acupuncture was used in the points as shown in Figure 9.11(a), with needles being retained for 20 minutes and rotated evenly after every 5 minutes. This procedure was repeated at 2 sessions, with a week's interval between them. Mrs C scored herself 3 out of 10 after these sessions.

At the second session, Mrs C was provided with a dual-channel TENS machine, and instructed to use it with the pads positioned over acupuncture points, as shown in Figure 9.11(b). Machine settings were: 30 minutes' stimulation at 2 Hz, pulse width 180 μs, an hour or more, according to patient need, at 110 Hz and 50 μs.

Mrs C was reviewed after 4 weeks, as she was on holiday for 3 weeks. At her review, she scored herself 0.5–1 out of 10, with only occasional reflection of referred pain into the left buttock. She had felt confident enough to return to gentle tennis. Mrs C was instructed in stabilizing-type exercises for both the abdominals and small spinal muscles around L5/S1 and shown potentially new TENS positions based on acupuncture points. She has remained pain free to date.

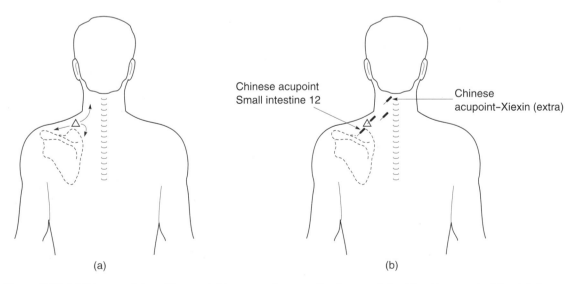

(a)   (b)

Chinese acupoint Small intestine 12

Chinese acupoint–Xiexin (extra)

Figure 9.10 (a) Trigger point position, and (b) acupuncture needle placement, for Miss H, – see text for details

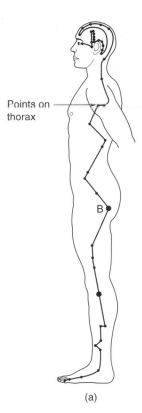

Points on thorax

B

(a)

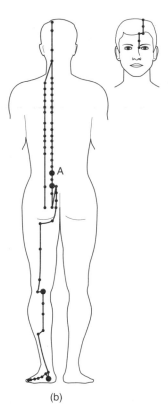

A

(b)

Figure 9.11 The acupuncture points used with Mrs C: (a) the gall bladder channel; (b) the bladder channel. The points used are drawn larger for ease of identification. See text for details of case history.

Case history 3

Mrs S, a 37 year old, presented with pain in the left scapula, left posterior arm and left side of cervical spine. Four years previously she had been involved in a road traffic accident and suffered severe whiplash. She was the driver in a stationary car, and had been leaning down to put something away in the driver's door compartment when she was hit from behind at approximately 20 mph. She is left handed and had taken a long time and a lot of treatment to reach the point where she could drive again. Previous physiotherapy had worked on the left cervical spine, but any direct treatment to the mid-thoracic region, particularly T5, would cause a severe flare in her symptoms, and she had been reluctant to pursue any direct approach.

At the time of her referral for acupuncture, Mrs S was complaining of a deep heaviness in the left arm, posteriorly, with occasional referral into the left side of the cervical spine and occasional left-sided headaches. She felt cold down the course of the arm and light touch over the skin to the left of T5 provoked a pilo-motor response on the skin surrounding T5 and into the lower forearm. Palpation of the area to the left of T5 also showed increased hydrosis.

The treatment from which she gained the most benefit involved acupuncture needles inserted as shown in Figure 9.12, with electrical current of 2 Hz attached to the needles marked A and B. Mrs S has stated that she felt the combination of acupuncture and electrical stimulation reduced her symptoms by 60%.

A possible explanation for improvement is that long-standing segmental disturbance is normalized with needles having an effect directly on muscle tone, capillary blood flow and local chemical release. The electroacupuncture, at 2 Hz, will have caused an endogenous opioid response, and stimulation from the distal referred area (C) will have provided a different afferent sensation.

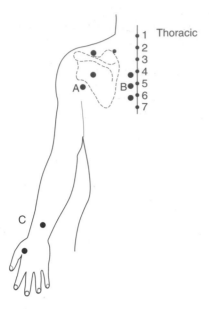

Figure 9.12 The position of acupuncture needles for Mrs S – see text for details of case history

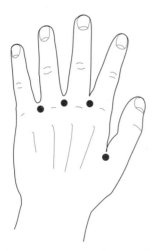

Figure 9.13 The acupuncture points used with Mrs L – see text for details of case history

Case history 4

Mrs L, a woman aged 67, was referred for treatment of arthritis of both limbs. She had worked in a furnishing fabric workroom for many years, initially as a cutter and subsequently as a curtain maker. Fabrics used were often very heavy. She had suffered with thumb pain for a number of years, and found it was always worse in cold, damp weather. She was right handed and the right thumb was the more painful.

X-ray examination had shown advanced osteoarthritic changes in both right and left carpometacarpal joints, with the right being worse than the left. All movements were generally limited, and pain was of a deep aching quality, often worse at night or in the early morning hours. Mrs L had been referred for physiotherapy in the past, and had received wax baths, interferential, general exercise, specific mobilizations to all finger and hand joints and TENS.

After gaining consent, acupuncture was used in the positions shown in Figure 9.13, with needles being retained for 10 minutes. The patient was shown how to use a moxa roll for home treatment. This involved holding a lit moxa roll over one of the acupuncture points previously needled, until the sensation of heat became too intense. The roll was then moved until it was over the next point, and the process repeated. In all, the stick was held over each point 8 times until the skin showed an erythema. The patient was asked to do this once a day.

At review, Mrs L stated she had felt much better with the moxa, and could use her hands much more freely. The stiffness she experienced in the mornings had reduced by 70%. She was quite happy to continue with this regimen as and when she needed, and was discharged direct treatment but left with a phone number contact to the therapist if she felt she needed further intervention.

Closing statement

The use of acupuncture within physiotherapy practice is already well established. The Chartered Society of Physiotherapy recognizes the use of acupuncture as a core skill in professional practice.

There is also an increasing interest being taken in the teaching of acupuncture at postgraduate level, and a growing demand for it to be included in the undergraduate curriculum. As the boundaries between therapies merge in the future, and truly integrated medicine is viewed as the way forward for health care, physical therapists should consider themselves well placed to utilize and explore the practice of acupuncture within mainstream medicine.

References

Alltree, J. (1993) Physiotherapy and acupuncture: practice in the UK. *Comp. Ther. Med.*, **1**, 34–41.

Baldry, P. (1993) *Acupuncture, Trigger Points and Musculoskeletal Pain*, 2nd edn. Edinburgh: Churchill Livingstone.

Bensoussan, A. (1991) *The Vital Meridian – A Modern Exploration of Acupuncture*. Edinburgh: Churchill Livingstone.

Chen Kuo-Gen (1996) Electrical properties of meridians. *IEEE Eng. Med. Biol.*, May/June, 58.

Cheng, R. and Pomeranz, B. (1980) Electroacupuncture analgesia is mediated by stereospecific opiate receptors and is reversed by antagonists of Type 1 receptors. *Life Sci.*, **26**, 631–39.

Darras, J.C., de Vernejoul, P. and Albarede, P. (1992) Nuclear medicine and acupuncture: a study on migration of radioactive tracers after injection at acupoints. *Am. J. Acupunct.*, **20**(3), 245–56.

Essentials of Chinese Acupuncture (1980) Compiled by Beijing College of Traditional Chinese Medicine, Shanghai College of Traditional Chinese Medicine, Nanjing College of Traditional Chinese Medicine, The Acupuncture Institute of the Academy of Traditional Chinese Medicine. Beijing: Foreign Language Press.

Han, J.S. and Sun, S.L. (1990) Differential release of enkephalin and dynorphin by low and high frequency electroacupuncture in the central nervous system. *Sci. Int. J.*, **1**, 19–23.

Hobbs, B. (1994) The application of electricity to acupuncture needles – a review of the current literature and research with a brief outline of the principles involved. *Comp. Ther. Med.*, **2**, 36–40.

Kaptchuk, T. (1983) *The Web that has no Weaver – Understanding Chinese Medicine*. New York: Congdon Weed.

Ken, C. and Yongqiang, C. (1991) *Handbook to Auricular Therapy*. Beijing: Foreign Language Press.

Maciocia, G. (1989) *The Foundations of Chinese Medicine – A Comprehensive Text for Acupuncturists and Herbalists*. Edinburgh: Churchill Livingstone.

Mann, F. (1998) A new system of acupuncture. In *Medical Acupuncture. A Western Scientific Approach* (Filshie, J., ed.). Edinburgh: Churchill Livingstone.

McMillan, C. (1994) Transcutaneous electrical stimulation of Neiguan anti-emetic acupuncture point in controlling sickness following opioid analgesia in major orthopaedic surgery. *Physiotherapy*, **80**(1), 5–9.

Nogier, P. and Nogier, R. (1985) *The Man in the Ear*. France: Maisonneuve.

Pontinen, P. (1992) *Low Level Laser Therapy as a Medical Treatment Modality*. Tampere: Art urpo.

Ropp, P. (1990) *Heritage of China – Contemporary Perspectives on Chinese Civilisation*. Berkeley, CA: University of California Press.

Stux, G. and Pomeranz, B. (1997) *Basics of Acupuncture*, 4th edn. Berlin: Springer.

Takeda, W. and Wessel, J. (1994) Acupuncture treatment for the pain of osteoarthritic knees. *Arthritic Care Res.*, **1**, 118–22.

Travell, J. and Bigelow, N.H. (1946) Referred somatic pain does not follow a simple 'segmental' pattern. *Fed. Proc.*, **51**, 106.

Travell, J. and Simons, D.G. (1983) Myofascial pain and dysfunction. In *The Trigger Point Manual*. Baltimore: Williams and Wilkins.

White, A. (1998) Electroacupuncture and acupuncture analgesia. In *Medical Acupuncture. A Western Scientific Approach*. (Filshie, J., ed.). Edinburgh: Churchill Livingstone.

10 Craniosacral therapy

Richard A. Harries

Definition

Craniosacral therapy (CST) is a non-invasive light touch therapy that uses the inherent mobility of the skull (cranium and facial bones) and pelvis, the integrity of body fascia and the craniosacral rhythm (CSR), sometimes referred to as the cranial rhythmic impulse (CRI), to facilitate and normalize body structure and promote well-being. At its most basic, CST is little more than adverse mechanical tension for the central nervous system (CNS) contained within the dural membrane, a purely physical system. At its most refined, it is a way of accessing long-forgotten conscious memory, communicating with specific groups of cells and cellular tissue memory and, if the patient's belief system is such, re-evaluating, if not re-experiencing, past-life trauma and memories that are relevant to this life. It requires a delicate touch, an awareness of subtle energy and the non-judgemental acceptance of anything the patient brings to the treatment session. The CST system is considered by craniosacral therapists to be the meeting place of Body, Mind and Spirit and as such allows the patient alternative access and insight to otherwise troublesome aspects of their life, should they require it. It is a therapy where the therapist's focus and intent is as powerful as their touch, and the weight of a thought can be crucial.

Much of what physiotherapists do is the restoration of normal movement. Whatever modality is chosen, the ultimate aim is pain-free function as normal as possible. Every structure within the body is capable of free movement with minimal disturbance to surrounding structures. From the free flow of air, obstruction-free circulation and drainage of body fluids, mobility of the gut, extensibility and movement of nerves, movement of muscle over muscle, muscle over bone and movement of bone on bone, every part of the human body is designed to move and to move freely. To craniosacral therapists, cranial osteopaths and a growing band of dentists the skull is no exception; it too is designed to move. They accept that free movement of the skull is essential, not just for the CNS but for a fully functioning body. The design is intricate. It allows the subtlety of regular cranial movement, in spite of the great forces produced by the muscles acting through the temporomandibular joint, which is a joint of prime importance to cranial function and to the whole body.

To any physiotherapist educated to a reductionist methodology, CST may come as a complete shock or blessed relief. Reductionism requires that one tests and retests, based on the patient's history, signs, symptoms, subjective and objective examination, to find the structures requiring treatment. The patient is undressed and the therapist observes, examines and palpates to test and confirm their findings. The therapist then actively treats and reassesses.

There are 22 cranial bones, 34 cranial sutures and 117 possible primary bony lesions at these sutures (Brookes, 1981). Temporomandibular joint function, the bite and the teeth are also implicated in cranial function (Blood, 1986). There are also bony lesions of the sacrum reflected through the dural tube and there is the effect on the craniosacral system from fascial disturbance anywhere in the body. A reductionist approach is possible but time consuming.

Fortunately CST does not require this. The patient remains clothed. A detailed history and examination is not required. Palpation is subtle, light and passive; it concerns the whole body and the problem, whatever and wherever it may be, and is perceived by the therapist as a disturbance in fascial mobility and of the CSR either physically and/or energetically. Whole-body evaluation, not just of the cranium and sacrum, by an experienced practitioner, takes less than 5 minutes.

In CST, the theory is that it is the patient's body that knows best what it needs to do to restore itself to full function. This may be a subtle release of tissue that takes place under the therapist's hands or an active whole-body realignment. As therapist, the role is that of a being-facilitator, not as a doing-therapist, allowing whatever is necessary to happen in order to facilitate the process of healing.

CST is gentle and non-invasive, requiring a sensitive, active, non-judgemental awareness, an intuitive right brain leading a semi-suspended left brain learning, the whole brain receptively attached to and trusting a perceptive intelligent pair of hands. Left brain learning is important to know where the therapist is in the body, and helps with visualization, but as a physiotherapist it can be all too easy to 'left brain' a treatment session, making judgements and evaluations as to how, where and why this resolution needs to proceed – leading the session instead of following the patient. A semi-suspended left brain is noticing, but passive, and right brain freedom allows intuitive action by the therapist's hands.

Historical background

Craniosacral therapy has its roots in, and evolved from, cranial osteopathy. William Garner Sutherland, in Kirksville, Missouri, an osteopathic student of A. T. Still, the Father of Osteopathy, began his development of cranial

osteopathy in the 1900s from his study of cranial bones (Sutherland, 1939). His interest came initially from the examination of a disarticulated skull. He was intrigued by the detail of the sutural surfaces, believing that the design allowed mobility between the bones. As he could find no reference to any hint of this idea, he began his own investigations looking for the link between form and function.

Sutherland's fascination with cranial sutures and mobility led him to experiment with a variety of ingenious devices based on leather football helmets and catcher's mitts to restrict such movement as he reasoned was there. He monitored his own physical reactions and his wife monitored his emotional and psychological changes.

From his work there slowly grew his Cranial Concept, the art and science of cranial osteopathy. Sutherland had to develop not only an understanding of cranial articulation in range and direction of motion, but the palpatory skill and sensitivity to test and verify his deductions. He then had to evolve a language to bring the Cranial Concept to his osteopathic colleagues who were, to say the least, sceptical if not hostile. Sutherland presented his findings to the American Osteopathic Association in 1932, having done 30 years of experimentation. In spite of a cool response he continued research and teaching for another 25 years. When he died in 1954 his work was still little recognized.

Sutherland's work was initially on the bones and articulations of the skull (a bony-osseous model), then later on the intracranial membranes and its reciprocal tension system (a membrane-structural model), then later still on the cerebrospinal fluid (the fluid model). Each development led him to a deeper understanding of the complexity of the system, and each development required a more exquisite sensitivity of touch (Sutherland, 1990). Osteopathy is usually associated with high-velocity manipulation. 'Manipulation' is much too powerful a word and completely inappropriate for the subtle, almost imperceptible, 5 g touch required for successful CST.

John Upledger, an osteopathic physician familiar with the principles of cranial osteopathy, describes his observation of a rhythmically moving dural membrane while assisting at the surgical removal of calcified plaque on the cervical dura. Finding no reference to any previous observation, he postulated the existence of a cerebrospinal fluid rhythm, leading to CST (Upledger, 1997). Sutherland (1939) had already postulated a vitality to the CSF, endowing it with mystical if not spiritual qualities, much as blood had been endowed by earlier generations.

Form and function

To understand how and why CST works there are various elements that need to be assembled: the cranium and sacrum, not just at a bony level but deeper to the dura mater, the intracranial dural membranes and the dural tube forming the reciprocal tension membrane system, then deeper still to the CSF and its circulation. CSF is produced and reabsorbed producing the craniosacral rhythm (CSR) (Upledger and Vredevoogd, 1983). The rhythm and the reciprocal membrane system are influenced by the freedom at the individual cranial sutures. Integral to the system is the fascial integrity of the body (Schultz and Feitis, 1996) and its intimate connection to every cell of the body (Oschman, 1981).

Since fascia is everywhere within the body and connects everything to everything and ultimately to the dura, any problem in the body can manifest anywhere, making CST a whole-body system. Dysfunction within the craniosacral system will affect body function, and body dysfunction, no matter how discrete, will affect the craniosacral system. At a deeper level, CST involves tissue memory and the concept of 'energy cysts' (Upledger, 1990), the body's attempt to minimize traumatic effects (see later section).

It is a fundamental maxim of anatomy and physiology that form follows function. They are interdependent. For cranial sutures this appears to have been largely ignored by English anatomists. The received wisdom was that in the adult skull the cranial sutures are immobile if not completely fused (Warwick and Williams, 1973). Spinero (1931) believes that fusion of cranial sutures in adults is pathological.

The acceptance or rejection of CST as a valid mechanical physical therapy depends on whether or not the skull is flexible structure.

For the majority of conventionally trained anatomists, the concept of cranial movement in an adult skull is, at best, still questionable, if not totally unacceptable.

There are studies to show that sutures do not fuse with age (Todd and Lyon, 1924, 1925; Kokich, 1976); that dissection and examination of surgically excised or fresh post mortem sutural material shows connective tissue, collagen, elastic fibres, blood vessels and neurological tissue with none of the calcification commonly found in material from preserved cadavers (Retzlaff *et al.*, 1975, 1976; Retzlaff and Mitchell, 1987), and that the skull is flexible (Frymann, 1971; Retzlaff *et al.*, 1975; Heifetz and Weiss, 1981; Jaslow, 1990; Heisey and Adams, 1993). Studies on cranial movement show vast differences between *in vivo* and post mortem subjects (Hubbard *et al.*, 1971; Pitlyk *et al.*, 1985; Kostopoulos and Keramidas, 1991).

If the skull were to be a rigid structure there would be no piezoelectric effect necessary for the healthy maintenance of that bone. It is proposed that the CSR manifests not only cranial bone movement but a piezoelectric effect within those bones. Examination of the bones of an 'exploded' disarticulated skull will show the variety of sutures not only from suture to suture but also within a suture from external to internal and for some sutures along their length. Craniosacral therapists have no doubt that the sutures allow and control movement.

As a flexible structure the cranium is capable of distortion, taking with it the intracranial membranes. Any suture not freely mobile locally restricts cranial movement and may maintain some degree of distortion. This may disrupt, or restrict, the underlying flow of CSF and possibly interfere with local brain activity. Tension or distortion of the intracranial membranes will have a more global effect on cerebral/cerebellar function.

It should be remembered that the majority of venous drainage from the brain is through the jugular foramen, formed at the junction of two bones. Some cranial nerves also exit via foramen similarly formed. Any misalignment between the bones forming these foramen will reduce the size of the aperture and compromise the function of structures passing through them, just as spinal lesions compromise nerve roots.

The dura 'contains' the central nervous system. Within the cranium the external layer of the dura is the internal periosteum of the cranial bones, the internal layer being reflected to contain the brain. This internal dura forms a four-leaved structure separating left and right cerebrum and cerebellum vertically, the falx cerebri/cerebelli, and the cerebrum from the cerebellum horizontally, the tentorium cerebelli, all centred on and forming the straight sinus. It is attached to the outer dura peripherally, with venous sinuses peripherally and in midline. This is the reciprocal tension membrane system within the cranium. Any tension or distortion will be reflected throughout this system and transmitted to the brain. Distortion may cause crowding of the quadrants, affecting the ventricles and their respective foramen, and to kinking or narrowing of the central aqueduct between the third and fourth venticles, affecting CSF flow.

Reduced venous drainage may also result from distortion of the membrane-walled central sinuses. Overall there may be pressure, congestion, stagnation and malnutrition, with consequent neurological dysfunction. The pituitary lies in the sella turcica of the sphenoid bone, roofed by a dural ring, the diaphragma sellae through which passes the infundibulum, an area ripe for potential distortion.

The dural tube, attached to the foramen magnum C2 and C3, is free until its sacral attachment at S2. Movement of the occiput by the CSR will affect the sacrum and vice versa, also forming a reciprocal tension membrane system. Since the dural tube and the cranial dura are continuous, they form and act as a single reciprocal tension membrane system.

The production, circulation and reabsorption of CSF forms a semi-closed hydraulic system (Upledger and Vredevoogd, 1983). Production takes place at the choroid plexuses in the ventricles. Reabsorption is via the arachnoid granulations found in the superior sagittal sinus and at the junction of the straight sinus with the great cerebral veins. Reabsorption is constant and production is intermittent and at twice the rate of reabsorption. Upledger and Vredevoogd (1983), in conjunction with Dr E. W. Retzlaff, describe a nerve connection between the sagittal suture and the third ventricle, proposing a feedback loop: as fluid is produced, the sagittal suture widens, stimulating a signal to the plexuses stopping CSF production. As the sagittal suture closes, production is restarted. This rhythmic rise and fall in CSF production creates the CSR. CSF pulse waves were recorded as long ago as 1966 (Dunbar *et al.*, 1966). Cardoso *et al.* (1983) showed CSF pulse waves related to intracranial pressure. Feinberg (1987) established CSF flow by magnetic resonance imaging.

As this CSR/CRI can be felt anywhere on the body, it has been proposed that it may be a soliton phenomenon (Oschman, 1993). A soliton wave is to fluid what a laser is to light – a coherent wave undiminished by distance from its source. Solitons carry information and can pass through each other undiminished and unaffected (Rebbi, 1979).

This rhythm is present before birth and clinical experience shows it can be felt by subtle palpation of the pregnant abdomen. It is also said to persist for some time after death. It is used diagnostically and therapeutically and, unlike other major body rhythms (respiratory, cardiac), can be artificially stopped for long periods, a still point, without any danger to life. It also stops spontaneously depending on what the individual is saying, doing or thinking. Its normal rate is 6–12 cycles per minute. Movement due to the craniosacral rhythm is described as 'flexion' and 'extension'. In CST, cranial flexion and extension does not refer to the accepted anatomical movements.

The terms derive from Sutherland's original work (Sutherland, 1939). He reasoned that the sphenoid is the keystone and drives the system. Therefore, all reference to cranial motion is related to the movement of the sphenoid. The sphenoid articulates with the occiput via the sphenobasilar synchondrosis. In *flexion*, as CSF is produced and the system *fills*, the angle between the sphenoid and the occiput increases, the skull becomes wider laterally, and shorter vertically and anteroposteriorly. The dural tube becomes shorter and fatter, as does the whole body, and the limbs rotate externally about their long axis. In *extension*, CSF is not produced and the system *empties*, the angle decreases, the skull narrows transversely, and lengthens both vertically and anteroposteriorly. The system becomes longer and thinner, as does the whole body, and the limbs rotate internally.

This is not normally a visibly perceptible movement, but is the CSR made palpable (Upledger and Vredevoogd, 1983) (Figure 10.1). The author has occasionally seen the effect of the CSR as the feet rotate and on the head as the ends of hair parted in midline move medially and laterally.

The skill of CST is in learning to 'listen'. Light and sensitive palpation is part of the art of CST, for it is more than just touch. The weight of the touch is about 5 g or less. Palpation is passive. The rhythm comes to the therapist.

Trying too hard to feel it is counterproductive. It is desirable to meld with the patient. Melding is the skill of tuning in to the patient, a matching and blending of energies, a therapeutic entrainment, becoming aware of the twist and pull of fascial tensions and the area from which they come and, perhaps, to the subtle ebb and flow of rhythms within. Therapists may experience the patient's pain and feelings in the process. This is not essential and is easily removed, yet serves as a reinforcement that the therapist is in the right place and space.

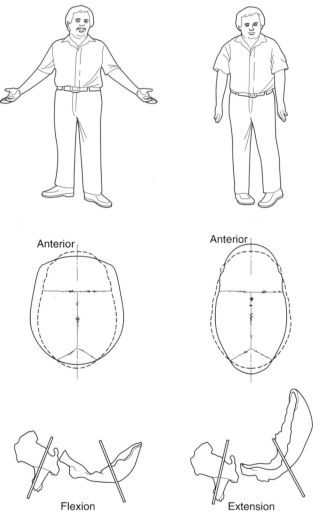

Anterior

Anterior

Flexion

Extension

Figure 10.1 Extreme ranges of cranial flexion and extension in the skull and sphenobasilar synchondrosis and habitual body posture in chronic flexion or chronic extension patterns (From Upledger and Vredevoogd, 1983, by permission from Eastland Press)

To the craniosacral therapist the human body is sensed as having an awesome plasticity. To sit cradling a head and feel it move and soften, becoming a flexible ball of a living fluid, the internal energies flowing under your fingers, is an amazing experience. To make contact with an ailing body and be drawn into the problem area from wherever is touched is thrilling. To feel bone, the densest and most solid of all body tissue, become plastic, softening, moving, changing and growing, feeling it remodel in moments is quite astonishing. To know that tissues are softening and reorganizing at a distance from the place of contact is incredible. To be in tune with the patient, melding, being aware of pain and emotions is wondrously aweful. All this, and more, is the province and privilege of the craniosacral therapist.

To watch a craniosacral therapist at work can be very dull. The therapist does not appear to be doing anything. Their hands do not appear to be moving. They may have their heads bowed and eyes closed and to all intents and purposes be meditating, in prayer or even asleep, as is the patient. Some appear to be intently listening, heads cocked to one side, hearing the sometimes faint and distant whispers of distorted tissue. It looks like the laying on of hands, like healing, but it feels more physical than healing. Its basis is in bodywork. To watch a craniosacral therapist at work can also be intriguing. The patient may be moving into some strange awkward and uncomfortable positions with contorted limbs and vigorous if not aggressive movements, enormous effort apparently being exerted by both therapist and patient. A treatment session may involve more than one therapist and treatment can be done anywhere on, and some say off, the body. Therapists may also make use of acupuncture meridians and Chakras. It is all still part of CST.

The contrast in treatments depends on how the patient chooses to work. In any case the release will be physical and there may, or may not, be an emotional release. CST, by its holistic nature, can be used to treat almost any physical condition and is useful in special needs education and psychiatry. It can be used from before birth to the point of death and can facilitate both processes.

Clinical indications

Any cranially-based problem from tinnitus, Bell's palsy, trigeminal neuralgia, sinusitis and migraine to endogenous depression, insomnia, visual problems, dental difficulties and facial asymmetry, epilepsy, allergy and any chronic condition can be alleviated. It has particular application to coma, head injury, cerebral palsy, autism, spinal cord injury and temporomandibular joint syndrome. Musculoskeletal, orthopaedic, rheumatic, respiratory, cardiac, gastric, pelvic, obstetric, gynaecological, neurological, paediatric, geriatric, oncological and chronic pain conditions will all manifest somewhere in the craniosacral system and benefit from appropriate CST. In children, CST has been shown to be effective in the treatment of autism, cerebral palsy, hyperactivity and attention deficit disorder, dyslexia and learning difficulties, epilepsy, colic, asthma, persistent crying, insomnia and glue ear.

Contraindications

There are some contraindications: acute intracranial haemorrhage, intracranial aneurysm, recent skull fracture, especially if it is unstable, and herniation of the medulla oblongata through the foramen magnum, i.e. any condition where a change in intracranial pressure would be dangerous. Cases of cranial iatrogenesis have been reported (McPartland, 1996; Greenman and McPartland, 1995) and some of them refuted (Upledger, 1996).

Technique

Treatment couches should be accessible all round and well padded. Treatment plinths are too firm, but feather pillows laid down the bed, or an air mattress, will give enough cushioning since the therapist may have a hand under the patient's body, taking their full weight, for some time. It is essential that the therapist is comfortable and relaxed.

CST is a process of finding, feeling, following and facilitating: finding and feeling the rhythm and fascial distortion, then following tissue movement to facilitate a release. Some therapists do not want to know about previous medical history or current complaints, relying on what they feel as a more useful indicator of the patient's present condition. Initial whole-body evaluation will give information about fascial disturbance and 'energy cysts', from differences in cranial rhythm as felt in different parts of the body. More localized evaluation will give specific information to the site and depth of the problem. Following the movement of the tissues into their direction of ease and then facilitating a release, allows the body the opportunity to realign and rebalance itself, after which re-evaluation will show if the problem has cleared.

The fascia of the body is primarily longitudinal and oblique, but there are regions such as the diaphragms, where the arrangement is primarily horizontal. As well as the respiratory diaphragm, the pelvic floor, the thoracic inlet, the region round the hyoid and the cranial base (CO/Cl), are all considered craniosacrally as horizontal diaphragms. These are all tensegrity structures, discontinuous rigid components under compression (bones), balanced against continuous elastic components under tension (connective tissue), as is the whole body (Oschman, 1987). Releases at soft tissue horizontal diaphragms are facilitated by gentle compression. By increasing the compression element of the tensegrity structure, the elastic element has the opportunity to rebalance itself. The compression element also has the opportunity to rebalance as the elastic component rebalances. Each peripheral joint also acts as a horizontal diaphragm.

Sutural restrictions may be felt as a bony block like a bony endpoint. A springy membranous restriction results in the bone returning to its original position. A release is felt in two phases. Lifting the suture initially feels as if all is lifting, and if let go would return unchanged. Holding against the spring soon results in an easing of the springiness as the suture spreads. It is like lifting out a full bin liner. On first lifting the liner the bin comes too, but as the liner is held the bin drops away.

Releases as described above result in a different quality of motion. There may be a softening, a release of heat, a change in the range of motion

or a therapeutic pulse – a phenomenon felt like an arterial pulse, but is unrelated, which crescendos then decrescendos as the tissues normalize. Borborygmus is commonly heard as releases occur, and is considered to be the result of a change in the balance between sympathetic and parasympathetic nervous system activity.

An extremely useful technique is the V-spread (Upledger and Vredevoogd, 1983), a technique originally developed by Sutherland. He used it on sutural restrictions, believing he was directing fluid flow to ease the restriction (Sutherland, 1939). It is very easy to do and only requires that you believe in the technique. It works on all joints, trigger points and pain as well as sutural restrictions. Patients can be taught to do it for themselves. Two fingers are spread in a V either side of the area. One or more fingers, usually of the other hand, are placed over the affected part directed towards the V. A stream of energy is visualized coming from one side through to the V. There is usually a marked relief in pain, a reduction in muscle spasm and an increase in joint range. It is extremely effective.

Energy cysts

When the body is physically traumatized it absorbs energy. The body then does its best to dissipate and normalize that energy. Some if not all of that energy will be dissipated. There will be increased circulation, heat, inflammation and repair. Should there be more energy than the body can dissipate, it will do what it does with any foreign material and wall it off, minimizing the area affected and creating a 'cyst' (Upledger, 1990).

Becker (1976) has a similar model referring to the balance of dynamic tension between the intrinsic biodynamic forces and extrinsic biokinetic forces. When extrinsic forces cannot be dissipated, they are 'centred', allowing the best possible compensation. Such areas of chronic dysfunction require that the body work around them, disrupting the normal flow and rhythm, and requiring energy to keep it encysted. Energy cysts can be remarkably persistent and often have a large emotional component.

This is a hypothetical construct. Craniosacral therapists believe they can locate and treat these cysts. Once removed, there is a remarkable improvement, particularly in long-standing chronic pain conditions.

Tissue memory

Since organ transplants began, the popular press has run stories of organ recipients taking on some of the characteristics and preferences of the donor. The clinical experience of many groups of bodyworkers, including craniosacral therapists, is that soft tissue holds physical kinesthetic and emotional memory. Recall of conscious, emotional, allegedly brain-stored memories, bring about physical changes, e.g. blushing, arousal. Emotional memory gets caught up in the physical trauma and may get locked in, preventing full recovery until the emotional content is dealt with. There is a growing acceptance of holographic memory not only throughout the brain (Pribram, 1969) but in every cell (Hammerhoff, 1988).

The limbic-hypothalamic system is old in evolutionary terms, but the cerebral cortex is a relative newcomer. The mind does not exist only in the brain. Biochemical messenger molecules, information transfer throughout the cellular network through microtubule cytoskeletal system, and the growing understanding of the complexity of individual cells, gives credence to the idea of mind and memory in the body, to the extent of the body being the manifestation of the mind. Trauma can occur on many levels and all are remembered. How troublesome they are depends on the individual's emotional state at the time of trauma (Upledger, 1990): 'Man is not disturbed by events themselves but by the view he takes of them' (Epicticus, 507 BC).

Craniosacral therapy in children

Since cranial bones in children are movable, CST for children has never been in question. In a newborn baby the mandible, sphenoid, temporal, frontal bones and occiput have still to ossify from multiple centres. As the occiput is in four pieces there are implications for the ultimate shape of the foramen magnum (Frymann, 1966). The younger the child, the easier it is to facilitate any corrections their system may want to make, yet the more difficult it can be to get in touch with their cranial rhythm. The nervous system is highly plastic and very susceptible to pressure changes. If newborn babies received CST as routinely as the APGAR assessment, though not immediately post partum, it is highly likely that, in the long term, they would be healthier, happier, more sociable and with fewer physical and emotional problems than at present.

A normal vaginal delivery is supremely important for the normal CSR of a gravity-bound existence. Babies with assisted deliveries still undergo the compression of the birth canal, but the decompression is disrupted by whatever mechanical device is used to help extract the baby, leaving them with a skull and underlying brain tissue distorted, if not disrupted, and an overstressed whole-body fascial system. If not corrected by external intervention there is a limit to what the self-correcting body systems can do, as cranial 'bony' lesions may already have been introduced. In spite of the largely cartilaginous nature of a baby's skull, deeply felt distortions can make their mark on the developing bone. It is possible for a cranial bone to ossify with unnecessary tension and distortion built in to it (Frymann, 1966).

Babies born by caesarean section are subjected to a rapid and uncontrolled cranial expansion as the intrauterine pressure collapses when the uterus is opened. Some such babies tend to have cranial problems, not of the discrete bony lesions that tend to occur with assisted deliveries, but more diffuse and diverse problems.

Babies who are breast fed for as long as possible, and encouraged to suck using anatomically correct orthodontic teats, tend to develop a wide maxillary arch with good dentition, and normalized sphenobasilar movement without craniosacral intervention. Babies and children who thumbsuck are often doing their best to correct their own cranial function. Thumbsucking in adults is no longer satisfying or necessary once normal sphenobasilar movement has been restored. When working with babies and young children, only very gentle forces are necessary and direct corrections can be made. It is especially useful to think of cranial bones as hard places in the dura, a concept that can be successfully carried over to the treatment of adults.

There are a number of schools of CST. They have differences of philosophy and understanding and each tends to make prime use of a different element of the craniosacral system. Some work primarily with bones, some with membranes, and some with fluid, yet they all derive from the original work of William Garner Sutherland. None of them uses their prime element exclusively, and there are large areas of overlap. The differences in philosophy and understanding may seem trivial, but lead to fundamental differences in the manner of work, especially with deeply-held trauma. This may be a cathartic release, or a quiet therapeutic re-evaluation, in each case supported by the therapeutic relationship. In spite of these differences they all work.

Case histories

Case history 1

Mrs A at 28 years old already had a 5-year-old son, and had been trying for a second child for 2 years. Tests and examination of both partners showed no reason why she should not get pregnant. Her previous pregnancy and delivery was uneventful. She had one session of CST and became pregnant within a month of treatment. At 5½ months she developed excruciating pain in her (R) sacroiliac joint. On examination the therapist's attention was drawn to her (L) maxilla. As the (L) maxilla was followed and facilitated into flexion the (R) ilium dropped backwards, and the pain in the (R) SI joint disappeared. The maxillae were rebalanced as was the temporomandibular joint. She was not seen again. Mrs A subsequently treated her own maxillae as and when the pain began to recur. At 9½ months she produced a healthy baby boy, 7 lb 4 oz, after 2½ hours' labour.

Case history 2

Mrs C is 48 years old. Since the birth of her daughter 27 years ago Mrs C has had constant low back pain (LBP) with vertex headaches. They were exacerbated pre-menstrually. Over the years she had tried exercise, physiotherapy, acupuncture, osteopathy, chiropractic and yoga with only temporary relief. Craniosacral evaluation led the therapist to her (R) abdomen over the (R) ovary. While working over the lower right abdomen she recalled a very unpleasant emergency appendicectomy at the age of 7. Her appendix was very inflamed and 'close to bursting'. The wound was large and unsightly and had been slow to heal. Over several sessions, deep fascial tension around the (R) ovary was released and the inferior ascending colon mobilized, resulting in considerable relief of her LBP. CST was also directed to the pituitary and produced a fascial release, after which her headaches disappeared.

Case history 3

Miss S, aged 17, was diagnosed with idiopathic scoliosis and sent for physiotherapy. Two years earlier she had had braces fixed to her upper teeth. The dentist had started at one side and worked his way around, crossing the midline with one side already fixed. She had worn the braces for about a year, during which time she developed diffuse back pain. The braces had been off for about a year. She now had beautiful teeth but chronic back pain and an increasing scoliosis. A CST evaluation showed that one maxilla had very limited mobility, mainly into extension, and the other had slightly more movement, mainly into flexion. Both maxillae were rotated to the left with a shear to the right. Freeing, rebalancing and realigning the maxillae, then rebalancing the temporomandibular joint, gave a rapid relief of pain. One week later the scoliosis had diminished and by the second week her spine was straight.

Discussion

Benor (1994) believes the whole craniosacral experience to be purely subjective and part of the healing continuum. In the experience of the author, having worked with craniosacral therapists who are purely bodyworkers, and craniosacral therapists who are healers as well as bodyworkers, there is often no discernible difference in treatment or outcome.

Clinical experience shows that when treating individuals who are aware of their body, only some of whom are bodyworkers or craniosacral therapists, they report feeling movement and physical changes in joints, cranial structure, soft tissue and fluid flow as treatment proceeds.

Benor also places great stress on the need to continually visualize whatever is necessary to be changed, be it the movement of the skull, the cessation of CSR or sutural integrity. Craniosacral therapists commonly report that changes often occur after their focus has drifted, their attention being refocused by the new restructuring.

There is a growing body of evidence for cranial, sutural and CSF movement (Rogers and Witt, 1997; Hornstein, 1998; Chaitow, 1998). As a physical therapy the mechanical effects are wide-ranging and long-lasting. CST is generally considered to be a safe procedure. At a more subtle level there is undoubtedly an interaction between the energy field of the therapist and the energy field of the patient, as in many bodywork therapies. The subtlety of whole body evaluation allows the therapist access to areas of distortion and disruption both energetic and physical. The unique combination of bodywork with emotional release makes CST a whole-body and whole-person therapy, powerful, subtle, effective, especially with longstanding and poorly-defined conditions.

References

Becker, R.E. (1976) Craniosacral trauma in the adult. *Osteopath. Ann.*, (yearbook) 213–25.

Benor, D.J. (1994) *Healing Research: Holistic Energy Medicine and Spirituality*, Vol. 2. Deddington: Helix.

Blood, S.D. (1986) The craniosacral mechanism and the temporomandibular joint. *J. Am. Osteop. Ass.*, 86(8), 512–19.

Brookes, D. (1981) *Lectures on Cranial Osteopathy*. Northampton: Thorsons.

Cardoso, E.R., Rowan, J.O. and Galbraith, S. (1983) Analysis of the cerebrospinal fluid pulse wave in intracranial pressure. *J. Neurosurg.*, 59(5), 817–21.

Chaitow, L. (1998) *Cranial Manipulation: Theory and Practice*. Edinburgh: Churchill Livingstone.

Dunbar, H.S., Guthrie, T.C. and Karpell, B. (1966) A study of the cerebrospinal fluid pulse wave. *Arch. Neurol.*, 14, 624–30.

Feinberg, D.H. (1987) Human brain motion and cerebrospinal fluid circulation demonstrated with MRI imaging. *Radiology*, 163, 793–99.

Frymann, V. (1966) Relation of disturbances of craniosacral mechanisms to symptomatology of the newborn: study of 1250 infants. *J. Am. Osteop. Ass.*, 65, 1059–75.

Frymann, V. (1971) A study of the rhythmic motions of the living cranium. *J. Am. Osteop. Ass.*, 70, 928–45.

Greenman, P.E. and McPartland, J.M. (1995) Cranial findings and iatrogenesis from craniosacral manipulation in patients with traumatic brain syndrome. *J. Am. Osteop. Ass.*, 95(3), 182–92.

Hammerhoff, S.R. (1988) Coherence in the cytoskeleton: implications for biological information processing. In *Biological Coherence and Response to External Stimuli* (Fröhlich, H., ed.). Berlin: Springer-Verlag, pp. 242–63.

Heifetz, M.D. and Weiss, M. (1981) Detection of skull expansion with increased intracranial pressure. *J. Neurosurg.*, 55, 811–12.

Heisey, S.R. and Adams T. (1993) Role of cranial bone mobility in cranial compliance. *Neurosurgery*, 33(5), 869–77.

Hornstein, S. (1998) *Craniosacral Therapy: A Report on the Evidence*. Vancouver: British Columbia College of Physical Therapists.

Hubbard, R.P., Melvin, J.W. and Barodawala, I.T. (1971) Flexure of the cranial sutures. *J. Biomech.*, 4, 491–96.

Jaslow, C.R. (1990) Mechanical properties of cranial sutures. *J. Biomechan.*, 23(4), 313–21.

Kokich, V.G. (1976) Age changes in the frontozygomatic suture from 20 to 95 years. *Am. J. Orthodont.*, 69(4), 411–30.

Kostopoulos, D. and Keramidas, G. (1991) Changes in the magnitude of relative elongation of falx cerebri during the application of external forces on the frontal bone of an embalmed cadaver. *Phys. Ther. Forum*, 5 April, 9–12.

McPartland, J.M. (1996) Craniosacral iatrogenesis. *J. Bodywork Move. Ther.*, 1(1), 2–5.

Oschman, J.L. (1981) The connective tissue and myofascial systems. In *Readings on the Scientific Basis of Bodywork and Movement Therapies* (Oschman, J.L. and Oschman, H.H., eds). Dover, NH: NORA.

Oschman, J.L. (1987) The natural science of healing. In *Readings on the Scientific Basis of Bodywork and Movement Therapies*, 2nd edn (Oschman, J.L. and Oschman, H.H., eds). Dover, NH: NORA.

Oschman, J.L. (1993) Sensing solitons in soft tissue. *Guild News* (the news magazine for members of the Guild for Structural Integration), 3(2), 22–25; also in Oschman, J.L. and Oschman, H.H. (eds) (1997) *Readings on the Scientific Basis of Bodywork and Movement Therapies*, 2nd edn. Dover, NH: NORA.

Pitlyk, P.J., Piantanida, T.P. and Ploeger, D.W. (1985) Noninvasive pressure monitoring. *Neurosurgery*, 17(4), 581–84.

Pribram, K. (1969) The neurophysiology of remembering. *Sci. Am.*, 220, 75.

Rebbi, C. (1979) Solitons. *Sci. Am.*, 240(2), 92–116.

Retzlaff, E., Michael, D.K. and Roppel, R.M. (1975) Cranial bone mobility. *J. Am. Osteop. Ass.*, 74, 869–73.

Retzlaff, E., Upledger, J.E., Mitchell, F. Jr. and Biggert, T. (1976) Structure of cranial bone sutures. *J. Am. Osteop. Ass.*, 75(2), 123.

Retzlaff, E. and Mitchell, F. Jr. (eds) (1987) *The Cranium and its Sutures*. Berlin: Springer-Verlag.

Rogers, J.S. and Witt, P.L. (1997) The controversy of cranial bone notion. *J. Orthopaed. Sports Phys. Ther.*, 26(2), 95–103.

Schultz, R.L. and Feitis, R. (1996) *The Endless Web. Fascial Anatomy and Physical Reality*. Berkeley, CA: North Atlantic Books.

Spinero, G. (1931) *Anatomica Umana*, Vol. 1, p. 203.

Sutherland, W.C. (1990) *Teachings in the Science of Osteopathy*. Portland, OR: Rudra Press.

Sutherland, W.G. (1939) *The Cranial Bowl*. Mankato MN: Free Press.

Todd, T.W. and Lyon, D.W. (1924) Endocranial suture closure. *Am. J. Phys. Anthropol.*, 7, 325–84.

Todd, T.W. and Lyon, D.W. (1925) Cranial suture closure – its progress and age relationship, Pts II–IV. *Am. J. Phys. Anthropol.*, 8, 23–71, 149–68.

Upledger, J.E. (1990) *SomatoEmotional Release and Beyond*. Palm Beach, FL: UI Publishing.

Upledger, J.E. (1996) Response to cranial iatrogenesis. *J. Bodywork Move. Ther.*, 1(1), 6–8.

Upledger, J.E. (1997) *Your Inner Physician and You*. Berkeley, CA: North Atlantic Books.

Upledger, J.E. and Vredevoogd, J.D. (1983) *Craniosacral Therapy*. Seattle, WA: Eastland Press.

Warwick, R. and Williams, P.L. (1973) *Gray's Anatomy*, 35th edn. London: Longman.

The Feldenkrais Method

Jill Wigmore-Welsh

Introduction

This chapter is written to give physical therapists a basic overview of the Feldenkrais Method. It begins with a history of the man behind the method and continues with an introduction and theoretical background for the techniques used. Included is an example of an Awareness Through Movement Lesson (ATM) and some of the author's own case histories.

The history

The Feldenkrais Method gains its name from, and was devised by, Dr Moshe Feldenkrais (1904–1984). Moshe Feldenkrais was born in 1904, in a small Russian town called Baranovitz. When he was a teenager he emigrated, by himself, and worked as a pioneer in the country that was then called Palestine (now Israel). He lived by his skills, teaching mathematics and doing all manner of manual work. He also had a deep interest in all aspects of the martial arts, and taught and wrote about self-defence. When he was 23 he matriculated, and moved to France, where he studied at the Sorbonne. He read for a doctorate in physics. While he was attached to the laboratory of Joliot-Curie he met Professor Kano, the creator of judo, and with his help and with help from his pupils Yotazo Sigimura and Kawaishi, he gained his Black belt. His interest in the martial arts was such that he formed the first judo club in France.

Feldenkrais escaped to England during the war years, and worked in the British Admiralty until the end of World War II. While in London he trained at the Budokwai. Finally, after the war he returned to Israel to be the first director of the Electronic Department of the Defence Forces of Israel (Feldenkrais, 1981).

This historical perspective of a man who travelled by himself from Russia to Israel at the age of 14, who had made his own way, supported himself and continued studying throughout his life, give us a clue to the curiosity and passion which Feldenkrais demonstrated through his lifetime. In the 1940s, as well as working and teaching martial arts, Feldenkrais was also exploring psychology, psychoanalysis, anatomy and neurophysiology.

Judo was a foundation for the development of Feldenkrais's movement classes. However, judo is not merely a sport or game, it is a principle of life, art, science, a means for personal and cultural attainment (Fromm and Soames, 1982). Within the Feldenkrais Method is the use of the circle, and this use of a circle is implicit in virtually all judo techniques. Jigoro Kano, who was inspirational to Feldenkrais, developed Itsutsu-no-Kata, the Kata of the five principles, symbolizing a circular movement in nature (Fromm and Soames, 1982). While teaching movement classes, Feldenkrais used methods which had come directly from Kano's refinement of the martial arts tradition. When a student was unconsciously resistant to freely performing certain movements, Feldenkrais would go along with the holding pattern of resistance that the student habitually performed. This process can be perceived within Functional Integration, and is skilfully used by experienced practitioners. It is reflected within the sensing which is developed during an Awareness Through Movement Lesson (ATM).

As well as his background of teaching martial arts, pivotal in Feldenkrais's development of the method was a knee injury which occurred when he was playing soccer. Surgeons informed him that there was nothing that could be done to help him, but instead of accepting this advice he took it as an inspiration. He used his injury as a stimulus to motivate his curiosity about easy efficient use of the self. All of this, combined with his thorough knowledge of mechanics, was at the origin of his Awareness Through Movement.

By 1949, Feldenkrais had published several books, including one on judo. However, *Body and Mature Behaviour* (Feldenkrais, 1949), with its chapters on 'The antigravity mechanisms', 'Erect posture' and 'Action', may be highly interesting reading for physical therapists. Here, his references to the practice of judo concomitant with his descriptions of physics principles demonstrate his core interests. At the conclusion of this early book he draws a clear distinction between

> . . . conditioning in animals and learning in men, as well as between adaptation, which is an evolutionary process correlating whole species to an environment, and adjustment through which individuals fit themselves to particular circumstances of a more temporary nature. (Feldenkrais, 1949)

The paragraphs below, taken from Feldenkrais (1981), illustrate the fundamental principles evolved in Feldenkrais's approach:

> To help ourselves, the victims of the passing social order, it is essential to realise fully that emotional instability and behaviour disorders are the result of faulty and exaggerated technique of habit formation. Even the motor activity, which is the centre of all activity, has been shown in the preceding pages to be considerably different in men and formed by the personal adjustment to the actual social and physical environment. In the ultimate analysis it is

little different from other habit formations. Radical changes cannot be expected without reforming muscular and postural habits. Indigestion, faulty breathing, crooked toes and feet, faulty sexual behaviour, postural rigidity and muscular tension go together with emotional disorders. The whole self, diet, breathing, sex, muscular and postural habits, must be tackled directly and concurrently with the emotional reduction.

> It should start with muscular and postural reduction . . . the whole procedure is that of adult re-education and not treatment . . . it is a question of teaching and learning and not of disease and cure. (Feldenkrais, 1981)

This procedure of teaching and learning as continuous evolution is witnessed in Professional Feldenkrais Trainings. Students accepted for training have a wide variety of backgrounds, professions and occupations. Because of this diversity of attitudes and beliefs the method continues to grow and develop to this day. Each practitioner is encouraged to develop and use the method in their own way, without losing the fundamental theories of the work. Through this approach the biomedical, scientific reductionist approach to health as absence of sickness or disease, is superceded by an encouragement for individuals to develop their own potential.

Introduction

The Feldenkrais Method is a behavioural-cognitive approach to learning. It is a means of enabling individuals to rediscover movements and parts of their body which may have become forgotten or excluded from their established actions or representations of behaviour. It is a 'power-with' approach: the practitioner and the student work together, an empowering process for the student. The student chooses which aspects of themselves they wish to explore, and the practitioner acts as a facilitator. The practitioner does not seek to correct the student, but to enable the student to learn. Practitioners take a stance which is congruous with the individual's own pattern of being. A student thus feels supported and safe, the environment non-threatening, encouraging free exploration. The individual's own patterns of being are first explored and, through the student accepting their own individuality, a sense of embodiment can be developed.

Learning is a creative process, with curiosity at the core. The state of mind which encourages a process of inquiry differs from wanting the right answers. In the author's experience, a physiotherapy training often leads therapists to search for the right technique, the right approach to correct dysfunctions. The body is often viewed as a machine to be fixed, with the therapist the mechanic. However, if individuals are given the answer, if something is fixed without an understanding of why that place caused distress, then a 'correction' has been made. When individuals are corrected, the fun of finding out has been lost, and an opportunity for learning missed.

Part of the process for individuals learning about how they have reached the point where they are at today is not by correcting, but by encouraging, individual self-exploration. Many forms of therapy aimed at the mind have this form of self-exploration as a first step. This stimulates the individual's natural animal curiosity. Visit any zoo, and you will see that the animals are given toys to play with. Humans are animals: we learn through exploration, through curiosity. However, what are your own memories of learning? Which teachers can you recall stimulating your learning? Within the Feldenkrais Method, in contrast to the classic therapy role, the practitioner does not provide packaged 'answers'. Instead, within a sequence of movements the student is offered many options and subtle opportunities to learn.

Our body is our home, and the place called home is usually considered to be the place where we are secure. However, most individuals dislike their own bodies; they separate themselves from their bodies. Embodiment and self-knowledge are interlinked and a sense of embodiment can lead to an acceptance that individuals have and are bodies.

Everybody has their own beliefs, attitudes, habits and patterns which enable individuals to cope with the challenges of everyday change. Feldenkrais believed that many problems with patterns of anxiety reproduce themselves in the body, and it is only through a safe exploration that individuals feel able to learn, and relearn, new options. If someone is forcibly taken away from their home, if a change is forced upon them, it can be distressing. Within the author's experiences as a therapist in a therapeutic setting, individuals continuously seek to return to what they know. Recent revivals of interest in muscle strengthening and balancing approaches frequently ignore the fundamental that movement is more than just a learned pattern. Movement is behaviour, and part of personality. The Feldenkrais Method provides individuals with the opportunity to explore and learn about themselves through movement.

The method of the Method

An individual choosing to attend for lessons in the Feldenkrais Method will encounter two terms: Functional Integration (FI) and Awareness Through Movement (ATM). These terms are used to describe the two main techniques which Feldenkrais practitioners use with their students. They are complementary parts of a somatic learning system whose medium is kinaesthesia. Kinaesthetic awareness is fundamental to our development (Laszlo and Bairstow, 1985) and by focusing attention on their patterns, subjects can learn to organize themselves to achieve increased clarity, ease and economy of use.

Functional Integration

Functional Integration is a one to one method. The teacher gently guides the student, physically, through patterns of movement. Sometimes verbal feedback is given, but the lesson gives a valuable opportunity for the student to experience and sense what their body does. Each lesson is composed for the individual, and involves subtle touch and direction. During the lesson the student is able to feel their own relative patterns of holding, to discover which areas of the body are included in their image.

FI enables the student to develop their own internal awareness through sensing and feeling. It is very safe because the practitioner moves with the student. They dance together. During the 4-year experiential training to become a practitioner, individuals learn about their own patterns. Thus the Feldenkrais practitioner is aware that there are many options for movements and being. Because the method is designed to enable the student to learn, one of the first principles is to provide comfort. Initially the student is positioned safely, perhaps using foams or rollers, with their patterns of self use supported. In later lessons the purpose of the lesson may change to enable the student to learn how to deal with the discomforts of everyday living. Rollers and blocks take on a different role, to act as supports to position the student's body. The practitioner frequently uses a specially-designed table and takes great care over his/her own organization. Unlike many therapy techniques where the comfort of the therapist is not considered, within the Feldenkrais Method ease of use is paramount. The weight of the practitioner and student is transmitted through the teacher's skeleton. Great care of the self is taken because even a subtle sense of imbalance within the teacher's organization can transmit to the student. Therefore the practitioner is able to move the student with effortless ease. The weight of the leg, trunk, and head may be lifted with virtually no strain and minimal expenditure of energy with maximum efficiency. Directions and pressures are aligned to give a skeleton-to-skeleton contact, directing the action from the contact with the ground. The practitioner takes a neutral, non-opinionated approach, not focusing directly upon areas of dis-ease.

During the lesson the student stays fully clothed; the practitioner is trained to observe patterns without needing to ask the student to undress. Lessons may focus on a particular function, action, anything which the student requests. This will vary from individual to individual. An athlete may be interested in learning how to move more powerfully, someone with degenerative joint disease may be interested in learning how to lie down without pain, while others may want to know more about developing their creativity, balance and flexibility. There are applications within the whole spectrum of human learning from disability and therapeutics to creative arts.

Hence, to understand FI beyond the aspect of it as a technique, means to accept it as a way of thinking about the learning process, psychology, self-image, self-education, self-direction, self-maintenance and so on. The title 'Functional Integration' gives a broader meaning to the word 'function'. Function may just be understood on the level of everyday movements, which can lead to satisfaction of basic needs and wants. However, function is not just about getting along or managing life to the end, it is about knowing oneself and leading a life which frees one's potential. Bringing into fruition one's curiosities, inspirations, projects and visions or, perhaps, leading to a state of self-acceptance. Motor functions, for example lifting the arm, may be performed in many ways, involving different joints, muscles, and with different intents. For example, lifting the arm to caress a loved one will be a very different action from lifting the arm in self-defence. Each is performed with a pattern of emotion influencing the use of self. Over time, patterns of movement become learned, and therefore the possibilities for performing a movement may become limited. Where a pattern of lifting could have been associated with protecting, that pattern of protecting may become a way of being. How many folk recognize their own ways of repeating patterns throughout their lives. Have you ever noticed a similarity between the friends you choose? The relationships you form? The words and syntax of your sentences? However, that aside, *Homo sapiens* has a great learning potential for the body to call back into use long-forgotten, or excluded, patterns of movement.

Awareness Through Movement

The other way in which individuals may encounter the method is through classes. ATM classes are verbally directed movement sequences primarily presented to groups. The lessons are highly structured, but emphasize the experience rather than the goal. They can be based upon developmental movements, functional activities or abstract explorations of joint, muscle and postural relationships. The lessons may start with gentle, comfortable, easy movements that gradually evolve into more complex ranges and movements. They are fun, and provide the student with an opportunity to explore by themselves. There is virtually no demonstration; each student is encouraged to find their own way. Unlike an aerobics, or step, class there is no teacher standing at the front demonstrating. Instead, the students are often placed with gravity eliminated, lying on the front, side or back. The instructions are given verbally, and although the classes often follow quite well-defined structures, the teacher attends to each student. Verbal instructions are directed to allow each student to progress and experience each step of the class without direct correction. Sometimes, audiotapes can be used, either at home or as a follow-up to attending classes. These can enhance physical and perceptual changes (Kegerreis and Ruth, 1992), but are most effective when the student already has some experience of the method.

During ATM lessons, constraints such as unusual skeletal configurations, unusual movement goals and proximity to the floor are introduced, and students explore their workspace. This type of exploration can lead to discovery of new types of movement forms or solutions. ATM is similar to FI, except that in an FI lesson the student is taken through the movement steps passively and in class the student explores dynamically. Within both ATM and FI lessons the teacher wishes to stimulate a learning experience. However, many lessons and classes can be restful and students may fall asleep. Nevertheless, every situation provides an opportunity for learning, and certainly the author soon realized that perhaps arriving at class tired could be a reason for falling asleep!

Feldenkrais spent many years developing his movement sequences. From the early 1950s to late 1970s he taught eight weekly public classes in Tel Aviv. In this way alone, over a period of 25 years, he perfected and recorded nearly 600 different lessons. Currently, thousands of planned lessons have been devised and have evolved as teachers introduce different approaches. Creating classes is an art form, with the complexity of an orchestrated piece of music.

An Awareness Through Movement lesson

This lesson is taken from the author's series of audio cassettes entitled 'The Thinking Body Series'. Working in clinic with people who have low back pain this lesson can be combined particularly effectively with strength and stability work for the base of the spine. Thus it can form a bridge between a prescriptive exercise session and an ATM class.

Lie on your back, and sense the contact you make. Observe where your back touches the floor, where your weight rests. Is your weight resting evenly on the surface beneath you? Do you feel a pressure or weight more on one side or the other of your back? What is it that you can use as a landmark, a way of knowing how one side of you is resting on the floor? Sense the heaviness, lightness, regularity of the weight. Now do this with your pelvis, then your rib cage. Take as much time as you wish to explore in your senses, the back surface of yourself. Really get to know your variations in pressure, weight and contact. Now bring your attention to your low back, what is the contact like here? Is there a part of your spine and back which is lifted away from the floor. Sense the shape of your low back. Where does the pressure start and finish? In your imagination could you draw this shape? Now, in your imagination, take a thick pen and draw the line of the low part of your back on a sheet of paper. What shape is it? Imagine the drawn line, and then to detect whether what you sensed in yourself is accurate you can check with your hand beneath you. How does your low back shape, what is the contact? Is it the same as you imagined? Is it more or less flattened? Now bring your attention to the back of your neck, again sense the contact which you are making at the back of your head, and then down into the ribcage. Again, mentally draw this shape and then once it is clear feel with your hand to compare the contact and get to know it intimately.

So now you have an image and a sense of your low back and neck, keeping these landmarks in mind bend up your knees and position your legs so that your feet are flat on the floor and the knees directly over them. Find an easy place where the foot supports the knee. Now in this position, with the legs bent, allow your knees to gently drop down to the right. Observe what you do. Do you strain to try to get your knees to the floor? Do you stress yourself and hold your breath? Notice how it feels to move your legs to the right. What happens in the rest of your body? What about your pelvis, does it roll, do you feel a movement in your ribs? Your head? Your neck? If you have back pain then take care to avoid straining, avoid your pain. Explore and find just how many ways you can move the legs to the side. Then leave it and rest.

Then once again return to this knees bent position and gently draw in the low abdomen, place one hand on the low belly and feel the muscles draw in. Allow yourself to contract your muscles this way without holding your breath, and then repeat the movement of dropping the knees to the right side. Observe how you do this, does this make a change to the way your legs move? How your rib cage and pelvis feel? Compare tightening the belly a few times and dropping the knees then leave the belly soft a few times and drop the knees. Sense the difference, is there a difference? Then draw your attention to your legs. As the legs are moving to the side are they staying close together as if tied to each other or do they move with their own life? Try just dropping the right leg, feel how it drops to the right. Now allow the pelvis to move to the right with the leg and feel where the left knee goes. What is the difference between the knees dropping as if tied together, and allowing the knees to move separately? What happens to your left side, can it lengthen? Compare these two movements. First the knees move together, then apart. Do the legs both take the same flight? Imagine a pencil attached to the right knee, what line does the pencil draw, where does it go? What about the left knee?

Now rest and digest, allow your legs to be long, sense how these movements have affected your contact with the floor. Spend a little time sensing yourself and how you feel after moving this way.

Once again return to the bent knee configuration, and imagine that you have a pencil attached to the tip of your right knee. The pencil is sticking right out from the tip of the knee towards the ceiling. Now gently, first in your imagination then in action, begin to draw a circle with the pencil on the ceiling. Move smoothly, languidly, and easily. Discover what different size circles you can draw. Where is it easy to move, which quadrant of the circle? Allow yourself to help with a gentle pressure through your foot on the floor. Repeat in both directions, exploring and allowing the pelvis to become involved. Now repeat this on the other knee, repeat the imagining, exploring the ease and fluidity of moving within your comfortable easy pattern. Now rest with your legs long and sense how your contact feels. Has this made any difference to the way you contact the floor?

Then return to the first movement of moving your knees to the side and sense how the movement feels now, compare again by including the tightening of the low abdomen. Now lengthen your legs and sense how your body contacts the floor. Check through your landmarks, are they the same? What has doing this work done to the contact you make with the floor? This same lesson can be done at different times of day, and through building up a bigger picture of your back's landscape on the floor, you may find a way to learn more about how you use yourself.

Case histories

Case history 1

Nick is 38, a clerical worker who is passionate about football and refereeing. He was referred by his orthopaedic consultant. He had been told that he should give up refereeing. He had pain after every match and had missed many matches. After reviewing the options available, my choice of approach was to work with Nick on his movement. He stood with an alert posture, as if ready to spring into action. His eyes were bright and his manner a little uncertain. When he walked, his patterns demonstrated a reliance on his ankle joints. Soon after starting to run his pain started. He was asthmatic and tended to wheeze when he ran. His muscle tone was pronounced, especially in the lower limbs. Over the next few weeks we worked together on his patterns of breathing and movement, using exploration and 'homework' tapes. Nick was a keen student, quickly taking interest in his own patterns and demonstrating an accurate ability to observe himself. He noticed that when he ran he kept his chest tight. His whole musculoskeletal system would tighten in sympathy. His wife was supportive; she noticed changes more quickly than Nick himself. As time progressed, his patterns of increased tone began to change. As he learned more about what he was doing, he became able to make the changes himself. Six months later, at the start of the next season, he wanted to referee again. He completed his training and has gone on to complete one, relatively pain-free season, and has now embarked on another. He still attends periodically for lessons.

Case history 2

The G's own a breeding and livery yard, Simon had fallen and sustained a painful ribcage. His acute strains responded to laser treatment. However, after the pain had settled it was apparent that he was restricted in his side flexion and rotation to the left. There was no apparent sign of injury, so we reviewed him and his horse. The horse also showed signs of limitation in bending to the near foreleg. Her neck was restricted, and it was not possible to take her chin to her chest. When Simon sat on the horse, the problems became more apparent. Simon was sitting over onto one sitting bone, and he found it particularly difficult to bend the horse around jumps. We worked with Simon on the horse, increasing his awareness of his sitting bones. As he became more balanced, and the weight more centred, so he found the horse easier to bend. Bringing his attention to the area in his thoracic spine, he was able to feel that allowing this part to move would translate through to the horse. After one more lesson both horse and rider were able to move more in tune with each other and have continued in competition. Movement has changed within horse and rider. Simon is still occasionally in contact for new lessons.

Conclusion

Training in the Feldenkrais Method is gaining popularity among health professionals worldwide. Nevertheless, the paradigms supporting biomedicine and Feldenkrais are divergent. The method is thought to work by imprinting new movement patterns into the central nervous system and motor cortex of the brain. Claimed benefits of the method are said to be increased awareness and ability to learn (Feldenkrais, 1949; Sharfarman, 1997), improvements in posture (Feldenkrais, 1985), changes in pain and feelings of well-being (Aum, 1996; Sharfarman, 1997; Little, 1997).

In Germany, Australia and America, studies on particular client groups using the Feldenkrais method have been published. Some studies have shown that increased range and ease of movement occur after individuals have practised Awareness Through Movement (ATM) classes (Kegerreis and Ruth, 1992). There are few contraindications to the method; the work is gentle and

within the individual's own patterns of behaviour. This method has much to offer any individual who wants to discover more about themselves.

This chapter has been written to provide a summary overview of the Feldenkrais Method. Perhaps the reader will take this as a starting point. Like any child who has been given a musical instrument, the student is encouraged to experiment with the many tapes and books available. However, although it is possible to experiment and learn alone, it is usually easier to learn to play wonderful music if one has an experienced teacher.

Acknowledgement

A special thank you to Timothy and Harriet, for their inspiration and support.

References

Aum, L. (1996) As young as you feel. *Yoga Hlth.*, July, 32–34.

Feldenkrais, M. (1949) *Body and Mature Behaviour*. Madison, CT: International Universities Press.

Feldenkrais, M. (1981) *The Elusive Obvious*. Capitola, CA: Meta Publications.

Feldenkrais, M. (1985) *The Potent Self*. San Francisco: Harper.

Fromm, A. and Soames, N. (1982) *Judo – The Gentle Way*. London: Routledge and Kegan Paul.

Kegerreis, R.S. (1992) Facilitating cervical flexion using a Feldenkrais Method; awareness through movement. *J. Orthopaed. Sports Phys. Ther.*, **16**(1): 25–29.

Laszlo, J. and Bairstow, P. (1985) *Perceptual-Motor Behaviour, Developmental Assessment and Therapy*. New York: Holt.

Little, T. (1997) The Feldenkrais Method; application, practice and principles. *J. Bodywork Move. Ther.*, October, 262–69.

Shafarman, S. (1997) *Awareness Heals: The Feldenkrais Method for Dynamic Health*. Reading, MA: Addison-Wesley.

Recommended reading

Feldenkrais, M. (1972) *Awareness Through Movement; Health Exercises for Personal Growth*. London: Arkana Penguin Books.

Feldenkrais, M. (1977) *The Case of Nora*. Tel Aviv: Harper and Row.

Feldenkrais, M. (1984) *The Master Moves*. Capitola, CA: Meta Publications.

12 Prenatal therapy, Metamorphosis and the Metamorphic Technique

Christine Jones and Hermione Evans

And therefore as a stranger, give it welcome.
There are more things in heaven and earth,
Horatio, than are dreamt of in your
philosophy. (*Hamlet*, William Shakespeare)

Introduction

To attempt to present Metamorphosis for a text
specifically directed to the physical therapist in
an age of 'evidence-based practice' is indeed a
challenge. The first hurdle is one of title. Is it a
technique, a defined therapy, a process, or
simply 'metamorphosis'?

In recent years the training of the health care
professionals has been directed to the analytical.
As such, it may be increasingly difficult to
explain the often unexpected and apparently
inexplicable response to gentle touch, unless
one accepts the interwoven, interconnectedness
of the body/mind and of the electromagnetic
network of all living forms.

Metamorphosis probably presents one of the
greatest challenges for the scientific mind, but to
be introduced to the process is usually a most
humbling experience. To have had this experience, and to witness the process of metamorphosis in the clinic and during courses, is most
thought-provoking. The approach insists on
'locate', 'acknowledge' and 'let be', in order to
allow only the individual's healing process to
proceed without any desires or expectations on
the part of the practitioner. It insists that the
practitioner must only support in a non-
attached manner, thus allowing any manner of
change, any time, anywhere, to come from the
recipient. And that is how it has to be in the
philosophy of metamorphosis.

It is a useful, and probably essential, exercise
to put the new learning into practice with a willing friend/colleague and commit oneself and the
philosophy to trial with regular sessions, to
inwardly reflect and evaluate the outcome
from a personal understanding. Personal experience is the best teacher, and courses which
encourage this process are invaluable in the
progress, health and balance of the therapist.
Flexibility is essential but also – a word of
caution before reading further – testing the principles, applying them in practice and observing
the effects of this approach will almost certainly
alter one's attitude to therapy and possibly to life
itself.

History and principles

Metamorphosis

The *Concise Oxford Dictionary* (1976) definition is 'to transform, change between immature
form and adult', and the *Collins English Dictionary* (1991) defines it as a 'complete change
of physical form or substance, character, appearance etc'. Robert St John (1979) refers to metamorphosis as

a method of approaching the prenatal or formative period of life. This is brought into focus, loosened and changed . . . a purely physical application which can initiate a complete metamorphosis of the attitudes to life and modes of living . . . a loosening of time and a releasing of the holds in time and a final freeing resulting in a natural and spontaneous removal of the barriers of consciousness and the use of the erstwhile faculties of the psychic.

Metamorphosis, or Prenatal Therapy

This technique was the innovative concept of Robert St John (RSJ), an English naturopath who, during the 1960s, became dissatisfied when he found that the beneficial effects of naturopathy were not sustained and seemed to have limited effect on mental stresses and emotional disorders. He considered that the majority of illness was created by inner mind stresses. He had a particular interest in autism and Down's syndrome, but noted that to a greater or lesser degree, within every person there was a variance in the tendency to be 'earthed' i.e. the tendency between being a thinker or a doer. Expressions such as 'air head' and 'down to earth' also acknowledge, perhaps subconsciously, these tendencies.

Reflexology was explored and found to be beneficial, although the improved health was not always sustained even though lifestyles had been adjusted. RSJ also noted correspondences of emotional and mental attitudes associated with the areas requiring attention, and superimposed a psychological profile on the physical reflexology chart. He was interested to find where the individual's problem originated. He noted that infant tendencies seemed to last into adulthood and considered that the gestation period could hold the answer. As the fetus develops from head to toe as the craniocaudal, manifested in the spine, he came to form his theory that the reflected spinal pattern along the medial border in the feet, hands and head (as described in reflextherapy) would reflect fetal development, a memory of the gestation period, together with the characteristics of the individual's personality. Investigating, he found

that it was as though different areas of the spine related to different time spans and influences during the gestation period. Thus the craniocaudal development (head to toe) in reflextherapy terms would be reflected from the great toe (head) to the heel (toe). The reflected spinal pathway by the side of the great toe was found to relate to the greater influence of the father at the time of conception and was termed the 'Father Principle', whereas by contrast, the part of the spinal pathway reflected in the heel, i.e. the pelvis, was found to contain what he called the 'Mother Principle' and was related to what happened to the child and/or the mother as a result of experiences previous to, and at the time of, birth. Thus the memories of the patterns of development during the time of gestation were laid down from the great toe (conception), to the heel (birth). Any influences beneficial or unfavourable to the healthy physical, emotional, mental and spiritual development of the fetus, would be held in the spinal memory and would begin, in turn, to influence the characteristics or tendencies of that individual's personality.

A hypothetical example might be as follows. A mother, fearing the actual birth process, could transmit that fear to her unborn child who, in turn, depending on the confidence and maturity developed during the previous stages of gestation (Figure 12.1), may begin to fear making the transition from the known safety of the womb to the unknown and possibly alien external environment. There may then develop a late or difficult birth. This lateness or difficulty in progressing through life's milestones, e.g. difficulty in 'earthing' (observed when the person with, or tending towards, autism will walk on the toes, so not 'earthing' through the heels), starting school, leaving home, changing jobs, may become a pattern of personality set down prior to and at birth and may inhibit the individual from achieving his or her potential in spiritual, mental, emotional or physical dimensions. RSJ called this a 'Block in Time'. Prenatal Therapy, in the metamorphic approach, is designed to allow the release of these time blocks in development to enable the individual to move forward from the restrictive patterns. This approach is simply a form of working with the principles of causation, but RSJ realized the correspondences.

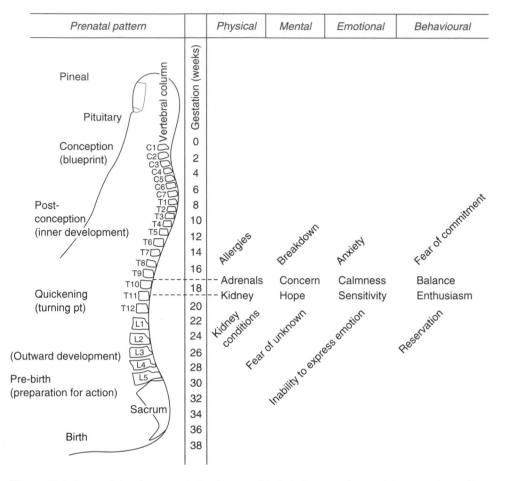

Figure 12.1 Prenatal development, indicating possible imbalance and potential connections with the Law of Five Elements

The principle of correspondence

The interrelatedness of all universal life forms and the mind is not a new concept. Eastern philosophy appreciates the integral relationships of all forms of universal energy. In this philosophy, The Law of Five Elements or Stages of Transition give substance to the interconnectedness of nature and that of the body/mind, linking emotional and mental attitudes to specific parts of all the physical body, giving rise to such connections as the 'irritable, liverish' person, or to 'vent one's spleen'. These laws link the health and balance of the individual with the twenty-four hour clock and the seasonal variations. Thus the person with 'liverish tendencies' may wake at 3 a.m. and find that unresolved

thoughts prevent further sleep. He/she will be worse in the morning and in the spring, until the body energies are brought into a better balance. Eastern philosophy considers ill-health to be out of harmony with nature.

Quantum physics also proposes theories on energy, which not only describe the material world in terms of energy–matter interchangeability, but also the influence of the mind and the interwoven body and mind relationship. Pythagorus (*c*.570–500 BC) searched for meaning in the physical and metaphysical worlds mainly through mathematics, whereas Plato (*c*.429–347 BC) claimed that the human intellect was not related to the material world, maintaining that mind, not matter, was the root of all reality.

RSJ called this interconnectedness the 'Correspondence Principle'. Following from this he postulated that where the human being or animal was concerned the skeleton, and in particular the spine, as the central most compact material, has therefore the greatest potential energy. He maintained it represented the primary patterns of life containing the genetic traits, the karmic patterns and all other factors present at conception and from which life begins. RSJ believed that the spine should be the focus for Prenatal Therapy. He also postulated that the three forms of activity, '*thinking*', '*doing*' and '*going*', were related to stages of gestation and contained within the patterns, in particular the head (thinking), and shoulder and pelvic girdles (doing and going), as these were the main body regions involved with these processes. Moreover, soft tissues allow movement, flexibility and change within the physical body and RSJ recognized that these phenomena correlate with the continuous movement and change of the mind itself. Thus he found correspondences between muscles, ligaments, fascia, skin and the mind itself. Increasingly, physiotherapists are considering more in-depth psychological links to muscles, ligaments, facial sheaths and organs of the 'physical body'. These somato-emotional relationships are particularly important in acupuncture, reflextherapy and cranial-sacral therapy. Spinal adjustments and massage may also facilitate unexpected emotional release which, on reflection, is identified with a particular traumatic event, tension or dis-order. RSJ further surmised that the fluids, blood, lymph, spinal fluids and water corresponded to the emotional aspects of the individual (from the Latin *emovere*, to move out), the emotional drive giving direction and expansion to the mental and spiritual consciousness. Such emotional responses are clearly observed in the sweaty palms, irritable bladder and in blushing, which often accompany nerve-racking situations such as exams or interviews.

The right side of the body, neurologically managed by the left brain, is expressed in Eastern philosophy as housing the more Yang tendencies, as it is energized by the morning sun in the customary practice of aligning to the east. Yang tends to be more masculine, logical, active and conscious in nature. Thus physical problems involving the right side of the body are seen to reflect those more 'Yang tendencies'. They may also be related to more recent issues. They tend to reflect the more explosive emotions and reactions and also reflect male influences and authority, for example the father, brother, son, male employer.

Conversely, the left side, managed by the right brain, is seen to mirror or reflect the more sensitive, deeper aspects and memories of the individual. Eastern philosophy acknowledges this as Yin. Therefore, the tissues in the left side carry within them the more Yin tendencies, deeper, sensitive thoughts and feelings. These may be of unconscious, past, deep sorrows or dormant patterns. The tissues of the left side tend to reflect the reactions to the feminine influences of the mother, sister, daughter.

RSJ saw the shape, texture and any 'abnormalities' of the tissues such as corns and calluses of the feet, hands, head and spine not only due to ill-fitting shoes and clothing but as a mirror of the restrictions of the mind blocked or limited in motivation and action. Support for these theories is expressed in the ancient science of chirology (the study of hands), in which the shape of the hands and nails as well as the depth, length and direction of the lines are recognized as indicative of the characteristics, desires and direction of the inherited traits as well as the individual's own conscious or unconscious desires.

Hence, the mind and body are appreciated in their entire integral interconnectedness, one immediately reflecting the other, and are approached as such, but without fixed analysis, only to locate the 'block', acknowledge the problem and let be of any direction for therapeutic results. This follows the assumption that, for example, within an acorn there is the blueprint of the perfect oak tree, within the caterpiller there is the blueprint for the perfect butterfly, and within the person is the blueprint for a perfect being. Each will mature in its own manner according to its own inbuilt code. The therapist is purely a catalyst to facilitate this normal process.

Prenatal Therapy to Metamorphosis

RSJ realized that Prenatal Therapy was only thought to be applicable to the time of pregnancy. He felt that this was too limiting and changed the name to 'Metamorphosis', indicating that this was an approach to life at any time, any age and also useful in the terminal stages of illness or the natural life span, giving increased quality to the process of dying.

Metamorphosis describes the process which occurs within the recipient facilitated by the practitioner, the latter working with the prenatal pattern as the representation of the gestation period when the weaknesses and strengths were first established. The principles apply to the entire process of development throughout life, each experience 'memorized' within the connected tissues.

Figure 12.2 indicates the reflected gestation period in the feet and hands, each indicative of moving and executing actions throughout life in metamorphic terms, the success of which is influenced by the maturity of development at the appropriate stage of gestation.

Sessions via feet, hands, head and spine

Sessions take the philosophy into practical application, that is to locate, acknowledge, but let be, any preconceived ideas which may have crept into the analytical mind. All direction must come from the recipient without prompting. This takes some discipline on the part of the practitioner. Strange at first, but it becomes surprisingly refreshing and then illuminating as the recipient takes charge of their process of change in all manner of ways, possibly developing unsuspected strengths in body or mind where negativity and sickness had prevailed. The position of the practitioner to the recipient is non-intrusive, that is, not 'eye to eye'. The recipient may be reclining or in any suitably comfortable position.

The area to be 'treated' is well supported, with the practitioner able to access the reflected spinal patterns in the medial border of the feet or hands, the central sulcus of the cranium or directly on the spine. The process takes the form of non-invasive or analytical assessment of any abnormalities along the appropriate

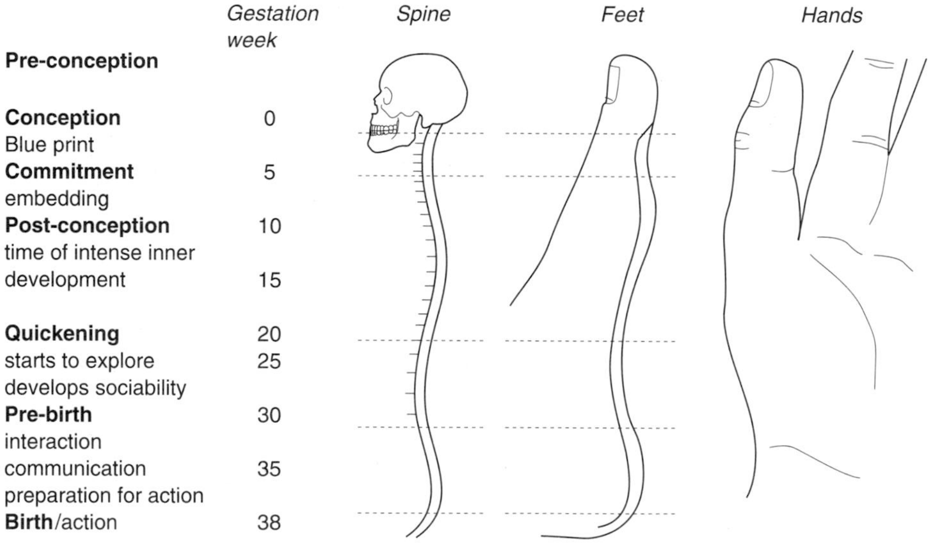

	Gestation week	Spine	Feet	Hands
Pre-conception				
Conception	0			
Blue print				
Commitment	5			
embedding				
Post-conception	10			
time of intense inner				
development	15			
Quickening	20			
starts to explore	25			
develops sociability				
Pre-birth	30			
interaction				
communication	35			
preparation for action				
Birth/action	38			

Figure 12.2 The prenatal pattern in the spine and as reflected in the feet and hands

areas. These may be mentally noted, but essentially the information is cleared from the mind, so as not to fix or confuse any possible change arising from the recipient, whether of a conscious or non-conscious nature.

The technique is simply applied, the practitioner lightly touching or massaging along the spinal reflected areas in a non-invasive manner, occasionally moving laterally to facilitate possible outward expression and movement. The sessions are usually limited to 1 hour per week and divided between feet, hands and head or maybe directly on the spine if preferred by the recipient. Usually the feet are approached first, the right foot containing the more conscious information of the present time, followed by the left with the deeper more dormant and potential patterns to allow movement of change in different time scales. This order may change, particularly with children, who seem to have their own healing ability more freely available than the conditioned adult. Subsequent to the initial treatment session, the recipient, not the therapist, decides which areas are to be 'treated' and also decides the interval between sessions.

Case histories

Undoubtedly, the only way to appreciate the nature of Metamorphosis is to see it in action and it is hoped that the following case histories will illustrate the main features.

Case history 1

Ian, 19 years old, was referred by his pastoral minister who had personally attended several reflextherapy talks and treatment sessions. Ian had had a 'mental breakdown' for over 2 years and had received considerable counselling from psychiatrists, psychologists and his pastor. His breakdown took the form of obsessive behaviour in hand-washing and the inability to continue a task after the initial stages; for example, he would fill the kettle but was unable to light the gas, or he could take the garden fork as far as the site but was unable to continue to dig. He had been very disturbed by a sermon on Original Sin two years previously. He felt that he had lived his life to date as another person and that his real self was trapped tightly inside his chest and was trying to break out.

As he was without problems physically, although facially pale, metamorphosis seemed to be the only appropriate approach, and counselling seemed almost contraindicated. Ian had no knowledge of reflextherapy or metamorphosis, nor why he had been sent to a physiotherapist.

Session 1: Commencing with light touch on the medial side of the right heel (RSJ's allotted birth area, to be found on both heels, but it is usual to start on the more conscious, less traumatic in intensity). This produced an active withdrawal and howl of pain; Ian explained that it was not the heel but the emotional pain that the touch had facilitated. He disclosed his traumatic birth in which, during the first stage of labour, he had disengaged and positioned himself high under his mother's diaphragm. A week later, after all manner of encouragement by medical intervention, he was suctioned out and placed in intensive care for a week with very little handling. The extent of other gestation patterns in his feet were not obvious at this first session. In practical physiotherapy fashion, swimming and active exercise were discussed, initiated by Ian.

Session 2: Ian was eager to proceed with more sessions and asked about each foot area as he felt it to be sticky, hot, cold, or numb to the touch. Ian was very enthusiastic about his swimming progress, as previously he had never had the courage to loose from the handrail and swim by himself. He also mentioned that as a toddler he was walking for nearly a year before he let go of his mother's hand.

Sessions 3–6 continued in a similar manner. At each, the disturbance in the patterns became more obvious and a main area of need was found in the early stages of gestation in the medial border of the proximal phalanx of the great toe (RSJ's area of commitment to the ongoing process of gestation, interestingly portrayed in Ian's 'breakdown' when he was unable to commit himself to the task in hand). Ian was now swimming and diving freely, but still felt trapped inside his chest and portraying another rather than his true self. Prior to the next session, Ian called in and insisted on a meeting. He was laughing uncontrollably – he was free, and was no longer Ian, he was to be called James. As he calmed down he described how he felt as though his chest would burst, and then felt it doing so, and then he felt freed from his wrong identity. He was so excited that he was oblivious to the fact that he had fallen off his bike in his enthusiasm to tell the world and he had knocked out two front teeth.

The sessions during the next months were very progressive but support was greatly necessary as Ian/James went through all the stages of child development because he had never felt natural emotions such as anger or love, having always portrayed the perfect child. He now felt the pain as a late teenager.

He retained communication when he took up his deferred place at university and returned at intervals when he felt the need; for example, when he went through the emotional pain of leaving his mother, as he had not allowed himself to feel such anxiety as a toddler, or anger when his new-found love decided to go with another. Ian/James came to realize that all these emotions were normal, but that he was experiencing them for the first time. Essentially, only his questions were reflected, allowing him to develop in his own timing so not to confuse him. Metamorphosis on feet, hands and head, and occasionally directly on the spine, was continued as, how and when he felt each need.

He changed from his chosen degree of physics (previously selected because he would be held in good stead in the community) to psychology. This became too much in light of his extensive counselling history and Ian/James took some time out with practical apprenticeship in catering and gardening. He is currently training as a physical therapist, having established himself as a person in his own right.

Case history 2

Request by a mother (ex-nurse) for treatment for her son with 'some coordination problems' (a gross understatement). John, 5 years old, diagnosed at 6 months as having tuberous sclerosis, an hereditary disease resulting in a developmental abnormality, in his case the brain, causing mental retardation. He was autistic and epileptic. John had extreme behaviour problems and was continuously disruptive and uneducable, but physically strong and able. His vocabulary consisted of 'No!', which was fairly continuous, while he ran amok with very limited heel gait. His family were knowledgeable, compassionate, stretched to the limit with his unsociable behaviour, and desperately concerned for his future as he became stronger and more violent.

Session 1: As John seemed unable to be still, the only approach was to follow him. Surprisingly, he elected to lie on the treatment couch and stretched his legs and feet to receive an approach which, in view of his complex and traumatic history, could only be gentle and minimal, so as not to facilitate an epileptic fit. In reflextherapy terms, the reflected brain pathways are mirrored in the toes and to be avoided until the individual's response can be assessed. A few minutes of gentle massage around the calcaneus (RSJ's birth, mother, earthing) was accepted, and extension of this to the base of the medial cuniform located considerable 'stickiness' in the superficial tissues. John decided to terminate the treatment session.

Session 2: Mother reported that change had occurred overnight following session 1. The usual 'No!' response to choice of cereal had prompted a 'No! Coco-pops' which was apparently the first time he had made any reasonable decision, had said more than 'no' or put two words together. The school reported that he was cooperative in a swimming session and had dived, retrieved a brick and presented it to the teacher rather than the customary practice of total disruption. The treatment session was conducted to John's direction as he availed himself and his feet for attention, stretching out in an indulgent manner.

Continuing sessions: Able progressively to extend the gestation pattern to include all areas. Only the lightest, non-intrusive massage was acceptable in the region of the great toe (over-enthusiasm on the part of the practitioner resulted in an epileptic fit – a learning curve). John's awareness of surroundings and relationships vastly increased, mostly greeted with a growing sense of humour and charm. John was also walking with a normal heel-toe gait which developed as his autism diminished.

Genetically, John was born into Irish nobility, and this was certainly exhibited in his behaviour throughout the times of our meetings, which were now more social. He was at his most charming, passing with a gracious smile, a kiss on the hand and then moving on. He continues to progress in ability and sociability, is enjoying his special education, and has the potential to be employable since he possesses a good sense of humour and a charming manner.

Conclusion

Evidence-based practice for Metamorphosis, in terms of controlled clinical trials, is sorely lacking. Instead, one may have to rely on the Uncertainty Principle proposed by quantum physics which may hopefully offer some credence for the unpredictable, particularly as regards the behaviour of the subatomic particles, which are the basis of all life forms and which do not behave in a manner explained by the classical laws of physics. The influence, quite literally, of mind over matter is explained by the 'observer effect', in which it is noted that waves and particles in the realms of the subatomic behave differently depending upon the attitude and expectation of the observer. Thus RSJ may be correct when he says 'observe and let be'. It may also be that if we can learn anything from the new physics and Metamorphosis, it must be to keep the mind compassionate, calm and unobtrusively observant in a non-directional manner. In this way the practitioner facilitates and supports the change which essentially proceeds from the individual's own making in degree, timing, direction, appropriateness and entirety. Essentially, the practitioner should be prepared to support the unexpected.

Even when there is little or no change in the presented symptoms, more subtle changes may be occurring. These may be facilitating a ripple of events which, on reflection, can be appreciated to be an obvious associated chain reaction. Thus, a change in a recurrent nightmare may alter in its pattern or be resolved at the same time that the dreamer alters the circumstances which have been causing an unexceptable degree of stress. Shortly afterwards the previously unresolved lower back pain seems to disappear without further treatment.

It is the clinical effectiveness that sells Metamorphosis – it is extraordinary for so many various and varied needs. The beneficial changes are a constant surprise; for those with spiritual trauma or need, or mental disability, emotional distress or physical symptoms, the process seems to facilitate a most unusual Metamorphosis.

The author's personal experience of Metamorphosis first occurred in 1978, following some years developing reflextherapy, and when she felt ready to investigate further extensions of reflexology. The course leader of the Metamorphic Technique, Gaston Saint-Pierre, seemed patient to the extreme while he dealt with a torrent of questions over three days, and these from the only physiotherapist of the group. It was only after some weeks of reciprocated 'treatment sessions' with a fellow course attendee that unexpected beneficial changes became obvious to family and friends. Some five years later, a course with Robert St John (who preferred the term 'Metamorphosis' as a process rather than a technique) gave further insights and his permission to include the teaching within the Midland School of Reflextherapy (see Appendix).

Postscript

Although 'Metamorphosis' is the name given by Robert St John to describe his work, the term 'Metamorphic Technique' was proposed by the Metamorphic Association (a charitable organization) to describe the actual practice. The Director is Gaston Saint-Pierre who has taught worldwide, written several books, and produced videos and tapes on the subject. The Metamorphic Technique is presented in seminars held at the Association, at international venues and also at several establishments.

The Midland School of Reflextherapy teaches the principles of Metamorphosis during its course 'Reflextherapy and Associated Studies for the Health Professional'. This course is credited by Coventry University, and endorsed by the Chartered Society of Physiotherapy. Courses are held in various locations in the UK, Israel and elsewhere.

References

The Concise Oxford Dictionary, 6th edn (1976) Oxford: Oxford University Press.

Collins English Dictionary, 3rd edn (1991) London: HarperCollins.

St John, R. (1979) *Metamorphosis: A Text Book on Prenatal Therapy*. London: The Metamorphic Association.

Recommended reading

Eastern philosophy and physics

Capra, F. (1992) *The Tao of Physics*, 3rd edn. London: Flamingo.

Kaptchuk, T.J. (1983) *The Web That Has No Weaver*. London: Rider.

Mind/body energy

Oschman, J.L. and Oschman, H. (1997) *Readings on the Scientific Basis of Bodywork and Movement Therapies*. Dover, NH: NORA.

Upledger, J. (1995) *SomatoEmotional Release and Beyond*. FL: UI Publishing.

Metamorphosis

Jones, C. (1995) Reflextherapy. In *Physiotherapy in Mental Health – A Practical Approach* (Everett, T., Dennis, M. and Ricketts, E., eds). Oxford: Butterworth-Heinemann.

Hummel, B. (1997) Metamorphic Technique. In *Medical Marriage* (Featherstone, C. and Forsyth, L., eds.). Findhorn: Findhorn Press.

Saint-Pierre, G. and Shapiro, D. (1993) *Metamorphic Technique – Principles and Practice*. Shaftesbury: Element Inc.

St John, R. (1979) *Metamorphosis: A Text Book on Prenatal Therapy*. London: The Metamorphic Association.

St John, R. (1976) *Prenatal Therapy and the Retarded Child*. London: Metamorphic Association.

Myofascial release – morphological change in the connective tissue

Mark F. Barnes

Introduction

Myofascial release is a whole-body treatment approach. Its focus is the identification of restricted soft tissue and the elongation of this foreshortened tissue. The goal of this treatment modality is the restoration of focal and global tissue health and subsequent functional gains in movement quantity and quality for the patient. Secondary to this treatment is patient instruction in self-directed myofascial elongation for home treatment. These home myofascial techniques are both passive and active release techniques.

It is imperative that manual therapists seek and understand a comprehensive and cohesive model of what is happening to the body's tissues with trauma, and how we are facilitating health in our patients. This greater understanding can lead to increased potency of treatment as well as encouraging a multidisciplinary approach. the conscientious bodyworker needs to ask: What am I trying to accomplish with my treatment, and what is happening beneath my hands to create these desired changes in tissue health and structural alignment? The facilitation of the body's self-correcting mechanisms, directing the tissues and systems toward metabolic and morphological efficiency, and ultimately gaining functional, pain-free movement, should be the primary goals of treatment.

Three major components to myofascial release treatment are:

- structural, soft tissue, and movement evaluations
- setting measurable clinical goals
- following the tissue as it releases into greater ranges of elongation which is time dependent
- allowing the body to find or 'slip into' positions of past trauma and unwind protective patterns of tightness and bracing.

The soma

The word '*soma*' (Greek) means the living body in its wholeness. Thomas Hanna has brought this term to the world of bodyworkers and considers the soma to be the body of life. The body of life, according to Hanna, is the original cybernetic system. Whether in an amoeba or the complex human form, it is a self-guiding system always striving to achieve stability and balance: 'A soma is neither static nor solid; it is changeable and supple and constantly adapting to its environment.' This viewpoint encompasses how we as individuals view ourselves, from the inside out. From the inside we are not aware of the body, but rather the feelings and the active processes of that body (Hanna, 1988).

Somatic pathology will encompass adaptive responses of the morphological and neuromuscular systems, reflected clinically as dysfunction and pain. These concepts are the very foundation of understanding the body's response to trauma, and treatment of subsequent dysfunction.

It is theorized that the alterations in tissue texture and tension resulting from myofascial release come from dynamic changes in the connective tissue and neuromuscular systems of the body. These two systems have been shown to be vitally interrelated in function and their response to therapy (Pischinger, 1975). This relationship is cellular, systemic and somatic.

This theoretical and clinical approach asks the individual to reflect on their view of the body; how it is structured, functions and communicates. It involves a conceptual shift from a biological systems infrastructure model to a self-organizing cybernetic biological systems model. Ideally, practitioners of various bodywork approaches are constantly updating their paradigm about bodily function, potentially leading them to a greater unified theory of somatic dysfunction and treatment. This conceptual shift is necessary to advance in the quality and efficiency of patient care. Over the last few years medicine has made many gains in the evaluation and treatment of musculoskeletal disorders, specifically chronic disorders of pain and movement. This has been slow in coming, but is very welcome. This chapter will discuss the connective tissue response to trauma and myofascial release, supported by a biocybernetic model of morphological function.

These concepts are the very foundation of understanding the body's response to trauma, and treatment of subsequent dysfunction. Utilizing myofascial release as a clinical modality requires knowledge of what is fascia, its response to trauma, and how we have a lasting permanent release of this tissue. Concurrently, the knowledge of the neuromuscular components to this tissue, the somatic adaptations and responses to trauma (present and future), and the facilitation of unwinding patterns of tone and bracing are essential. The three aspects of myofascial release are passive, active and spontaneous release of the myofascial tissue.

Myofascial concept

The term 'myofascial' now has potent clinical meaning, *myo* representing the neuromuscular elements, and *fascial* representing the connective tissue components of the body. It is a term denoting a major body system, the intact functioning of which is vitally important to the health and economy of the individual. It is a dynamic, integrative system that is at the most basic level responsible for intra- and intercellular communication (Pischinger, 1975). This system is ubiquitous, affecting and responding to every aspect of bodily function. The myofascial system provides support, resilience, communication, protection, biomechanical linkage and movement. It is the suprastructure and infrastructure of every other system, creating the foundation of form and function. The tissues of this system, connective and neuromuscular, make up the bulk of the body's tissue and it is logical that there should be communication between these components. It is suggested that we can no longer separate the nervous, muscular and connective tissue systems if we are to be successful in our attempts to facilitate change in any one of these parts. They work together and are inseparable.

The extensive work of the author's father, John F. Barnes RPT, in myofascial release has always empirically used this comprehensive view of the body in treatment. Both fascial release and tissue unwinding are intimately related, having a tissue elongation and release of neural holding patterns as a solid foundation for making profound changes in tissue health. The whole-body results seen with myofascial release are due to this interrelationship and stem from both micro and macro changes to this ubiquitous system.

The work of Lawrence Jones DO (1981), for example, utilizing positional release of trigger points, can be more greatly understood. Korr (1978) explained the treatment efficacy of this approach as a product of resetting the proprioceptive receptors of the muscle spindle, although mechanically shortening the collagenous ligamentus structures through positioning joints, shortening the muscular components, inhibiting the neuromuscular input and, to be later explained, changing the ground substance state from a crystal to a gel, are all a part of the many techniques being used today to create positive change in the myofascial system. The myofascial structures are a part of a system and are best viewed as components of a communication network that are extremely responsive to input, either negative (e.g. trauma) or appropriate therapeutic facilitation. The word 'myofascial' denotes the vitally inter-related nature of the connective tissue and neuromuscular systems. A model of the way these tissues communicate within and between their surroundings, the rest of the body, should be incorporated into our paradigms of operation. This process is termed 'biocybernetics' and best describes the somatic events involved with tissue trauma and the reversal of the somatic response to this trauma.

General cybernetic principle in organisms

The basic concepts may be summarized briefly as follows:

- A system science perspective recognizes the cybernetic nature of all physical, physiological and psychic processes as being subject to uniform laws.
- These laws apply to both living and inanimate matter which are based on identical principles of control, coordination and regulation.
- These processes also make use of homeostatic feedback mechanisms (circuits) to produce continual reciprocal checks and balances among intermeshed levels of organization.
- Dis-ease symptoms, such as chronic pain in the soft tissues, can be regarded as regulatory disturbances and are considered to be a biocybernetic problem of persistent malfunction of the information and feedback mechanisms, as in the example of fibromyalgia.

Cybernetics regards man as a highly-developed, self-regulating system, always attempting to reach homeostasis and equilibrium. The principle of linear causality, a mechanistic philosophy of cause and effect, of which, in fact, much of Western medicine is based, no longer applies to the treatment of musculoskeletal disorders, especially diseases chronic in nature. An example: fibromyalgia being both a connective tissue and neuromuscular syndrome having fascial tightening and hypertonus points. This syndrome has proved to be self-perpetuating and to date has perplexed much of the medical community.

Ground regulation system and cellular communication

In 1975, Alfred Pischinger published *Matrix and Matrix Regulation. Basis for a Holistic Theory in Medicine*. This work offers the basis for an understanding and explanation of the morphological and physiological events occurring with manual therapies such as myofascial release, joint mobilization and various movement therapies. Pischinger founded his observations on the works of Wiener (1963) who propagated developments in cybernetics and thermodynamics, and Von Bertalanffy (1952) who described biological systems as non-linear, but highly integrated and subject to biological vital flow equilibrium. The biological system exchanges energy and material with its surroundings as 'open systems'.

According to Pischinger, open systems are in contrast to the classical Newtonian closed systems. Open systems show that when there is an influx of non-chaotic energy, this energy can spread suddenly through the entire system. The essential points in this phenomenon are the transmission and dissemination of information. The body acts as an open feedback system like a thermostat, in contrast to a light switch only having an on and off mode. The body has available many varying states which are receptive to input and has the ability to adjust itself accordingly for homeostasis. Pischinger concerned himself with investigating and describing the communications that the connective tissue uses to spread itself over the entire organism.

Pischinger's system of Ground Regulation (Figure 13.1) is defined as the functional unit of the final vascular pathway, the connective tissue cells and the final vegetative-nervous structure. The entire field of activity and information exchange of this triad is the extracellular fluid, forming a matrix. The lymphatics and lymphatic organs are also connected, constituting the largest system penetrating the organism completely. It regulates the 'cell milieu', determining the extracellular environment, providing nutrition to the cells and eliminating waste; at

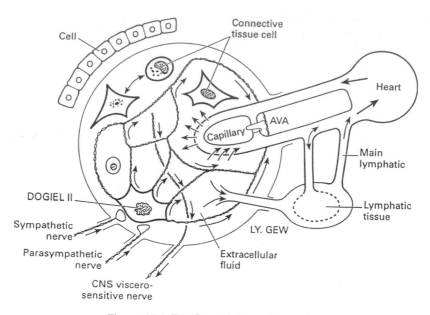

Figure 13.1 The Ground Regulation system

the same time it is a part of every inflammatory and defence process and is therefore responsible for all basic vital functions of the organism.

According to Pischinger, it is in this extracellular environment that all the primary regulating processes occur which make life possible. The basic concept is as follows:

- it is a medium for the oxygen, water and ion balance (the basic autonomic system) to indirectly produce energy, and all the other conditions essential for the organ cell to live
- all external stimuli must pass through this basic tissue to reach the organ cell
- the autonomic fibres have no synaptic connections to the parenchymal cells; they must form mediating chemicals which have to pass through the extracellular fluid to act upon the cell
- therefore the cell and its environment are continually interacting with each other, forming a tri-level intermeshed circuit of cellular, neural, humoral control, attempting to maintain homeostatic functional equilibrium
- if the functions of the interstitial connective tissue are impaired by interference fields (trauma), the defence system is subject to

permanent stress and the defensive capability of the organism is constantly reduced
- as long as this situation can be compensated, the body remains apparently healthy
- if the noxious stimuli of the interference field exceeds the tolerance of the autonomic system, functional disturbances and objective pathological changes will occur (Kellner and Kleine, 1976)
- as a consequence, the organism will be forced to further compensate, overwork and break down – this is seen clinically as physiological, neuromuscular and mechanical loss of efficiency and function.

Connective tissue (fascia)

Connective tissue is analogous to fascia; they are one and the same. In much of the osteopathic and physical therapy literature, fascia is considered to be sheaths of connective tissue (primarily collagen) that forms cavities and muscular septums, and covers organs. It is necessary to shift this concept of fascia to the ubiquitous and multifunctional system of connective tissue.

The very term 'connective tissue' denotes its primary role; a tissue that interrelates every part of the whole, creating an integrated body. Connective tissue comprises collagen, elastin and ground substance. The collagen gives support, shape and stability, the elastin gives dynamic flexibility, and the ground substance provides cushion and surrounds every cell, determining its functional capacity. The ground substance makes up the bulk of the extracellular matrix and it is towards this environment surrounding the cell that the work of Pischinger is directed.

Connective tissue response to trauma

The moving body depends on connective tissue for support and biomechanically efficient movement. Connective tissues make a major contribution to the dynamic properties of the body. Movement depends on connective tissue being functional and properly distributed. Tightening of the fascial system due to trauma is a protective mechanism that will arise from either microtrauma over time or acute injury such as a contusion or tendon strain. The fascial components lose their pliability, become restricted and are a source of tension for the rest of the body. This is specifically evident at the ground system/cellular level (Ingber and Folkman, 1989), as well as mechanically from collagenous tinsegrity (Klebe, 1989; Levin, 1990) in which the ground substance solidifies, the collagen develops cross-links, is fibrous and dense, and the elastin loses its resiliency (Figure 13.2).

Stauber *et al.* (1990) reported disruption in the extracellular matrix following post-traumatic eccentric exercise, with resultant inflammatory response and pain (Figure 13.3). Stauber *et al.* (1996) later reported a 44% increase in non-contractile tissue (expansion of extracellular matrix and fibrosis) after 4 weeks of repeated muscular strain (Figure 13.4). Many researchers have identified the loose and dense connective tissue response to trauma (Forrest, 1983; Rennard *et al.*, 1984; Hunt *et al.*, 1985), demonstrating the tendency of the connective tissue to solidify and develop adhesions, and become less resilient both physiologically and mechanically with trauma. The effects of this, in the long term, are detrimental to the functioning and efficiency of the myofascial tissues. At the cellular level, Heine (1972, quoted in Pischinger, 1991) states:

> Phylogenetically the extracellular matrix is older than the nerve and hormonal systems. In its formation and breakdown it is appropriately regulated by a very basic cell system in a compensatory way by the fibroblasts' macrophage system. Since the fibroblasts are not able to differentiate between the good and the bad situation, the result in chronic alterations is the development of an extracellular matrix whose structure is not physiologically efficient, which can make an important contribution to the development of chronic diseases.

Mechanical stress due to connective tissue tightening

Fascial restrictions can create abnormal strain patterns that can crowd, or pull, the osseous structures out of proper alignment, resulting in compression of joints producing pain and/or dysfunction (Figure 13.5). Neural and vascular structures can also become entrapped in these restrictions, causing neurological symptoms or ischaemic conditions. Shortening of the muscular component of the myofascial fascicle can limit its functional length, reducing its strength, contractile potential and deceleration capacity. Facilitating positive change in this system would be a clinically relevant event.

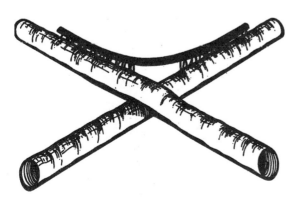

Figure 13.2 A fibrous cross-link at the junction of two collagen fibres forming from trauma and inflammation

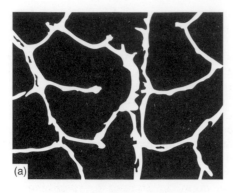
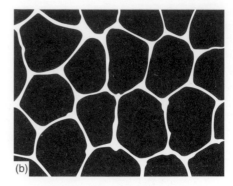

Figure 13.3(a, b) Diagrammatic representation of extracellular matrix disruption and thickening, with resultant inflammation

Cellular and CNS stress due to connective tissue response

Hans Selye (1956) has clearly demonstrated a specific and stereotyped reaction of the hormonal system to 'the stress of life'. Due to the bioelectric information capacity of the extracellular matrix, any situation that alters the electrical tone of the matrix can be encoded, and reciprocally spread and processed through the entire organism, a potential by-product of cellular shock. Therefore, the solidification of the extracellular matrix with trauma and inflammation will produce a signal of cellular shock, transmitted via the neurovegetative pathway to the brainstem and higher regulatory centres. In lung biopsies of severely traumatized accident victims, Heine and Henrich (1980) showed severe disturbance in extracellular matrix and significant increase in collagen in the alveolar septa within 30 minutes, producing shock lung syndrome weeks later. This is a clear depiction of the interrelated nature of the fascial and neuromuscular systems in regards to trauma response; both a local and global somatic response.

A drawing from Selye's (1956) *The Stress of Life* has been adapted to demonstrate this cellular response to trauma and depict the CNS reaction (Figure 13.6). A chain of neurophysiological events is proposed that are commonly observed clinically, stemming from local to diffuse cellular and tissue damage:

- a patient may have sustained a severe 'whiplash' injury resulting from a motor vehicle accident
- the anterior cervical soft tissues would have been traumatized, with resultant inflammation

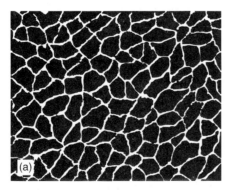
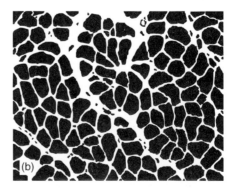

Figure 13.4(a, b) Diagrammatic representation of extracellular matrix disruption, collagen fibrosis and a 44% increase in non-contractile tissue

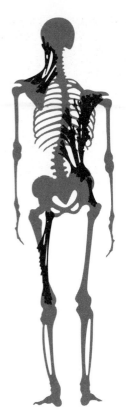

Figure 13.5 Three-dimensional myofascial restrictions

- the connective tissue will have responded with solidification of the extracellular matrix and collagen
- this cellular environment will have become toxic, leading to poor nutritional support and elimination of waste, sending a signal to the higher centres of tissue shock
- in response, the CNS would have increased segmental tone, creating spasm and neuromuscular holding patterns as a protective reaction.

This chain of events corresponds to the exhaustion phase as described in Selye's general adaption syndrome (Selye, 1956). The patient would now be dysfunctional as well as in pain.

Neuromuscular response to trauma

The extraordinary stimuli (trauma) that are the cause and origin of much illness act as specific stimuli for the defence mechanisms of the body. Illness can be considered as a general reaction by the organism as a whole, mediated by the cerebral cortex, reacting to any pathogenic stimulus which brings into disorder the equilibrium within the organism and its relations to the environment (Pavlov, cited in Dosch, 1984). Life can be considered to be cybernetically self-sustaining and dependent on the formation, modulation and maintenance of its optimum bioelectric potential. The whole of neurovegetative regulation, at centre and periphery, in its neural and hormonal components, can be seen to ultimately serve the main purpose of all regulation and control, namely to maintain certain bioelectric potentials (Dosch, 1984).

Adaptive neuromuscular reflexes

Adaptive neuromuscular reflexes represent and reflect the physiological responses to stress outlined by Selye. They are inscribed in our central nervous system and critically affect function over time, creating what we see clinically as solidification and pain syndromes. These responses are protective adaptations to subtle disturbances in our equilibrium, over time viewed by the soma as microtrauma. As in the connective tissue response to trauma, they seem to be cumulative and excessive. The cybernetic cycle of dysfunction involves chronic shortening of the neuromuscular element produced by tone (stress from outside environmental input), and reciprocally increased tone of the neuromuscular element produced by solidification of the extracellular matrix resulting from trauma (stress from the internal environment; tissue/cellular damage).

The interference-field effect changes the cell environment in such a way that higher order neural, hormonal, psychological and cellular control systems can also become involved (Selye, 1956; Keidal, 1970; Drischel, 1973; Pischinger, 1975; Hildebrandt, 1985). This phenomenon should be considered a total somatic response to trauma, a positive reaction necessary for homeostasis, although which left unchecked can lead to chronic dysfunction. Hoff (1960) studied the neurovegetative aspect

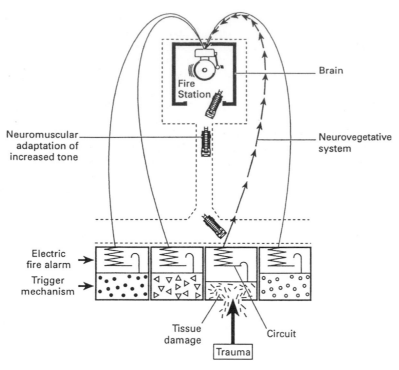

Figure 13.6 A representation of the cellular response to trauma and the CNS reaction (After Selye, 1956)

of the non-specific defence shock reaction of the body. Hoff related his findings of an initial sympathetic reaction to a negative stimulus (stress or trauma) and a subsequent parasympathetic reaction of the CNS to the hormonal reactions found by Selye. Pischinger related these findings to the disturbance of the Ground Regulation system focally and globally. The fundamental stability of bodily functions in humans, and their ability to maintain upright posture and move through their environment, all result from regulating processes. Somatic therapies have to incorporate these processes into their modes of operation in order to be able to affect the entire organism.

Myofascial release

Evaluation

Comprehensive treatment includes an evaluative process that makes treatment goal directed.

A major aspect to myofascial release treatment is the proprioceptive nature of the three-dimensional tissue release that follows therapy, which can be confirmed by documenting the resulting diminution of symptoms. Evaluation, both prior to and after treatment, includes a standing static postural analysis, noting the position of bony landmarks, spinal and extremity range of motion, and tissue texture. The soft tissues should be just that, soft. Tissue that is hard, fibrotic and tender should be treated. It is important to view the body as its integrated whole, looking at not just symptoms but also pathomechanics. Causal relationships are made apparent to the practitioner by problem-solving mechanics. Always correlate the soft tissue analysis to the objective findings. A good place to start would be to ask the question: What is the soft tissue region that could be so excessively tight that it would produce this clinical presentation? Symptoms and restrictions may be only mechanically related, existing in adjacent or distant regions of the body.

Treatment

Connective tissue is colloidal in nature, having elastic, plastic, viscoelastic and piezoelectric properties. Its morphological state is determined by proportions of energy input and temperature. Deformation is well described by the Spring and Dashpot model (Upledger, 1983), and stress/ strain curves (Zachazewski, 1989). The Spring and Dashpot model depicts the viscoelastic functional properties of connective tissue of deformation over time (90–120 s). The stress/strain curve represents the same viscoelastic properties, but also depicts the failure of the tissue when rate of deformation exceeds the tissue tolerance to the amount of load. The goal of myofascial release is to elongate and soften the connective tissue, creating permanent three-dimensional length and width.

Fascia is the tissue which spreads throughout the body in a three-dimensional web from head to toe. The fascia is ubiquitous, surrounding every muscle, bone, nerve, blood vessel and organ, all the way down to the cellular level. Generally, the fascial system is one of support, stability and cushion. It is also a system of locomotion and dynamic flexibility, forming muscle.

Tightening of the fascial system is a histological, physiological and biomechanic protective mechanism that is a response to trauma. The fascia loses its pliability, becomes restricted, and is a source of tension to the rest of the body. The ground substance solidifies, the collagen becomes dense and fibrous and the elastin loses its resiliency. Over time this can lead to poor muscular biomechanics, altered structural alignment and decreased strength, endurance and motor coordination. Subsequently, the patient is in pain and functional capacity is lost.

Myofascial release is a hands-on soft tissue technique that facilitates a stretch into the restricted fascia. A sustained pressure is applied into the restricted tissue barrier; after 90–120 s the tissue will undergo histological length changes, allowing the first release to be felt. The therapist follows the release into a new tissue barrier and holds; after a few releases, the tissue will become soft and pliable (Figure 13.7). The restoration of length and health to the myofascial tissue will take the pressure off the pain-sensitive structures like nerves and blood vessels, as well as restore alignment and mobility to the joints.

Most important to our discussion is the change of the ground substance from a sol to a gel. This occurs with a state phase realignment of crystals exposed to electromagnetic fields. This may occur as a piezoelectric event,

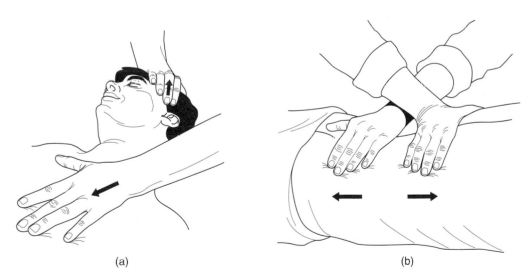

(a)   (b)

Figure 13.7 Myofascial release: (a) release of the anterior cervical region; (b) cross-hand release to the lumbar region

changing a mechanical force to electric energy. The electrical charge of collagen and proteoglycans within the extracellular matrix is changed affecting the ionic state of the ground substance (Schmitt *et al.*, 1955; Athenstaedt, 1974; Linsenmeyer, 1983). This provides the opportunity for electrical signal processing locally and globally throughout the somatic system. Due to the web-like structural matrix of the soma, piezoelectric phenomena can be local or spread to distal regions along the uninterrupted connective tissue mechanical and bioelectrical network throughout the body. Indicative of this phenomenon are the appearance of vasomotor responses, fasciculations of the neuromuscular elements and heat. These responses may be seen in the region being treated or in other regions of the body, either during or after treatment. In addition, symptoms may be felt during or after treatment in adjacent or distant regions from the treated area. It is always interesting to have the patient report an increase of chief complaint symptoms while the therapist is working on distant areas. Treatment of the posterior scalene often reproduces temporomandibular joint pain and headaches.

Athenstaedt states:

> The entire organism is interwoven with chains of piezoelectric dipolar molecules which are capable of oscillation due to their spiral nature. Thixotropy is the change of phase state of the ground substance to become more fluid when stirred up and more solid when left sedentary. Mechanical energy and subsequent friction from myofascial release or exercise has the effect of changing the gel portion of connective tissue to fluid from a dehydrated crystalline state. Alterations in the functional capacity of this three-dimensional, ubiquitous network provides further reason for degeneration in the movement system and that regulatory processes can be affected by varied techniques facilitating change in the polarity potential of the tissue [myofascial release to acupuncture].

The molecular form of proteoglycans is particularly suitable for binding water, creating the viscoelastic, shock-absorbing and energy-absorbing behaviour of the extracellular matrix (ECM). It is at this level that energy flow throughout the organism is most apparent. Functional morphology (the prime mover of energy flow) is based in the interaction between water and the ECM. More specifically, the liquid–crystalline water and the sugar molecules determine the degree of organization and structural proportions in the ECM. It was stated earlier that all vital functions are mediated by the ECM and that this ECM is a dissipative system. The states of organization are not stable, oscillating far from thermodynamic stability (Pischinger, 1975). Biological energy is quantitatively and qualitatively tangible.

The special suitability of these networks of water molecules and proteoglycans for information conduction and storage between cells is optimal at 37.5°C (normal body temperature). False information stored within the liquid crystals could therefore be cancelled by temperature increase (and piezoelectric events) and transferred back to a homogeneous fluid (Trincher, 1981). This process ideally depolarizes the interstitial tissue and resets the ground regulation system to be more efficient in information transmission and eliminating any false signals produced by the crystalline dehydrated matrix.

In light of this information, the introduction of a mechanical force, myofascial release, following the low load, long-duration principle of the Spring and Dashpot model, would be sufficient to change the phase state of the ground substance, creating an extracellular environment of a healthy and efficient fluid gel. Barnes (1990) has described myofascial release as having a three-dimensional quality with a sustained pressure (90–120 s) into the colloidal/viscoelastic fascial tissue, having the goal of restoring length, dimension and health to the tissue environment.

Myofascial release is now widely taught and practised with impressive claims of benefit in terms of pain reduction and functional improvement. The underlying biophysical somatic principles described in this chapter may help to demystify this therapeutic approach and so help to explain its well-documented results, in terms which mainstream practitioners and therapists find acceptable.

Myofascial unwinding

The therapeutic effects from the human touch are fascinating and can be profound. John F. Barnes has taken myofascial release to such refined levels, utilizing an open awareness of proprioception to detect and facilitate inherent fine motions in our bodies. The first step is to quiet our mind and body and gently touch the patient. Our ability to breath deep and slow, decreasing our heart rate and entering into a more parasympathetic state, has a great effect on our patients. This also allows us to feel into the tissue system for restrictions and subtle movements within the patient. Feeling this motion will allow us to take our patients into the three-dimensional position or sequential positions necessary for more total structural and neuromuscular release and, for many, bringing disassociated traumatic memories to the conscious level.

Myofascial unwinding is a component of the release process that encompasses, to a greater extent, the release of patterns of bracing and memories of trauma, this memory being cellular, tissue and somatic. These patterns are contained within our central nervous system (Levine, 1997), neuropeptide system (Pert, 1997), and the connective tissue (Hammerhoff, 1994). This is integrated with the release of the connective tissue aspect of the myofascial complex. The framework in understanding this process is the retaining, remembering and releasing of trauma to the somatic system. In fact, this is happening all the time, but under our conscious level of perception. Cumulative and acute trauma can be so involved and multilayered that this process of treatment is considered facilitory in regards to accelerating a natural process inherent to our self-correction.

Resetting the nervous system/sequence of regulation

The following should be noted:

- Sensorimotor disturbances are considered to be the tip of the iceberg, representing stress symptoms of the underlying ground regulation system.

- The regulatory response to functional pathomechanics or pathogenic information from the ground regulation system consists of changes in muscular tone.
- Muscular tone is regulated at the tissue, spinal and cerebral levels having, as their primary response to a stimulus, increased tone.
- Each component is also connected indirectly or invested into the extracellular matrix completing a feedback loop between the CNS and the connective tissue.

Somatic education

The soma is a functional system that will rebalance and reharmonize itself if given the chance. In functional disorders, what is required is not the exchange of words with the 'mind', nor is it the exchange of chemicals with the 'body'. The requirement is a change in the living human system's awareness of its own functioning. The somatic system needs more information of itself and more efficient control. In sum, the distorted human soma needs sensory information and new motor control (Hanna, 1979) through therapist facilitation and education.

Myofascial unwinding, as in many movement therapies, has the element of awareness as a learning tool – a tool that offers possibilities of new body postures and quality of movement. It seems that when we lose this awareness we fall out of accordance with our environment. As we go through life, with its major and minor traumas, emotional and physical, we tend to fall into habitual patterns of posture and movement. These patterns, over time, may not be beneficial. We actually lose sight of their existence, literally struggling, pulling ourselves through our day, week and life, unaware of our dysfunctional patterns of use.

During myofascial unwinding the patient may experience positions of trauma, the recognition of both tissue and tonal release, and the advancement into new positions. This process may continue through many positions and sensations of release. As mentioned above, the remembrance of trauma may also be accompanied by an emotional release either during, or after, treatment. This process of release comes by experiential learning from the patient, not intellectual learning. In the hands of the practitioner, these moments feel like still points in the subtle, fluid movements of the patient. It is believed that these still points are minute, but potent positions, where the somatic reorganization or resetting of the myofascial system is occurring.

A little insight or recognition of a new possibility facilitated by the practitioner can start to break down these patterns, helping to free the body. This distinction between the new and the old, over time, can re-educate, helping in the abandonment of old habits and acquisition of new functional ones, thus improving control over the body, and ultimately a more pleasurable relationship with the environment.

The Arndt–Schultz law of physiology states that the body responds to a greater extent when the stimulus is subtle compared to abrupt suddenness. The body and mind seem less threatened by this approach, with less need to protect themselves, thus learning through distinctions of free movement, less pain and awareness of new positions. Any improvement in functional alignment tends to have the effect of relaxation, decreased energy expenditure and positive changes in pathomechanics.

Every biological control circuit has a large number of sense gauges which, on the one hand, monitor the physiological processes by acting as proprioceptors and, on the other, signal any threatened or actual damage by acting as nociceptors or pain receptors (Dosch, 1984). By restimulating the sensorimotor system and resetting its efficiency, myofascial unwinding, in effect, lowers the tonal input segmentally or globally from all three centres of tonal control. Having their roots firmly planted in the extracellular matrix, the entire biological system will have improved homeostatic information coming from the neurovegetative end of the cybernetic loop, establishing for the individual greater quality and quantity of movement.

Case histories

Chronic postoperative low back pain

A 32-year-old man who worked as a choker setter, a job that involves dragging large heavy cables and wrapping them around trees so they can be hauled, had a lumbar laminectomy in 1983, followed by decompression surgery at the same level in October 1985. Five months after his second operation, he was referred to physical therapy by his surgeon for 3 weeks of treatment for chronic low back pain and bilateral anterior thigh pain. His treatment included hot wet packs with concurrent interferential electrical stimulation, a home exercise programme and myofascial release to the low back area as well as to the surgical scar. After two treatments, the man experienced no further leg pain and only mild low back pain with movement. After four treatments, he cancelled further appointments because he was no longer having any pain and had returned to work. At follow-up by telephone 3 months later, he reported having low back discomfort at times and never any leg pain. He is pleased with his ability to continue his strenuous job.

Chronic dislocating patella

A 15-year-old girl had a history of a chronically dislocating right patella for 3 years. At age 11, she fell and hit a kerb, injuring the lateral aspect of the right knee. Approximately 1 month later, her patella began dislocating. Dislocations gradually became more frequent. She stated that even with normal walking, the patella would dislocate and she would fall. She had had constant pain at the lateral aspect of the knee for the past 2 years. Originally, her patella dislocated about twice per week, progressing to daily for a year before she came to us for therapy. The only previous treatment given her was quadriceps and hamstring 'sets', and a trial of two types of brace.

The referring physician requested straight-leg raises, quadriceps strengthening and iliotibial band stretching. We treated her five times with ultrasound to the lateral retinacular area of the right patella, followed by myofascial release of the iliotibial band and lateral retinaculum. She was also given straight-leg raises against theraband, with some external rotation of the hips to emphasize strengthening of the vastus medialis obliques.

After the first treatment she had no further dislocations, even when running up and down stairs. On follow-up 9 months later, she reported having no further problems at all with her right knee. This patient was a possible candidate for surgical release of the lateral retinaculum of the right knee. Because she had done exercises in the past without eliminating chronic dislocation of the patella, we feel that the rapid resolution of her problem was due primarily to non-invasive release of the scarred and adhered lateral retinaculum with myofascial release techniques.

Myofascial syndrome after open heart surgery

Three months after a 73-year-old woman had open heart surgery, she came for physical therapy complaining of excruciating pain at the sternal surgical scar region that spread up the left sternocicidomastoid and into the left upper extremity to the elbow. She also complained of paraesthesia of the left side of the face, episodes of dizziness, difficulty breathing when tilting the head back, and lack of pulse in the left side of the neck.

Four treatments were given in a 10-day period, including moist heat, myofascial release and a home programme of stretching the neck and shoulders. Myofascial release was performed over the surgical scar, left chest, left neck, cranial base and left side of the face. A left arm pull was also performed. At the end of the fourth and final treatment, she reported feeling 100% improved. She had no pain, she could feel a pulse again in the left side of her neck, her breathing was unrestricted with cervical extension, she had normal sensation in her face, and experienced no further episodes of dizziness. Her six standard cervical motions have improved a total of 40 degrees, including a gain of 15 degrees extension.

On follow-up by telephone 4 weeks after her final treatment, she reported feeling as well as after the last treatment. She only had 'soreness' in the left neck and left axillary region when stretching while doing her home exercises, which were recommended that she continue daily.

Status post right mastectomy and radiation burn

A 73-year-old woman came for her initial physical therapy treatment in July 1987, 1½ years after a right mastectomy. She underwent 1 year of chemotherapy after surgery, and then 6 weeks (30 treatments) of radiation therapy. She had an irregular-shaped radiation burn with hypertrophic scarring over the distal third of the sternum (approximately 6–7 mm diameter). It still had a small area of scab. Her right shoulder was drawn forward. Her right shoulder and chest were extremely hypersensitive to mild touch and minor movement of the right shoulder. She was referred to us as soon as the physician felt that the burn was sufficiently healed to begin physical therapy. Right shoulder external and internal rotation ranges of motions were within normal limits. Active flexion and abduction (standing) were, respectively, 0–130 degrees and 0–97 degrees. The woman was given a home exercise programme with a cane and treated 15 times with moist heat and myofascial release to the chest, right upper extremity and neck. At the final treatment she had 160 degrees of motion of both right shoulder flexion and abduction (equivalent to the contralateral motions). She had no further discomfort except for mild tenderness when pushing her motion exercises to the end of the range.

On follow-up more than 7 months later the patient had maintained her range of motion and reported no limitations of function and no pain. She felt fully recovered in every way other than some tightness at the site of radiation. She was thoroughly grateful for the remarkable increase of motion and reduction of pain that occurred with such gentle and relatively painless techniques.

Self-care utilizing myofascial techniques and dynamic stretching

Treatment results of fascial elongation and decreased neuromuscular tone are better kept when the patient continues treatment at home. By instructing the patient in simple home techniques and giving them a basic working knowledge of myofascial release, the amount of control the patient can have over symptoms and reversing the body's compensations to trauma can be great. The two basic components to the home programme are dynamic stretching and passive myofascial elongation.

Dynamic stretching is a self-stretch that is three-dimensional and has both a myofascial elongation component and a neuromuscular action. This self-stretch is performed for at least 90 s, taking into account the mechanisms of the myofascial complex characteristics of elongation. The concept of tissue elongation has been shaped by the ideas and theories of stretching. These concepts are inadequate in explaining morphological lasting change in tissue length. Traditional stretching wraps and pulls tissues around the joint fulcrums and is typically taught as a 30-second process. Myofascial relief elongates the structures three-dimensionally, telescoping the myofascial tissues and subsequent bony spacers. The use of a counter-pressure, depth into the tissue, and the time factor, are major differences between the two approaches.

Stretching is commonly prescribed to patients and athletes to prepare tissue for exercise and lengthen foreshortened tissue. An aspect usually not taken into account with the typical prescription of stretching exercise are the histological properties and mechanisms of change for tissue elongation. Active elongation is a combination of a passive stretch and neuromuscular work. This is accomplished through activating one side to stretch myofascial structures on the other side, and also to inhibit the neuromuscular elements of the inactive side (Figure 13.8).

Patients are taught to utilize fulcrums such as the Swiss ball, smaller diameter balls for more focal treatment, and padded wedges for anchoring tissue. The home treatment programme is tailored from the clinical goals in the office setting and are specific to the hands-on treatment.

Summary of concepts

Fascia is a ubiquitous, three-dimensional weave of connective tissue throughout the body that spreads from head to toe. This system is one of support, movement and communication down to the cellular level. There is an intimate relationship between the fascial system and the neuromuscular system, denoting the name myofascial. This system tends to become adhesive, solidified and dehydrated, with microtrauma over time, poor posture and acute tissue damage. This response is a somatic process of protection. Fascial restrictions and tonal patterns of bracing are concurrent with trauma, and are the focus of myofascial release treatment. Fascia/connective tissue has the same viscoelastic properties as plastic. Permanent deformation and subsequent elongation of this tissue occur after greater than 120 s of light mechanical force. This phenomenon is considered a piezoelectric process of changing mechanical energy into bioelectric cellular changes. The high clinical efficacy of myofascial release is due to the time factor and the conscientious hands of the practitioner.

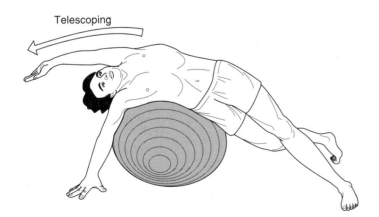

Telescoping

Figure 13.8 Active elongation using the Swiss ball as a fulcrum

References

Athenstaedt, H. (1974) Pyroelectric and pieziolectric properties of vertebrates. *Ann. N.Y. Acad. Sci.*, **238**, 68–110.

Barnes, J. (1990) *Myofascial Release: The Search for Excellence*. Paoli, PA: Rehabilitation Services.

Bertalanffy, L.V. (1952) *Perspectives of General Systems Theory*. New York: Braziller.

Dosch, P. (1984) *Manual of Neural Therapy According to Huneke*. Heidelberg: Haug.

Drischel, H. (1973) *Einfuhrung in die Biokybernetic*. Berlin: Akademie Verlag.

Forrest, L. (1983) Current concepts in soft tissue wound healing. *Br. J. Surg.*, **70**, 133–46.

Hammerhoff, S.R. (1994) Quantum coherence in microtubules: a neural basis for emergent consciousness. *J. Consciousness Studies*, **1**(1), 91–118.

Hanna, T. (1979) *The Body of Life: Creating New Pathways for Sensory Awareness and Fluid Movement*. Rochester, NY: Healing Arts Press.

Hanna, T. (1988) *Somatics: Reawakening the Mind's Control of Movement, Flexibility, and Health*. New York: Addison-Wesley.

Heine, H. and Henrich, H. (1980) Reactive behaviour of myocytes during long-term sympathetic stimulation as compared to spontaneous hypertension. *Fol. Angiol.*, **28**, 22–27.

Hildebrandt, G. (1985) *Therapeuticische Physiologie, Grundlagen der Kurotbehandlung in Balneologie. Medizinische Klimatologie*. Heidelberg: Springer Verlag.

Hoff, F. (1960) *Behandlung Innerer Krankheiten*. Stuttgart: Thieme Verlag.

Hunt, T.K., Banda, M.J. and Silver, I.A. (1985) Cell interactions in post-traumatic fibrosis. *Clin. Symp.*, **114**, 128–49.

Ingber, E. and Folkman, J. (1989) *Tension and Compression as Basic Determinants of Cell Form and Function: Utilization of a Cellular Tensegrity Mechanism*. London: Academic Press.

Jones, L.H. (1981) *Strain and Counterstrain*. Newark, OH: American Academy of Osteopathy.

Keidal, W. (1970) *Lehrbuch der Physiologic*. Stuttgart: Thieme Verlag.

Kellner, G. and Kleine, G. (1976) Richtlinien zur Synovialzytologie. *Z. f. Rheumatologie*, **35**, 141–53.

Klebe, R.J. (1989) Cells transmit spatial information by orienting collagen fibers. *Matrix*, **9**, 451–58.

Korr, I.M. (1978) *The Neurobiological Mechanisms in Manipulative Therapy*. New York: Plenum Press.

Levin, S.M. (1990) The myofascial-skeletal truss: a system science analysis. In *Myofascial Release: The Search for Excellence* (Barnes, J.F., ed.). Paoli, PA: Rehabilitation Services.

Levine, P.A. (1997) *Waking The Tiger: Healing Trauma*. Berkeley, CA: North Atlantic Books.

Linsenmeyer, T.F. (1983) Collagen. In *Cell Biology of Extracellular Matrix*, 2nd edn. New York: Plenum Press.

Pert, C.B. (1997) *Molecules of Emotion*. New York: Scribner.

Pischinger, A. (German edn 1975, English edn 1991) *Matrix and Matrix Regulation: Basis for a Holistic Theory in Medicine*. Brussels: Haug International.

Rennard, S.I., Bitterman, P.B. and Crystal, R.G. (1984) *Current Concepts of the Pathogenesis of Fibrosis: Lessons from Pulmonary Fibrosis. Myofibroblasts and the Biology of Connective Tissue*. New York: Liss.

Schmitt, F.O., Gross, J. and Highberger, J.H. (1955) Tropocollagen and the properties of fibrous collagen. *Exp. Cell Res.*, suppl. 3, 326–34.

Selye, H. (1956) *The Stress of Life*. New York: McGraw-Hill.

Stauber, W.T., Clarkson, P.M., Fritz, V.M. and Evans, W.J. (1990) Extracellular matrix disruption and pain after eccentric muscle action. *J. Appl. Physiol.*, **69**(3), 868–74.

Stauber, W.T., Knack, K.K., Miller, G.R. and Grimmett, J.G. (1996) Fibrosis and intercellular collagen connections from four weeks of muscle strain. *Muscle Nerve*, **19**, 423–30.

Trincher, K. (1981) *Die Gesetze der biologishen Thermodynamik*. Vienna: Urban u. Shwarzenberg.

Upledger, J. (1983) *Cranial Sacral Therapy*. Seattle: Eastland Press.

Wiener, N. (1963) *Kybernetik oder Regulung und Nachrichtenubertragung im Lebewesen und der Maschine*. Dusseldorf: Econ Verlag.

Zachazewski, J.F. (1989) *Phys. Ther.*, **39**, 698–732.

14 Reflextherapy

Josephine Smith Oliver and Linda J. Skellam

To see a World in a Grain of Sand,
And Heaven in a Wild Flower,
Hold Infinity in the palm of your hand,
And Eternity in an hour (William Blake)

Introduction

Physiotherapy courses lay heavy emphasis on anatomy, physiology and pathology of disease. At postgraduate level, clinical skills are incorporated into practice, where techniques based on rational knowledge can be used to treat a wide range of conditions. Reflextherapy is one form of specialist physiotherapy which extends beyond these boundaries into a sphere of awareness encompassing alternative views of health and healing. It gives a fascinating insight into the theories regarding the interaction of body, mind and spirit and differing views on the causation of disease. Taken to its full potential, reflextherapy can thus be used in a truly holistic manner.

Theoretical base

Reflextherapy is essentially a form of micro-acupressure (which could be described as a form of acupuncture without needles, stimulating relevant points with the use of finger and thumb pressure). It involves the application of a form of touch on certain points around the feet. The feet are considered as 'mirrors' of the body, with reflections corresponding to each system and structure.

In fact, it is possible to superimpose an image of the head, neck and torso directly onto the feet, with the limbs to be found along the lateral borders. Each foot represents the same side of the body. The inner borders of the feet including the middle phalanx reflect the spine, with the toes representing the head area. (The whole of the head is reflected by the distal phalanx of both great toes and can also be interpreted as a whole by the corresponding areas of the other toes put together.) Shoulder points are to be found at the distal head of the fifth metatarsals, with the elbows at their proximal extent. The hip reflexes are found on the lateral borders of the calcaneum and talus bones. Other structures round the pelvis, including the sacrum, uterus, fallopian tubes and sciatic nerve, are mirrored on the medial, anterior and inferior aspects of the heel (Figure 14.1). In the early stages of pregnancy, a local redness can be seen over the reflex to the uterus. As the baby develops, this area becomes swollen and taut.

The theory is, that any imbalance can be apparent in the feet as reflected areas of tenderness or altered sensation. The role of the therapist is to locate these areas and to treat them in order to facilitate a change. This then produces a reflex response within the corresponding area of the body which encourages relaxation, allowing healing processes to take place.

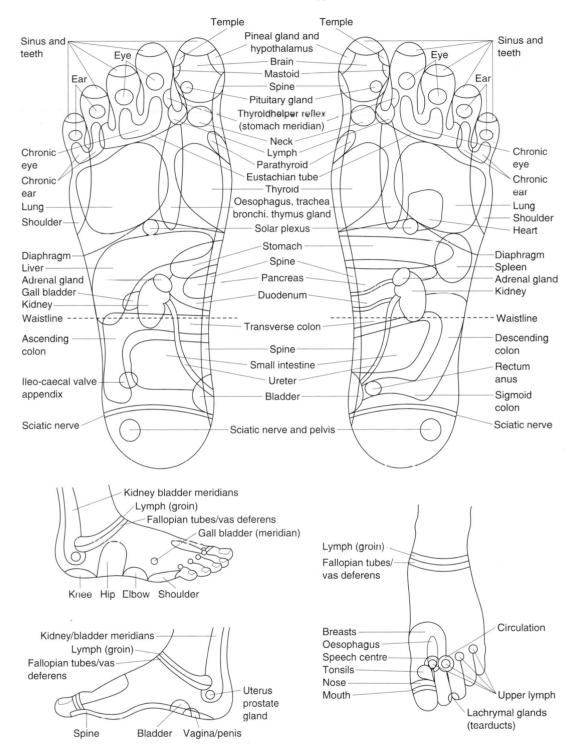

Figure 14.1 Superimposition of body structures onto foot surfaces according to reflextherapy theory (reprinted with kind permission of Inge Dougans, PO Box 68283, 2021 Bryanston, Republic of South Africa)

Historical background

Evidence of the value of foot acupressure has been depicted in Egypt, India and China, in writing and through art, with records dating back to 2500 BC. It is thought that this knowledge was spread by Ptolemy from Egypt into the Greek and Roman Empires and information also passed by Buddhist monks travelling from India into Japan. Records of specific massage techniques, many of them relating to the feet, have been found in ancient Chinese literature dating back 5000 years. It is also known to have been practised by some North American Indian tribes, and contemporary Cherokee chiefs claim skills passed down over hundreds of years.

There are many gaps in the history of this fascinating subject. Christine Issel notes (1990), in her review of the literature of reflexology, that 'zone therapy' (a similar form of acupressure) was practised in Europe in the sixteenth century. Issel points out that the term 'reflex' was first used in 1771 by a German physiologist, Johann August Unzer, who used the term in reference to his study of motor reactions. In England in 1833, the physiologist Marshall Hall described it in neurophysiological studies, demonstrating differences between conscious and unconscious movement.

At the turn of the century, Dr Alfons Cornelius (1902) published a manuscript on the significance of pressure points. Through personal experience of a course of massage for an infection, he noted that treatments he received which concentrated on tender and painful areas were more beneficial than those applied generally. Through this experience he was prompted to incorporate the use of pressure points in his practice. He felt that the effect was produced by a mechanical effect upon the neurons of the sympathetic nervous system. He noted that all conditions produced sensitive reflex points, which '. . . introduced the picture of an illness long before it is to be recognised as an expression of a neurological problem'. He also noted that varying qualities and degrees of sensitivity existed, indicating differences in severity and type of condition.

Issel also pointed out that, at a similar time, the Neurological Society of London was founded to study theories regarding the workings of the human brain and nervous system. The neurophysiologist Sir Charles Sherrington (1861–1952) found that the whole nervous system adjusted to the application of an isolated stimulus. A colleague of his, Sir Henry Head, wrote a paper stating the relationship between specific areas of the skin with internal organs and spinal segments (Head, 1893). These became known as 'Head's zones'. Tissue innervation was then divided into dermatomes, myotomes and sclerotomes as they developed from their embryonic relationships, thus helping to explain why pain is sometimes felt at a distance from its source. The surgeon John Hunter described referred pain in 1835 as a disorder occurring in the mind, and this approach was emphasized by Cyriax (1979), who also stated that it depended upon the nature of the structure, the strength of the stimulus and its position within the dermatome.

Throughout history there have been several examples of subdivision of the body for medical purposes. The Chinese devised the longitudinal meridian system in 2500 BC. Issel also notes that in 1913 a Japanese psychologist, Dr Kurakichi Hirata, divided the body into horizontal zones of influence.

In the early 1900s an American ENT surgeon, Dr William Fitzgerald, divided the body into 10 longitudinal zones. Zone One included an area around the midline of the body, extending into the limbs as far as the thumb and the great toe. The four adjacent zones on either side were then defined by parallel longitudinal lines, which terminated in the spaces between the fingers and toes (Figure 14.2). During his investigations he found that prolonged pressure on one area could have an anaesthetic and therapeutic effect on other areas within the same zone. He went on to use pressure point techniques with his patients for pain relief, and in place of anaesthetic during surgery.

Fitzgerald's ideas met with fierce scepticism and were not accepted by the medical profession, but were taken up by Dr Joe Shelby Riley in Washington, who was the first to produce simple diagrams of the feet reflecting areas of the body in 1919. With his wife he taught Fitzgerald's work, and one of his students, Eunice Ingham (1879–1974), extended the work further, calling it 'reflexology'. She published several books (e.g. Ingham, 1938, 1951). With

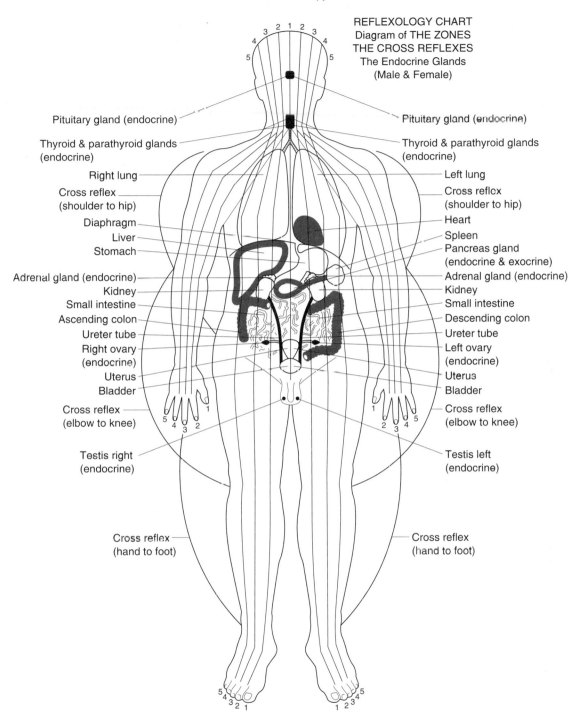

REFLEXOLOGY CHART
Diagram of THE ZONES
THE CROSS REFLEXES
The Endocrine Glands
(Male & Female)

Pituitary gland (endocrine)

Pituitary gland (endocrine)

Thyroid & parathyroid glands (endocrine)

Thyroid & parathyroid glands (endocrine)

Right lung

Left lung

Cross reflex (shoulder to hip)

Cross reflex (shoulder to hip)

Diaphragm

Heart

Liver

Spleen

Stomach

Pancreas gland (endocrine & exocrine)

Adrenal gland (endocrine)

Adrenal gland (endocrine)

Kidney

Kidney

Small intestine

Small intestine

Ascending colon

Descending colon

Ureter tube

Ureter tube

Right ovary (endocrine)

Left ovary (endocrine)

Uterus

Uterus

Bladder

Bladder

Cross reflex (elbow to knee)

Cross reflex (elbow to knee)

Testis right (endocrine)

Testis left (endocrine)

Cross reflex (hand to foot)

Cross reflex (hand to foot)

Figure 14.2 The body divided into ten longitudinal zones according to Fitzgerald (reprinted with kind permission of Earthkinds, London)

encouragement from Riley and other doctors of a similar outlook, she began lecturing to the public and non-medical community, as well as teaching other fellow therapists. This later led to some difficulty, as some of her students began practising without a State licence and caused reflexology to became outlawed in America in 1955. It is now only accepted in certain States.

Hanne Marquadt (1974) followed, restricting her work to pressure points within the feet. Ann Lett, a registered nurse, continues this work, teaching in London. Inge Dougans (1995) believes there to be a link between the recognized zones and the Chinese meridian system. She has developed a method which encompasses these theories.

Christine Jones, a chartered physiotherapist, began practising reflexology in 1972, after having trained with Doreen Bayley (an English nurse who studied with Ingham). After using the therapy for some time, she decided to develop it, and renamed it 'reflextherapy' in order to reflect the change in approach. Subsequently, in 1976, she established the Midland School of Reflextherapy (MSR), based in Warwick, England, teaching reflextherapy with associated studies. Courses are now also run at selected national and international venues.

Her work was finally accepted as part of mainstream physiotherapy practice by the Chartered Society of Physiotherapy (CSP) in 1992. In 1994, Jones set up the Association of Chartered Physiotherapists in Reflex Therapy (ACPIRT), a clinical interest group which also includes other health care professionals. All those who have completed a recognized training in reflexology or reflextherapy are eligible for membership. In 1997, she was awarded a fellowship of the CSP in recognition of her innovative work.

Terminology

The difference in terminology between 'reflextherapy' and 'reflexology' can be muddling. Eunice Ingham herself interchanged these terms with 'zone therapy', so the confusion is not new. There is the obvious difference within the derivation of the suffix 'ology' meaning 'study' and 'therapy' meaning 'treatment'. However, 'reflex therapy' (two words) is a collective name agreed by ACPIRT that could be applied to therapies concerned with treatment involving the system of reflexes in the body as is postulated in complementary medicine. This includes reflexology, reflex zone therapy and reflextherapy as taught by the Midland School.

Principles of reflextherapy (MSR approach)

In reflextherapy, the procedure always considers the physiological systems in an order which allows the body gradually to adjust to changes which take place both during and between treatments. The procedure begins with foot effleurage, to encourage relaxation and to enable the practitioner to gain an insight into the general condition. This assists in identifying any areas of imbalance or differences in sensation perceived by patient or therapist. The reflected area to the solar plexus is the first structure to be specifically worked upon. In the body, this lies just beneath the diaphragm and consists of a network of sympathetic nerves. In the foot, this is found in line with the third toe, just underneath the ball, on the plantar surface, at the level of the middle third of the metatarsal. This encourages relaxation, as well as facilitating diaphragmatic breathing. From here, treatment progresses through the circulation and lymphatic systems, the organs of elimination, digestive tract, heart, spleen and musculoskeletal systems as found on the feet. The nervous and endocrine systems then follow. To conclude the treatment, techniques are used to encourage gentle balance where imbalance has been found, plus mobilizing movements of the feet.

The length of the session can vary, lasting from a few minutes to an hour, according to the patient's condition and the time available. It is always tempting to think that time is directly proportional to the rate of recovery, in line with intensive rehabilitation procedures, but great care must be taken not to over-treat. This allows equilibrium to be restored naturally, and in its own time.

It must be remembered that although there is a recommended order, it is always important to tailor treatment to the requirements of the patient. This is ascertained by taking a thorough case history, including all medical conditions as well as past and present physical disorders. It is important that the patient feels free to discuss any emotional, family or work stresses with the practitioner. These often have a direct bearing on the presenting problems.

The emphasis is placed on a *gentle* approach, with the tender pressure point being eased into a state of relaxation, rather than being forced. In fact, it seems that factors similar in nature to homoeopathic principles are at work here. In the making of remedies, substances are diluted and potentized in order to produce the therapeutic effect. The greater the dilution, the stronger the dosage effect. In reflextherapy, it is often found that the more gentle the approach, the greater the effect of treatment.

It is important to bear in mind the 'observer effect' which occurs in quantum physics. Here, it is recognized that the expectation of the 'observer' in any quantum-type experiment (performed at the subatomic level) can have an effect upon its result (Capra, 1975). The more gentle and subtle a therapy becomes, the more likely it is that the treatment enters the realms of bio-energies when it is probable that a phenomenon similar to the 'observer effect' exists. In other words, the mind of the therapist can have a profound effect on the outcome of treatment. It is important that his or her mental attitude becomes centred and observational, rather than being specific and directional. The outcome can then follow its own pattern, and is not in any way affected by preconceptions, attitudes or moods of the therapist.

Clinical indications and contra-indications

Reflextherapy can be used in any condition normally covered by physiotherapy, provided that no contraindication exists. Because of the depth of relaxation induced, it is of particular value in any condition associated with adverse stress. Conditions giving rise to panic attacks and depression, for example, respond particularly well. Caution is employed in early pregnancy, unstable blood pressure, carcinoma, acute infectious diseases, unstable psychological conditions and with some medications and metal implants, such as cardiac pacemakers, etc. It is contraindicated in cases of deep vein thrombosis and internal bleeding, syncope, malignant melanoma, and in conditions where the rationale of treatment is uncertain.

How reflextherapy works

In 1965, Melzack and Wall proposed that touch could induce pain relief by activating the large A beta afferent nerve fibres from the receptors in the skin as they connect with the cells in the dorsal horn of the spinal cord. Stimulation of these fibres by stroking the skin has been found to affect the activity of these nociceptive cells in the dorsal horn and 'close the gate' on the barrage of painful stimuli reaching the brain. This could help to explain why many experience pain relief during treatment.

Issel informs us that the early pioneer, William Fitzgerald, considered that prolonged pressure applied to the relevant reflex points could have the same effect. He also thought that the massage could improve circulation to an area, preventing bruising. In addition to this, he gave great importance to the effect of the interaction between patient and therapist, and to the empathetic rapport which resulted. He saw this as being due to the effects of animal magnetism, a theory which would seem to be in line with current thought and research findings regarding the effects of directed healing techniques.

Eunice Ingham, on the other hand, believed the effects to be associated with reflex action on the autonomic nervous system and on hormonal balance. There are those who support the theory of the existence of micro-crystals within the reflex points. Doreen Bayley (1986) was of the view that pressure on these points can break up and disperse the crystals, causing an electrical impulse and energy flow. This is backed up by Barbara Zeller-Dobbs (1985), who describes her hypothesis of the existence of lactic acid crystals within the reflex points. More therapists now place a greater emphasis on reflexology as an energy therapy. Gillanders (1987) believes that the human body operates as an electrical circuit, where the treatment acts upon energy centres in the body, creating a harmonizing flow between all cells.

Coghill and Oldfield (1988), have put forward the theory that the brain acts like a radio transmitter and receiver, capable of communicating directly with the cells, as well as indirectly via the nervous system. According to them, the pyramidal cells in the brain's motor cortex oscillate between positive and negative polarities, sending signals into the electromagnetic field which surrounds the body. These signals are then received and recognized by individual cells and tissues, which adapt according to the information received. This allows for a much faster form of communication than that allowed by the CNS. They postulate that any adverse condition such as stress could alter this signalling, and that if unfavourable conditions are of sufficient duration or intensity this can cause malfunctioning of the cells, resulting in imbalance or dis-ease. They have suggested that many complementary therapies work by 'retuning' or replacing the missing signal. This occurs as the correct 'energy wavelength' is produced by an appropriate stimulus.

In 1972, an American neuroscientist, Candace Pert, discovered evidence of an intercommunicating network linking all systems. In particular, she found that receptors exist on the cell membrane which connect with certain chemical messengers found in the brain, nervous, endocrine and immune systems. These messengers, or neuropeptides, move freely through extracellular space in blood and cerebrospinal fluid connecting all systems. As they bind to the appropriate receptor molecule they can dramatically change the function of the cell. Pert believes that it is this network that can give a deeper, emotional view on the understanding of pain symptomatology and a key to the understanding of disease (Pert, 1997).

With this evidence, and with the knowledge that massage can produce both physiological and psychological effects, we can begin to understand how touching reflex points on the feet, hands and the head can enhance this effect. In our view it is unlikely that any one system is responsible, but that a combination of changes take place, involving electrical, chemical, neurological, circulatory and hormonal systems.

Research literature

A reasonable amount of literature is available covering many subjects and conditions. Kunz and Kunz (1997) have produced an alphabetical list of studies. A booklet of research reports and ongoing projects is also available from the Association of Reflexologists. Five abstracts of case studies are used here as examples. In a small-scale study by Berker (1993) at Exeter University, a sample of 4 patients with non-cardiac chest pain were given a series of 7 weekly and 2 follow-up sessions of reflexology. Nine months later 3 of the 4 participants were clear of previous symptoms, with the fourth having experienced an improvement.

A randomized double blind trial including 91 patients, entitled '*Neuro-Reflextherapy Intervention in the Treatment of Non Specified Low Back Pain*', was conducted by Kovacs *et al.* (1993). The 48 patients in the treatment group showed statistically significant improvements in pain of $p < 0.0001$, i.e. 10 000 : 1 against chance in pain, muscular symptoms and mobility. This allowed them to cease medication and kept them pain free during the period of the study.

A trial concerned with the treatment of asthma was conducted at the Health Centre for Women and Children, at Haimen, China (Hui-Xian, 1994), examined the effects of reflexology in infantile bronchial asthma. Forty-five children were selected, ranging from 5 months to 7 years of age. Daily treatments were applied, for periods ranging from 2 to 12 weeks. Results showed improvements in clinical symptoms in all 45 cases, with a clinical cure rate of 100%.

Central and Cecil Housing Trust (1995) published a pilot study entitled '*Health Alternatives for Older People*,' which examined the benefits of the use of complementary therapies in residential homes. Results were monitored with the use of questionnaires completed by either the staff, clients or therapists. Results were positive, with clients reporting varying degrees of improvement in symptoms in cases of osteoarthritis, stress and neurological conditions.

Although there is a reasonable amount of research literature available, there are few conditions which are covered by more than one or two studies. Many projects do not report sufficient data, which leads to difficulties when conclusions need to be drawn using current protocol.

Associated studies

As an assistance to developing the use of reflextherapy as a holistic method, it is important to have an understanding of other related philosophies. The Law of Cure (especially recognized by homoeopaths) gives an understanding of the reactions that are likely to be produced within a patient as healing takes place. Within this philosophy, it is recognized that the treatment is directed at the whole person and not solely at the presenting symptoms. Past ailments can re-emerge temporarily, in an order which progresses backwards in time. Symptoms may also be transferred from the inside to the outside of the body, such as from the lungs to the skin, or as a release in the form of a cough or a cold or increased elimination from the bladder or bowels.

The Chinese Law of Five Elements also gives an understanding of broader views on health and healing, where there is a recognition of the links between emotions and the physical body. Each element (water, wood, fire, earth and air) is taken to be a manifestation of universal energies and is associated with corresponding seasons, times of day, sounds, colours and other factors which relate to them. Each element is linked to a major emotion and is associated with a pair of organs. For example, the wood element is associated with the liver and gall bladder, and with anger.

Knowledge and understanding of these elements and their paired relationships gives the reflextherapist a useful tool in the understanding of a patient's overall condition, and in the application of the therapy. For example, on encountering an obviously angry person, it will be important to examine the liver and gall bladder area for signs of imbalance as compared with the rest of the body. Also, through the pairing of the organs it is possible to indirectly treat a problem area, by stimulating the reflex points to its opposite partner. For example, the air element relates to the lungs and the large intestine. In the case of a patient with lung dysfunction,

the large intestine reflex points can be used to treat the lungs.

An increasing number of books are available discussing various aspects of body and mind connections, some of which have a particular relevance to reflextherapy. Avi Grinberg (1993a,b) has developed a technique of foot analysis where detailed examination of the physical shape and characteristics of the feet is combined with an understanding of the elements as above. Somagi (1997) and Stormer (1995) have developed theories and systems of analysis of toes and feet, respectively, that represent a mirror to the personality.

Others expand the view that imbalances within mental and emotional spheres are mirrored in physical illness. Shapiro (1990) provides a dictionary outlining the mental and emotional links with each. Dethelfson and Dahlke (1990) give an in-depth understanding of this link, encouraging the reader to be their own interpreter of symptoms.

Case histories

Low back pain

A lady in her mid-40s, who worked as a shop supervisor, presented with acute low back pain and sciatica of 13 weeks' duration. She had previously been advised to take 1 week of bed rest, with a further 7 weeks off work, neither of which had resolved any symptoms. On examination, pain extended across the base of her spine at L3–4 level, radiating to the left knee and extending to mid-thoracic level. There was an alteration in her posture, with side-flexion and rotation on weight-bearing. From this and other evidence presented, it was considered that the patient was suffering from a prolapsed intervertebral disc. She had now returned to work. Direct manual pressure on the spine was too painful and therefore inappropriate. It was agreed that reflextherapy would be the most suitable treatment, especially as her job was particularly stressful. The feet were noticeably deep pink in colour and very immobile.

Treatment 1: Treatment was applied, including all systems. Her feet were very tender, particularly around the lumbar spine and large intestine reflexes. Postural advice was also given, with attention paid to the importance of maintaining a normal lumbar lordosis at all times.

Treatment 2: Three days later, the patient reported that there was a significant reduction in the level of discomfort and that the leg pain now only radiated to the left hip. On examination it was noted that her posture had now straightened and that she was moving more naturally. Treatment followed as before. The lumbar spine reflexes on the feet were much less tender.

Treatment 3: Seven days later, the discomfort was now reduced to an area on the right side of the lower lumbar spine. All reflexes were now much less tender, especially at the lumbar and sciatic nerve areas.

Subsequent treatments: Four further weekly sessions followed, during which time the pain continued to reduce in accordance with similar findings on the reflexes on the feet. At her last attendance she reported that her only remaining problem was that of a slight discomfort on overstretching, although lumbar movements were now of full range.

This case illustrates how reflextherapy can directly affect symptoms associated with lumbar dysfunction in a similar way to that which one might expect with other more physical therapeutic modalities. It is interesting to note that gentle pressure on the reflex areas appears to trigger a mechanism of self-healing in the patient, rather than specific treatment being applied to a patient by the physiotherapist.

Low back pain and asthma

A 49-year-old textile worker presented with chronic debilitating low back pain, which came on in 1968 as a result of lifting heavy paving stones in a manual job. He also had a long-term history of asthma, for which he received regular medication. At the beginning of treatment he had been experiencing regular episodes of acute back pain occurring in a 6-weekly cycle. This would consist of 2 weeks of acute pain, 2 weeks of recovery and 2 weeks pain free. Symptoms were located centrally in the lower lumbar spine radiating on occasions to thoracic levels and into both legs. General mobility was affected, and the patient was unable to walk far. He also stated that it could take him 10 minutes to put on his socks. Surgery had been suggested, but the patient was not

keen to pursue this if at all possible. At this time he was also needing to take inhalers on a regular basis, during the day and night, and would wake most nights with an asthma attack. The patient maintained regular 6-weekly chest examinations at the local surgery. On examination, lumbar movements were severely limited, particularly flexion.

Treatment 1: A complete treatment was given. Tender areas were noted around the reflexes to the solar plexus, spine, and large and small intestine. The patient was extremely sensitive to treatment and was likely to respond well. Possible effects were explained to him, and an appointment was made for a few days later. Results proved to be dramatic. Approximately 10 minutes after arriving home, while sitting relaxing, he experienced what he described as 'The sensation of an energy layer being lifted from his body, in a similar way to that of a snake shedding its skin'. It was a comfortable, and in no way alarming, sensation for him and it was following this that quite profound changes occurred.

Treatment 2: Four days later, the patient reported that he had much improved 'in every way'. He had experienced no asthma attacks in the night, pain levels were reduced and there was an increased mobility of his lumbar spine. Forward flexion measuring fingertips to floor had progressed to 10 inches (4 cm) and he was now able to put on his socks without discomfort.

Subsequent treatments: It is now 18 months since his first appointment. Since then he has continued attending on a regular basis. His progress has been maintained, although it has continued rather more slowly and gradually than that following the first session. Over the last 12 months he has experienced minor twinges in his back only. His chest capacity has increased from 300 to 500 cm^3 and has improved so much that he has now been discharged from further attendance at the surgery. His capacity for physical exercise has improved and with it his quality of life which he estimates has increased from 40% to 95%. Subsequently he is better able to live life to the full, with longer walks and gardening, and normal work no longer posing a problem.

This study illustrates how reflextherapy can also identify and treat other areas of imbalance in the body which may be resulting from, or contributing to, the presenting condition. Many patients often report that they feel significantly different after treatment, and although unable to describe exactly how, are subtly changed in a profound and moving way that allows them to face life with greater optimism.

Conclusion

Clearly, much work is to be done, particularly if reflextherapy is to be fully integrated into physiotherapy and the medical profession. Research to date has been limited, as it is difficult to apply the normal protocol. There are many who subscribe to the fact that scientific knowledge somehow dampens our deep intuitive sense, which is an invaluable and important tool within the application of any complementary therapy. Reflextherapy is a very deep and profound treatment, with enormous potential for development. Somehow, a balance must be found between the intuitive and scientific in order to fully prove its true value. As the feet are associated with moving forward, so the knowledge of reflextherapy be advanced, thus encouraging the development of a greater understanding of humanity and its place in the universe.

References

Bayley, D. (1986) *Reflexology Today*. New York: Thorsons.

Berker, M. (1993) *Is Chest Pain Affected by Reflexology Intervention?*, AOR Research Reports, 4th edn. Henfield: AOR.

Capra, F. (1975) *The Tao of Physics*. London: Flamingo.

Central and Cecil Housing Trust (1995) *Health Alternatives for Older People*, AOR Research Reports, 4th edn. Henfield: AOR.

Coghill, R. and Oldfield, H. (1988, reprinted 1995) *The Dark Side of the Brain*. Shaftesbury: Element.

Cornelius, A. (1902) *Pressure Points, their Origin and Significance*. Berlin.

Cyriax, J. (1979) *Textbook of Orthopaedic Medicine*. London: Baillière Tindall.

Dethelfson and Dahlke (1990) *The Healing Power of Illness*. Shaftesbury: Element.

Dougans, I. (1995) *The Art of Reflexology*. Shaftesbury: Element.

Fitzgerald, W. (1917) *Zone Therapy*. Mokelumne, CA: Health Research.

Gillanders, A. (1987) *Reflexology: The Ancient Answer to Modern Ailments*. Harlow: Gillanders.

Grinberg, A. (1993) *Foot Analysis to Self Discovery*. Wellingborough: Thorsons.

Grinberg, A. (1993) *Holistic Reflexology*. Wellingborough: Thorsons.

Head, Sir H. (1893) *On Disturbance of Sensation with Especial Reference to the Pain of Visceral Disease*.

Hui-Xian (1994) *A Clinical Analysis of Foot Reflex Massage for the Treatment of 45 Cases with Infant Bronchial Asthma*, AOR Research Reports, 4th edn. Henfield: AOR.

Ingham, E. (1938) *Stories the Feet Can Tell*. St Petersburg, FL: Ingham Publishing.

Ingham, E. (1951) *Stories the Feet Have Told*. St Petersburg, FL: Ingham Publishing.

Issel, C. (1990) *Reflexology: Art, Science and History*. Sacramento, CA: New Frontier Publishing.

Kovacs, F.M., Abraira, V., Lopez-Abente, G. and Pozo, F. (1993) *Neuro-Reflexotherapy Intervention in the Treatment of Non Specified Low Back Pain*, AOR Research Reports, 4th edn. Henfield: AOR.

Kunz, B. and Kunz, W. (1997) *Alphabetical List of Research in Reflexology* (Internet web pages).

Marquadt, H. (1974) *Reflex Zone Therapy of the Feet*. Wellingborough: Thorsons.

Melzack, R. and Wall, P. (1991) *The Challenge of Pain*. Harmondsworth: Penguin.

Patel, M. (1987) Problems in the evaluation of alternative medicine. *Soc. Sci. Med.*, 25(6), 669–78.

Pert, C. (1997) *Molecules of Emotion*. London: Simon and Schuster.

Shapiro, D. (1990) *The Bodymind Workbook*. Shaftesbury: Element.

Shelby Riley, J. (1919) *Zone Therapy Simplified*. Mokelumne, CA: Health Research.

Somagi, I.(1997) *Reading Toes, Your Feet as Reflections of Your Personality*. Saffron Walden: C.W. Daniel.

Stormer, C. (1995) *Language of the Feet Headway*. London: Hodder and Stoughton.

Zeller-Dobbs, B. (1985) Alternative health approaches. *Nursing Mirror*, 2, 41–42.

Recommended reading

Botting, D. (1997) Review of literature on the effectiveness of reflexology. *Comp. Ther. Nurs. Midwif.*, 3, 123–30.

Connely, D. (1987) *Traditional Acupuncture: The Law of the Five Elements*. Columbia, MD: Centre for Traditional Acupuncture.

Frankl, B.S.M. (1997) The effect of reflexology on baroceptor reflex sensitivity, blood pressure and sinus arrhythmia. *Comp. Ther. Med.*, 2, 80–84.

Gerber, R. (1998) *Vibrational Medicine*. Santa Fe, NM: Bear.

Kapchuk, T. (1987) *Chinese Medicine: The Web that has no Weaver*. London: Rider.

Kushi, M. (1993) *The Book of Do In*. Tokyo: Japan Publications.

Shiatsu with physiotherapy – an integrative approach

Andrea Battermann

Introduction

This chapter describes the history of Shiatsu, its theory and practice, and presents a detailed case study in which a Western medical approach is combined with the Traditional Chinese Medicine (TCM) approach. Since it is beyond the scope of the chapter to explain the TCM terminology and TCM organ functions fully, interested readers are referred to Chapter 9 and the reference list.

What is Shiatsu?

Shiatsu is a Japanese word meaning 'finger pressure'. It is a healing art and a manual therapy which has its roots in TCM and uses Eastern philosophy as its theoretical framework.

TCM incorporates a system of acupuncture and moxibustion (application of heat), acupressure, herbalism, diet and therapeutic exercises. These exercises are known as **T'ai Ji** (**T'ai Chi**) and **Qi-Gong** (**Ch'i Kung**) breathing exercises.

The concept of **Qi** (the body's vital energy, known as **Ki** in Japanese) is fundamental to understanding TCM theory and its application in practice. Like acupuncture, Shiatsu aims at stimulating and encouraging a free Qi flow in the **meridians** (energy lines) in the body as well as improving the patient's general constitution. In disease and illness, Qi energy becomes excessive or deficient in the meridians and moves into a state of imbalance (Masunaga and Ohashi, 1977).

A detailed investigation of all the physical and psychological expressions and phenomena of the body is used in TCM for diagnosis leading to treatment. The practitioner diagnoses patterns of disharmony in the Qi, **Blood**, **Yin**, **Yang** and fluids usually long before they become somatized or develop into a disease. The type of treatment is chosen according to the phenomena observed in the patient, rather than following a causal or linear approach of treating a specific disease. For this reason, TCM plays a major role in preventative medicine and can complement the Western medical model.

In Shiatsu, mainly thumbs, fingers and palms of the hands are used to apply different depths of pressure to acupuncture points (**Tsubos**) and meridians. The patient is sitting or lying in various positions. A variety of techniques are used, e.g. stretching, slow sustained holding pressure, and mobilization of joints and soft tissue. Physically, this has the effect of stimulating the musculoskeletal, neural and hormonal systems and improves the circulation of all body fluids (Dubitsky, 1997). Mentally, Shiatsu allows the receiver to relax deeply. This engenders a feeling of calmness and well-being and improves the self-awareness of the body.

Traditionally, Shiatsu is carried out on a futon (cotton mat) at floor level with the client remaining fully and comfortably clothed. **Do-In** exercises (literally 'leading and guiding' Qi energy in the body), **Makko-Ho** meridian stretches (similar to Yoga) and **Qi-Gong** are sometimes taught to clients to practise between sessions, to support the Shiatsu treatment.

Similar to acupuncture, Shiatsu is recognized as a complementary therapy by the Chartered Society of Physiotherapy in the UK. It is seen as a manual application of acupuncture and practitioners can be registered in the special interest group of acupuncture.

The history of Shiatsu

About 5000 years ago, the Chinese discovered that pressing certain points in stiff and sore areas, relieved pain locally and distally and influenced the functioning of certain internal organs. This form of massage is called **an mo** (literally 'pressing and rubbing') and is acknowledged as one of four classical forms of medical treatment, along with acupuncture, moxibustion and herbalism (Lee and Whincup, 1983). The Chinese physicians developed a system of curing certain conditions by stimulating specific points and meridians. Menstrual pain, for example, seemed to improve by stimulating points and meridians in the legs and feet.

This system evolved over centuries through precise observation and experience. It was practised by people whose awareness and sensitivity was so highly developed that they could localize constriction in a patient's body. They were therefore able to treat the appropriate points which alleviated the problem.

In order to understand the principles and theory behind Shiatsu, we have to study TCM which was introduced to Japan in the sixth century AD by a Buddhist monk Jian Zhen. A few well-known practitioners developed Shiatsu in Japan early in the twentieth century: Tamai Tempaku, Serizawa Sensei, Tokyjiro Namikoshi and Shizuto Masunaga who, with W. Ohashi, published *Zen Shiatsu* in 1977 and created a unique synthesis of TCM, Western physiology and psychology. Masunaga's approach is known as Zen Shiatsu. He developed a system based on treating the meridian system of the entire body. He also developed a system for abdominal diagnosis and extended the location of classical TCM meridians throughout the body (Dubitsky, 1997).

The Japanese Minister of Health and Welfare defines Shiatsu as

. . . a form of manipulation administered by the thumbs, fingers and palms, without the use of any instrument, mechanical or otherwise, to apply pressure to the human skin, correct internal malfunctioning, promote and maintain health and treat specific diseases. (Masunaga and Ohashi, 1977)

Shiatsu in theory and practice

Diagnosis and treatment

There are several diagnostic techniques: observation, questioning, hearing and smelling and palpating which elucidate the states of disharmony in the body. The **Hara diagnosis** often used in Shiatsu, prior to and after a session, is the palpation of specific zones on the abdomen which mirror the state of Qi in the meridian related to each zone (Masunaga and Ohashi, 1977).

The most common theories used in TCM and Shiatsu to describe the movement and pattern of Qi are the Five Elements cycles, the Eight Principles or the **Kyo-jitsu** theory.

Kyo is the condition of deficient energy manifested as an area of weakness or stiffness sensed through penetration. The technique used to treat Kyo areas is called tonification which requires a holding touch to encourage Qi flow. **Jitsu** is the condition of excess energy, which appears hard but elastic in a state of resistance in the body tissue. The technique used to work with Jitsu areas is called sedation and requires a more active technique to disperse excess energy.

The Hara diagnosis will identify the meridians to be worked on. During a treatment we concentrate on tonifying and sedating the acupuncture points, and relating them to the whole meridian line in order to balance the Qi in the entire body (Masunaga and Ohashi, 1977). Figure 15.1 gives the principal Hara zones of the abdomen.

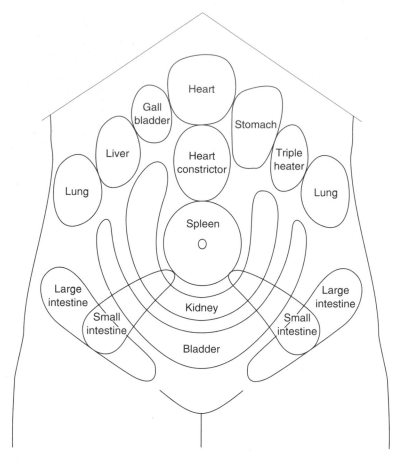

Figure 15.1 The main Hara zones of the abdomen (After Masunaga and Ohashi, 1977)

Conditions responsive to Shiatsu

The following conditions respond well to Shiatsu:

- headaches/migraine
- sinus congestion
- insomnia
- lower back pain
- neck/shoulder problems
- fatigue/low energy
- stress/depression/anxiety
- menstrual/menopausal/hormonal problems
- low resistance to infection
- arthritis
- digestive disorders.

Clinical experience shows a positive outcome and effect in these chronic conditions.

Shiatsu works well in combination with spinal manipulation techniques, by relaxing muscles before or after using manipulation techniques. It also promotes muscle relaxation before the use of proprioceptive neuromuscular facilitation (PNF) techniques.

A national survey carried out by Harris and Pooley (1998) shows that musculoskeletal and psychological problems are the most common conditions treated with Shiatsu. The most frequent musculoskeletal problems are neck/shoulder problems, followed by lower back problems and arthritis. Depression is the main psychological problem, followed by stress and anxiety.

Contraindications

Shiatsu is contraindicated in the following conditions (Dubitsky, 1997):

- haemorrhage
- shock
- acute appendicitis and peritonitis
- cerebrovascular accident (not yet stabilized)
- diabetic coma
- myocardial infarct (MI, not yet stabilized)
- pneumothorax
- severe asthma attack
- severe atherosclerosis
- severe, unstable hypertension
- fever
- systematic/contagious infections
- any acute inflammation
- thrombosis
- acute inflammatory arthrides (rheumatoid arthritis, ankylosing spondylitis).

Precautions

Generally, the following precautions apply:

- treat the abdominal area carefully with a light touch, especially if somebody is severely ill or has a very advanced or complicated chronic organ disease
- use light touch on lymphatic areas such as the throat, below the ears, the groin, and near the armpits
- do not work directly on a serious burn, an ulcerous condition, an open wound or an area of inflammation
- do not work directly on new scar tissue, skin rashes or varicose veins
- take special care in pregnancy – gentle work is recommended on the lower back and sacrum (acupuncture points to avoid are GB 21, LI 4, SP 6, BL 60 and LIV 3).

Techniques and principles

The following techniques and principles are adopted:

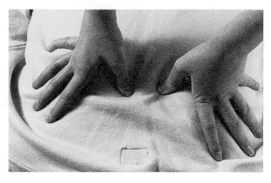

Figure 15.2 Perpendicular pressure on the Bladder meridian

- use body weight to apply pressure on to the body without muscular power
- pressure is perpendicular and stationary in order to access meridians and points (Figure 15.2)
- work along the whole length of the meridians to find points of deepest penetration to access directly the Qi energy
- use two hands simultaneously (Figure 15.3)
- treat the receiver as a whole, considering their mind, spirit and emotions as well as the physical body
- move with a steady rhythm throughout the treatment
- stay relaxed, working from the most comfortable position.

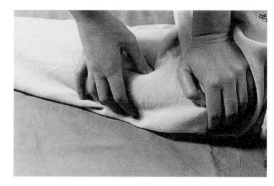

Figure 15.3 Two-handed technique: one hand is holding and the other is tonifying the Lung meridian

Case study

The following case study will show how Shiatsu benefited a patient who reported no improvement following a course of physiotherapy. It was a complex case, using TCM diagnosis and Shiatsu treatments combined with physiotherapy.

Lorna, 29 years old, was referred by a physiotherapist for Shiatsu therapy. She received physiotherapy regularly, including manual traction, heat application, spinal mobilization techniques, acupuncture, and exercises for shoulder and neck, but all were of little benefit. She lives with others and works in an office as a PC operator.

Past medical history

Lorna had had an accident 10 months previously, in which she fell on the stairs of a bus. She tried to prevent the fall with her left arm. Nothing else of note.

Main symptoms reported by client

Severe muscle spasms with muscle tremors and pain on the left side of neck and face, thoracic spine and abdomen. Recent deterioration, leading to severe and constant muscle twitching which mainly affected her neck and resulted in increased muscle tone and pain in her upper body.

(i)   *Sleep:* Waking up several times a night with pain and muscle spasms. Sleeping on her left side and more in extensor than in flexor pattern due to pain.
(ii) *Vertigo:* Suffering from dizziness in sitting, standing or while walking. In the past, had only suffered from dizziness when she had a cold.
(iii) *Body temperature:* Heat rushes in the whole body.
(iv) *Chest:* Production of whitish phlegm and flu-like symptoms since her injury; increased frequency of colds and sore throats.
(v)   *X-ray for shoulder and neck:* Did not show any abnormalities.

(vi) *Consultations:* Consultant neurologist reported no neurological abnormalities and normal reflex activity. Her condition was characterized by muscle spasms with an overproduction of adrenaline.
(vii) *Medication used:* diazepam, co-dydramol, ibuprofen and propranolol.

Physical assessment

(i)   *Visual:* Right shoulder lower than left, head and facial muscles constantly twitching, head protraction, left scapula area elevated with spasm, walking very rigid, decrease in muscle bulk around left shoulder joint, particularly deltoid.
(ii) *Cervical spine and shoulder range of movement:*

neck movements:
- flexion: $\frac{1}{4}$ range
- extension: $\frac{1}{4}$ range
- right lateral flexion: nil, block, and no pain
- left lateral flexion: $\frac{1}{4}$ range
- right rotation: nil, block, and no pain
- left rotation: $\frac{1}{4}$ range
- protraction: full ROM
- retraction: full ROM.

(iii) *Shoulder movements:*

- flexion/elevation – 30° limited by pain
- extension – 30° limited by pain
- abduction – 20° limited by pain
- adduction – 20° limited by pain
- internal rotation – $\frac{3}{4}$ range
- lateral rotation – $\frac{3}{4}$ range.

(iv) *Passive movements:* Same as active, pain at end of range.
(v)   *Sensation problems:* Occasional paraesthesiae from mid-deltoid muscle down into left arm, reduced sensation in C7 dermatome, intermittent burning pain at base of skull, hot burning sensation around neck and left scapula.
(vi) *Palpation:* Painful around left shoulder and increased muscle tone in the deltoid muscle, C4 and C5 painful in supine, increased muscle tone in general, severe muscle

spasm of the paravertebral muscles of the left cervical region and the trapezius muscle in cervical and thoracic spine.

(vii) *Pain:*

- pain eases following: heat application, rest (lying down for 1 hour), pain-killers, better in the morning
- pain worse following: after a working day, any shoulder movement; deep-seated pain is constant in neck and shoulder and varies in intensity
- perceived level of pain: 1 (0 = extreme pain, 10 = no pain)
- perceived level of energy: 2 (0 = extreme fatigue, 10 = no fatigue).

Other relevant factors in TCM diagnosis

(i) *Appetite:* Following the accident it became erratic at times, especially when the pain was greater.

(ii) *Stools:* (Pre-morbid) irritable bowel syndrome constipation, normal stools and diarrhoea alternate.

(iii) *Urination:* Increased frequency, large amounts, pale colour.

(iv) *Digestion:* Occasionally vomited.

(v) *Taste:* Craved sweet food at time of menstruation, otherwise preferred salty taste.

(vii) *Thirst:* Prefers to drink a lot of warm drinks more often (pre-morbid).

(viii) *Climate:* Preferred warm and hot temperatures.

(ix) *Perspiration:* Since the accident, suffered from day and night sweats (drenching sweat on torso at night).

(x) *Eyes:* Sensitive to bright light, stares when in pain, sometimes dry eyes, dark patches under eyes, watery in the wind and easily tired.

(xi) *Ears:* Tinnitis in both ears, worse in left ear when tired.

(xii) *Voice:* Tired and weak.

(xiii) *Spleen:* Bruises easily (the Spleen in TCM regulates the blood in its pathways).

(xiv) *Nails:* White flecks.

(xv) *Hair:* Sometimes lank, lifeless, soft and thin when in pain (since accident), loose head hair (pre-existent).

(xvi) *Headaches:* Occasional above eyes, particularly right side.

(xvii) *Circulation:* Cold hands and feet (pre-existent), more on left side of body and hands since accident.

(xviii) *Menstruation:* Pre-menstrual pain and cramps, dark clots in menstrual blood; since accident, more painful with breast distention, cramps and lower back pain.

Aims of treatment

Physical

- To reduce muscle spasm and tremor with Shiatsu techniques.
- To relieve pain.
- To increase mobility in cervical and thoracic spine and left shoulder.
- To re-educate: self-mobilization techniques, postural advice, ergonomics and pain management.

Mental

- To re-educate: relaxation techniques for stress management, establish a positive body image.

Energetical

- To remove obstruction of Qi flow in traumatized area and thus relieve pain.
- To promote free flow of Qi circulation throughout the whole body to restore energy and vitality.

Emotional

- To reduce anxiety and calm the mind.

Diagnosis and interpretation of symptoms from the TCM point of view prior to the accident

(i) *The Kidney, Liver and Spleen Qi:* These are mainly involved in the underlying energetical pattern of Lorna's constitution prior to her accident.

(ii) *Kidney Qi deficiency manifests in the following symptoms:* Tinnitus in both ears, worse when tired, loose head hair, increased frequency and large amount of urination, preference for warm drinks and salty food.

(iii) *Liver Qi stagnation manifests in the following symptoms:* White flecks on nails, occasional lateral headaches, vertigo, and painful periods with dark blood clots and cramps. Psychologically, it manifests in stubbornness and suppression of feelings (Kaptchuk, 1983).

(iv) *Spleen Qi deficiency manifests in the following symptoms:* Poor digestion, occasional nausea and vomiting at times, diarrhoea, preference for sweet taste around menstruation due to Liver attacking Spleen, intermittent menstrual blood flow at the end of period instead of a clean cut-off. Psychologically, it manifests in worrying.

Diagnosis and interpretation of symptoms from the TCM point of view following the accident

Various physical symptoms were aggravated after the accident. Due to pain she had a white face with staring eyes. Lack of sleep led to an exacerbation of Kidney and Spleen Qi deficiencies, manifesting as dark rings under her eyes and a weak voice.

The Liver Qi had been out of balance before the accident. The shock of the accident and pain increased muscle tension in her body. In TCM, the Liver controls the sinews. The muscle twitching which appeared several weeks after the accident could be explained by Liver-Blood failing to nourish and moisten the sinews due to spasm impeding supply (Kaptchuk, 1983), and giving rise to endogenous Liver wind.

In general, pain causes constraint and stagnation in Qi flow which aggravated Lorna's Liver Qi stagnation. Lorna reported that her menstrual problems had become worse. Psychologically, she pushes herself beyond her physical capacity to maintain her full-time job. She overworks despite feeling tired and in pain. In TCM terms, the increased Liver Qi stagnation attacks the Spleen, further depleting it

and aggravating pre-existing gastrointestinal symptoms. The accident injured the meridians located posterior and lateral in the head, neck and shoulder area. Lorna's pain was relieved by rest, with her head positioned towards her affected side indicating a deficiency problem.

The three-arm Yang meridians (Large Intestine, Triple Heater and Small Intestine) flow to the head. The physical trauma to these meridians had caused obstruction in the Qi flow to the head and face. Lorna developed a deficient Qi flow in her head, especially in the left side of her face. In TCM terms, it is said the 'Qi moves the Blood' (Veith, 1949). Impeded Qi flow means impeded Blood supply to the sinews and muscles which then start to twitch. The area around C7 and T1 was affected by the accident. This is the localization for the GV 14 point through which all the Yang meridians of the body pass. The trauma to this area could affect the Yang functions in the whole body. This could explain the heat flushes and abnormal day-sweating symptoms. These might be related to the Kidney Qi deficiency.

Lorna's tinnitus had become generally worse due to the increasing Kidney deficiency. The Triple Heater meridian which supplies Qi to the ear was reduced in its function due to the trauma, specifically exacerbating the problem at that side.

The treatments

First session

As mentioned previously, the author works with the extended meridian system from Masunaga.

According to the characteristics of the symptoms and location of the injury, the following meridians are involved: Liver (LIV), Large Intestine (LI) and Kidney (KD), Triple Heater (TH), Conception (CV) and Governing Vessel (GV).

Lorna was lying in supine position with her body twitched continuously. Physical palpation of the Hara diagnostic zones revealed a deficiency (Kyo) in the Kidney energy and an excess (Jitsu) in the Liver energy. The upper Hara (proximal abdomen) was very tight which indicates stagnation of Liver Qi.

Treatment commenced on the chest with an even holding touch tonifying her Kidney

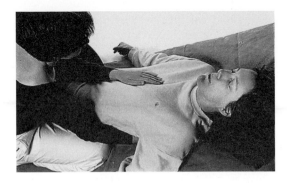

Figure 15.4 Stimumlating Qi flow by holding points on the Kidney and Bladder meridian in the upper back

meridian beside the sternum on either side and dispersing the accumulation of Liver Qi energy with the other hand on the chest. Then continued on the following points: GV 13, GV 14, GV 15, GV 16. Two points were held at the same time on the Governing Vessel meridian to establish the Qi energy flow between these points and in Governing Vessel meridian. Then one hand was moved on the chest, finding points of deepest penetration on the Kidney meridian. The other hand was holding points on the Kidney and Bladder meridian in the upper back at the same time (Figure 15.4). Working locally in the chest and upper back area, the author tried to establish an energetic connection between hands placed anterior and posterior on the upper body.

Lorna's muscle spasms and tone, as well as the twitching intensity, visibly decreased. By working along the spine with the patient lying in side position (Figure 15.5), the muscle tone on the left side in the thoracic spine was signifi-

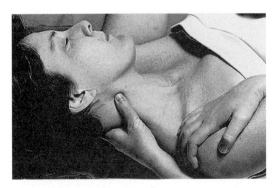

Figure 15.5 Sedation technique on the Large Intestine meridian in side position

cantly increased with very limited spinal mobility. The author then held and contacted the Liver meridian on the chest while applying a more dynamic and active Shiatsu technique with the other hand to disperse the Qi stagnation in that area. Eventually, a better Qi flow was established, resulting in more muscle relaxation and spinal mobility. The muscle tone in Lorna's left leg and foot was increased and painful to the touch.

Second session

Lorna reported less muscle spasm and twitching after her treatment and she felt more relaxed. In this session, work was given on head, neck, shoulder girdle and along the spine on the Kidney and Large Intestine meridians.

Third session

Lorna reported that the muscle twitching had disappeared. There was increased pain in her left shoulder and neck. The author worked locally on Large Intestine and Small Intestine meridians to improve the Qi flow throughout the left shoulder. This resulted in reduced pain and increased energy (using LI 4, LI 11, LI 15 and SI 9, SI 10, SI 11, SI 12, SI 14, and GB 20, GB 21).

Summary of sessions

In further treatments the author worked more intensively on Lorna's neck, trying to establish the Qi flow between head and torso while working on dispersing local Large Intestine and Liver Qi stagnation and tonifying the Kidney energy (Figure 15.6).

The energetical connection between head and torso, especially the thoracic spine, was always blocked and stagnated. Treatments were often finished by working down the Bladder or Kidney, Liver or Large Intestine meridians into the legs and feet to encourage the Qi flow downwards from the upper body into the lower half.

The technique used initially was a very light energetic touch until the patient tolerated more physical pressure, with the author constantly having to readjust and align her own posture to work with the most physical techniques (Figure 15.7).

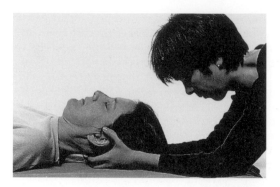

Figure 15.6 Neck release by holding acupuncture point BL 10

Several months later the patient suffered a severe flare-up when bending forward repetitively for filing in the office. The severe muscle spasm and twitching recurred which was successfully treated with two further Shiatsu sessions.

Throughout the course of treatment, Lorna was taught relaxation techniques, postural exercises and ergonomics, stretches for her neck, shoulder and thoracic spine. Additionally, advice was given on pain relief by using Do-In (self-Shiatsu). Initially, the treatment consisted of 3 one-hour sessions every fortnight and later this was reduced to 1 monthly session.

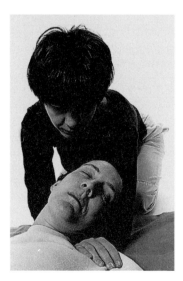

Figure 15.7 Stretching technique for the cervical and upper thoracic spine

Treatment outcome

Outcome of treatment was as follows:

- the pain in Lorna's neck, shoulder and upper back eased immediately after the sessions
- the neck mobility has increased by 50% in range of movement immediately after treatment
- the paraesthesia in Lorna's left arm, shoulder and neck area has disappeared
- Lorna was able significantly to reduce her pain medication
- the range of movement in the neck is normal in extension, flexion, rotation and side flexion to the left; the rotation and flexion to the right has improved by 50%
- the range of movement in Lorna's shoulder has generally improved, but there is still limited movement in flexion, and external rotation at the end of the range due to increased muscle tone
- the deltoid muscle is slightly wasted and the muscle power in her left arm remains reduced
- Lorna's vitality and general health have improved
- Lorna practises a daily exercise programme and she avoids activities that might aggravate her condition.

Feedback from the patient

Feedback from Lorna, after treatment, was as follows:

- the whole body was treated and not just the local area of pain and injury
- long-lasting benefits reduced the number of appointments
- additional to several positive treatment outcomes, Lorna experienced Shiatsu as very relaxing
- she felt that the most important factor was the length of the appointments, which allowed enough time for feedback and physical work – this reduced the number of appointments in that the benefit (outcome) lasted longer

- Lorna commented that Shiatsu might prevent injury from turning into a chronic pain
- she is able to pace her physical activities better by allowing for frequent rest times in between
- Shiatsu should be available on the NHS and is a competitive cost-effective treatment.

Conclusion

This chapter conveys that Shiatsu is an approach requiring considerable skill and training, i.e. its remit lies beyond a merely mechanical stimulation of acupuncture points. It takes years to trust one's own perception and develop a proprioceptive sense to feel the Qi flow in the body, as well as gain an understanding of TCM. In order to comprehend Shiatsu fully you have to receive it. It is a therapy which is based on a non-verbal communication through touch between giver and receiver, affecting the whole being. Each Shiatsu session is unique and cannot be exactly repeated. The relationship between practitioner and client is particular to that interaction and only those involved can really know the effect of this very personal process.

Each traditional therapy, as offered in the NHS in the UK, has its own principles of practice and success rate. Due to the increased development of alternative therapeutic approaches, more and more people are turning to these as a means of alleviating their problems. Furthermore, in some places, alternative therapies are being integrated within the medical system. It is important, therefore, as practising health care professionals, that there is openness, understanding and acceptance of alternative therapies.

Training in Shiatsu

The Shiatsu Society in the UK is the regulating body which can be contacted by anyone interested in this form of therapy. The Society holds a register of practitioners and provides a list of training schools. Registered practitioners are entitled to use the letters MRSS (Member of the Register of the Shiatsu Society).

Acknowledgements

I would like to thank Stephane Erviel for the photography, and Anne Crawford, Mark Wright, Marietta Birkholtz, Clifford Andrews and many colleagues, teachers, students and clients for their encouragement and inspiration.

References

Dubitsky, C. (1997) *Bodywork Shiatsu*. Rochester, VT: Healing Arts Press.

Harris, P.E. and Pooley, N. (1998) What do Shiatsu practitioners treat? A nationwide survey. *Comp. Ther. Med.*, 6(1), 30–35.

Kaptchuk, T.J. (1983) *Chinese Medicine*. London: Rider.

Lee, H. and Whincup, G. (1983) *Chinese Massage Therapy: A Handbook of Therapeutic Massage*. Boulder, CO: Shambhala.

Masunaga, S. and Ohashi, W. (1977) *Zen Shiatsu*. Tokyo: Japan Publications.

Veith, J. (1949) *The Yellow Emperor's Classic of Internal Medicine*. Malaysia: Pelanduk Publications.

Recommended reading

Beresford-Cooke, C. (1996) *Shiatsu Theory and Practice*. Edinburgh: Churchill Livingstone.

Liechti, E. (1998) *The Complete Illustrated Guide to Shiatsu*. Shaftesbury: Element Books.

Lundberg, P. (1992) *The Book of Shiatsu*. London: Gaia Books.

Masunaga, S. (1987) *Zen Imagery Exercises*. Tokyo: Japan Publications.

Namikoshi, T. (1981) *The Complete Book of Shiatsu Therapy*. Tokyo: Japan Publications.

Serizawa, S. (1976) *Tsubo: Vital Points for Oriental Therapy*. Tokyo: Japan Publications.

Part IV

Mind–body therapies

16 Stress counselling – a practical overview

Anna Corser

Introduction

Stress is, alongside virus, a current 'buzz' diagnosis. There are many ongoing arguments about its validity as a cause of various symptoms and resulting lost working days and, more importantly, human suffering.

Dr Stephen Palmer, Director of the Centre for Stress Management in London, was recently interviewed on this subject on BBC Radio 4 (Palmer, 1998). He explained that pressure is, up to a certain optimum level, beneficial. It gets us out of bed in the morning, is generally stimulating and drives us onwards and upwards in all sorts of ways. However, when that pressure becomes excessive and our coping strategies are insufficient to deal with it, pressure then becomes stress, with its associated detrimental and far-reaching symptoms which are referred to in more detail later in the chapter.

Stress counselling is an intervention which uses training in different techniques to enable clients to recognize and minimize the detrimental effects caused by the stressors encountered in their daily life.

Any therapist considering studying stress counselling as an adjunct to their other skills also stands to benefit greatly personally. The author has never taught a client any technique which has not been tried and tested personally. As a physiotherapy manager working in an NHS Mental Health Trust through all the continuing and threatening changes, depleted resources and vast workload, trying impossibly to provide a needs-led service, using these strategies has been invaluable. It is wonderful to share with clients anything you believe in and watch the change in them and the progress they make as they take more informed responsibility for their own physical and mental state.

It may seem strange to include a chapter on stress counselling in a book relating to the other complementary therapies. Learning to use and encourage positive energy and to repel and discharge negative energy is very much part of the background basis of the various interventions when training people to minimize the destructive effects of stress.

Like other modalities, comprehensive certificated training is essential to protect both practitioner and client. This chapter is based upon the author's experience, and the techniques to be discussed have all been used and found to be beneficial.

Psychophysiological effects of stress

Clients usually present with physical symptoms. These have often been investigated to rule out any obvious pathology. At first they find it difficult to accept that these distressing, and sometimes very acute, problems are stress related. Once this is explained and understood, the rest of the training can begin. The body's reaction to stress mirrors the 'flight and fight' mechanism. Initially the stressor is perceived by ears, eyes, nose or skin, the message being relayed to the brain. The hypothalamus reacts by transmitting the message to the autonomic nervous system. It is the sympathetic part of the system which evokes the 'flight' response. It is the first line of defence and prepares the body for action. If the stress passes quickly, it may be the only part of the system to be involved. The adrenaline production from the adrenal glands, which it stimulates, has an immediate effect on the body's organs, producing acceleration of heart action, dilatation of respiratory passages, inhibition of abdominal function, relaxation of the bladder, increased sweating, increased mental activity and increased tone of skeletal muscles.

If the stress passes quickly, with the help of the parasympathetic division which conserves energy, most of the organ functions would settle down. In extreme stress, mainly adrenaline is released producing very marked anxiety symptoms. If the stressful episode lasts more than a few seconds, the endocrine system reacts and augments and prolongs the responses. The pituitary gland acts on the adrenal cortex releasing cortisol, sensitizing organs and blood vessels to both adrenaline and noradrenaline. The immune system can be affected in the longer term; hypertension and fluid retention are other effects. The thyroid gland releases thyroxin which increases the basal metabolic rate, blood sugar, gastrointestinal activity, depth and rate of respiration, heart rate and blood pressure. Oxytocin is also released from the posterior pituitary and this can be detrimental during pregnancy.

All these changes mean that clients can present with some or all of the following: sweating, chest pain, palpitations, abdominal symptoms, headaches, breathlessness, trembling, insomnia, poor concentration and premenstrual tension. Long-term stress can encourage, due to the continuation of these processes, conditions such as coronary heart disease and, it is thought, some forms of cancer.

Assessment

It is, of course, essential to assess the client to try to deduce the main stressors involved and the reasons they have reacted as they have done to them. Obviously the detail of this will evolve as they get to know the therapist and begin to feel more confident in them and also as they learn more about the mechanism of the stress response. Changes in their behaviour noticed by them and/or others are also important to note, e.g. increased smoking and caffeine and alcohol intake; over- or under-eating, slower reaction time, poor concentration, irritation or aggression, loss of interest in things, cynicism or inappropriate humour, poor timekeeping and poor sleeping. It is useful to ask about life events too and general lifestyle.

This helps to place clients into their context or story. Ask too what are their normal coping strategies. These could be appropriate or potentially detrimental. The latter are, for example, smoking, drinking to excess, driving fast, going on an over-extravagant spending spree; more positive ones are, for example, walking, sport, yoga, music, meditation, dancing or sharing time with family or friends. It is useful to find out what a client's social support network consists of, and their home and work atmosphere and environment, and how well they fit into them both. How much people have control over their lives is a very important factor. Some clients have developed a defence mechanism to help them mind less when their level of control is low: apathy or sometimes suppressed anger. The other factor, often related, is how much their value as a worker, friend, partner or relative is acknowledged. When this does not happen, clients often become very withdrawn and frequently have a very low opinion of themselves and their role in the general scheme of things.

Some assessments have a scoring system so that, following treatment, a comparison can be made. An example of this is found in Burns (1989). It is useful to note whether they have any phobias or obsessions, as these will need a specific approach. After assessment it is possible to deduce whether stress counselling is the approach of choice or whether 'in depth' counselling, psychology or psychotherapy are indicated. If, following discussion with the client, stress counselling is chosen, it is important to choose the most appropriate technique to start with. Clients are presented with a 'menu' and find that, after the first couple of sessions, the order evolves naturally depending on their reactions to the modalities already explored. Quite often a very commonsense practical approach helps, as it is sometimes easier to make changes in a client's lifestyle, relationships, work dynamics, etc., than to alter their attitudes and behaviour. However, if longer term intervention is the choice, the best results are achieved by doing both.

Breathing techniques

Many clients choose to start with breathing exercises, as there can be some fairly rapid results, particularly with a technique which the author gives as a kind of first aid intervention. It is a useful preparation before going on to other more comprehensive ones. It involves breathing out gently and letting go, thinking and visualizing a chosen word, such as waves, water, breeze, and allowing the anxiety, tension or anger to flow away. This should only be repeated twice without a break, as sighing can lead to hyperventilation which people trying to combat stress have a tendency towards anyway. If clients do this exercise often enough to become fully proficient at it when they do not need to use it, they can apply it much like a light switch being flicked on when things begin to build up. If hyperventilation is occurring, the technique to combat it involves focusing the breathing on the diaphragmatic area and lessening the rise and fall apically. This needs frequent and regular practice and monitoring. Acute hyperventilation is relatively easy to pick up, but often chronic hyperventilators are less obvious. The results from this work are encouraging once the client has recognized the problem and mastered the necessary changes in breathing pattern. A comprehensive handout should be given. An excellent one is produced by Lesley Seaton (1995).

Even when actual hyperventilation is not occurring it is still calming to breathe diaphragmatically and rhythmically, gradually and comfortably slowing down and increasing the depth. One method of this is an old Eastern pattern called 'the mother's breath'. It involves the breathing being focused abdominally: breathing out counting seven, holding empty counting one, breathing in counting seven and holding for one. Naturally, to start with counting is fairly rapid and then slowed down gradually. As a further adaptation clients can then breathe out tension or a negative thought or emotion and breathe in well-being, calm or some appropriately positive countering state or emotion.

Relaxation

This is a natural follow-on from breathing techniques, but may be contraindicated for certain clients, e.g. those with paranoia, flashbacks (initially) or asthma – as relaxation is a respiratory depressant. Also, sometimes it is better introduced once the client has perfected some cognitive techniques to diminish the intrusive effects of their negative thinking.

The two methods that the author has found to be most effective are, as an introduction, the Laura Mitchell approach and then progressive relaxation. The Laura Mitchell approach involves reciprocal relaxation, i.e. moving the part of the body in the opposite direction from the tension in it and then letting go. It is useful to enable people to see where they are most tense and also to feel the contrast between tension and relaxation. It is also found very beneficial as a way of reducing locally-recognized tension, particularly in the neck and shoulders. Some clients who find progressive relaxation difficult to do, use it as a full method adding in breathing focusing and visualization at the end.

The mental relaxation taught involves, first, good preparation. Anybody else in the house should be made aware of the client relaxing, in order to keep the noise down. A comfortable warm position should be chosen, knowing that this can be changed as necessary during the session. Noise should be listened to and accepted and the mind prepared for its level to fluctuate. The relaxation starts at the head and neck and works down the body in fairly large blocks, e.g. head and neck, shoulders and arms, but always keeping the hands separate as they need extra concentration. Very detailed relaxation is wonderful to be talked through and a deeper level can be reached, but not many clients set aside sufficient time regularly to do it. This shorter version seems to be more acceptable and more frequently done.

Having been through the body once, the client is asked to check through and concentrate on any remaining tense areas. They then do some breathing focus, on the abdominal area, and finally individually chosen visualization. All clients receive a handout and a tape and they add their own music to the end of it, to fit in with their personal taste.

Progressive relaxation (Jacobson, 1938), where muscles are contracted, held and relaxed, is particularly likely to adversely affect people suffering from high blood pressure, heart problems, anxiety, panic attacks, asthma, diabetes, substance misuse, epilepsy, schizophrenia and paranoia (Palmer, 1992). Therefore, it appears preferable that, in these conditions and in group work, where less detailed diagnosis is sometimes given, and less close supervision is possible, this type of approach should be avoided.

There is a beneficial cumulative effect from regularly practising relaxation or meditation. This is because it encourages the production of noradrenaline which, as previously stated, counteracts the effects of adrenaline.

There are physical ways of measuring physiological changes caused by relaxation. Blood pressure can be measured before and afterwards. Biodots are small circles of thermally sensitive material which can be stuck on the hand, a good place being on the dorsum, between the base of the thumb and first finger. They change colour to show different temperatures. The ones that the author uses react to a temperature range of 89.6° F to 94.6° F. They remain their original black outside that range:

Amber	89.6° F	Tense
Yellow	90.6° F	Unsettled
Green	91.6° F	Involved (normal)
Turquoise	92.6° F	Relaxed
Blue	93.6° F	Calm
Violet	94.6° F	Very relaxed

These visual changes are popular with clients and, like other methods discussed, can also be used during or following other stress-reducing techniques. Another, more mechanically sophisticated method of measurement is biofeedback (Palmer and Dryden, 1995).

Problem-solving

These are very useful techniques and once learnt can be applied to almost any situation. First, of course, the actual problem must be to take stock of the situation. Decide which things have to be dealt with that day and list them under **A** – most urgent; under **B** – less urgent and under **C** – things which can wait. (Some people even file **C** items in the wastepaper basket, but this can have unfortunate consequences if somebody else expecting these things actioned has a different prioritizing scale.) Then decide whether things under **B** are **A** or **C** and just start by doing all the items listed under **A**, and going on to the **C**'s if there is time. Other considerations are: grouping and preparing for outgoing telephone calls; making sure that requests and instructions have been heard and understood correctly; preparing for meetings and encouraging focusing and brevity; do one thing and think about one thing at a time; allow flexibility and time to tackle the unexpected; do not put things off; learn to say 'no' and try to handle each piece of paper only once. The author keeps a list of these things on her office wall as a reminder and encourages clients to do the same.

Assertion, communication skills and confidence building

The above skills are very much interrelated. Many highly-stressed clients have lost their confidence, both in their own abilities and in themselves. To rebuild this, or in some cases, to introduce a more confident attitude to life, must be done carefully. It is important for clients to get support and understanding, if this is possible, from friends, partners and families.

This can be a real problem, because many of the reactions leading to loss of confidence may be based on not having this support in the first place. Male partners, particularly, become very concerned if 'assertion' is mentioned. It seems to conjure up the picture of a convenient 'doormat' becoming an aggressive, challenging and grossly feminist individual with a complete personality change. When assertiveness training is being done, it is therefore important for handouts to be shared and sometimes it could usefully be preceded by sharpening up and deepening communication skills. The lack of one of these skills is often revealed when working on assertion anyway.

Assertion is frequently confused with aggression. It is necessary always to emphasize how positive assertiveness is when trying to put over a point of view or need. By use of the techniques the outcome should be one acceptable to both parties, sometimes involving some agreed compromise. There should not be the sense of a winner or a loser, more one of resolution. Everyone has the right to be treated with respect and consideration; to be listened to and have the opportunity, space and time to set personal priorities, to change minds, to make mistakes, to say 'no' and to express constructive criticism, and also to be able to enjoy life. A person should receive, in addition, a response when asked for, and also understanding and not derision when expressing feelings and opinions.

Teaching these skills is often easier in a group with opportunities for role-play. When working individually, it is useful to request a list of ways in which they want to become more assertive. Having listed these, they are arranged in order with the easiest first. The least challenging scenario is recreated and, using rehearsal, the client is shown how to be assertive in those circumstances and then asked to put it into action, bearing in mind another right – the right to fail should be accepted by all concerned. It is then suggested that they work through the other examples with a debriefing between each one. Preparing phrases such as: 'I know you may not like this but . . .'; 'Knowing how much these things mean to you, I was wondering . . .'. If each person expects respect and understanding when they state their point of view, then they must extend the same to others with whom they may disagree or when assertion does not work. Each person needs good listening as well as speaking skills for this. In situations of conflict, it is important to take one issue at a time and not to become side-tracked, and to try to look together for creative ways to sort things out – brainstorming can be useful in these circumstances. Use of eye contact and appropriate body language is also important. It can be seen that by building up communication skills and assertiveness, clients can gradually improve their self-confidence.

Cognitive and behavioural approaches

Some of the techniques that the author teaches are purely cognitive and some behavioural, but throughout there are many links and one (rational emotive behavioural therapy), particularly, marries the two approaches.

To deal with phobias and obsessional behaviour clients often respond best to a very hierarchical approach, involving listing the manifestations of their problems and tackling these one by one in order of threat. In this method they expose themselves deliberately to these situations or limiting of checking, etc., dealing with the anxiety using taught techniques or simply 'sitting it out' until it passes. The biggest challenge and obstacle is dealing with the resulting anxiety, and sometimes panic, which becomes more and more marked as the list of obsessions and/or phobias are progressed through. Repeated reassurance before and during this work must be given so that severe anxiety and panic attacks do gradually subside with or without intervention. The mechanism must always be explained properly to anyone embarking on this difficult, but frequently rewarding, set of tasks or omissions which is usually referred to as exposure therapy. A great deal of work is done in this way at the Maudsley Hospital in London and the interventions are very accessibly recorded, for both clients and therapists (Marks, 1978). People's choice whether to tackle phobias and obsessions is usually based on the level at which they have a limiting effect on the rest of their lives.

Some of the most empowering approaches are those involving teaching the client about the power of thought and how they can learn to modify their reactions to things. As mentioned earlier, many people feel they have no control over what happens to them, so being able to understand and deal with some of their thoughts and linked behaviour and resulting strong emotions gives them the sense of being slightly more in the 'driving seat'. When people are anxious, depressed, angry or guilty these emotions are often fed by negative filtering which only emphasizes and acknowledges thoughts which add to their anxiety, depression, anger or guilt. Once this is pointed out, they are able to recognize the patterns and learn to change them. One of the ways to change thinking is through positive self-talk. This is a way of reasoning with themselves to lessen or discount negative thinking and will tend to change the filtering system to a much more positive approach with raised awareness training and practice.

Rational emotive behaviour therapy is a method which, as its title suggests, clearly illustrates and exploits the association between the cognitive and the behavioural. Professor Windy Dryden has done a great deal to develop and teach this approach in this country (Dryden and Gordon, 1990). It is based on the premise that it is not *what happens to us*, but *what we think or believe about what happens to us*, that produces our emotions or behaviour. As in some other cognitive methods, it uses the **ABC** model of Activating Event or Situation (**A**), Thoughts or Beliefs (**B**), and Behaviour or Strong Emotion(s) (**C**) (Consequences). It then goes on to use the other lettering [**D** (Disputing), **E** (Effective approach) and **F** (Formulation of less acute response)], forming a framework to focus on changing the amount of reaction so that it is not out of proportion, or so gross that it interferes with other aspects of the client's life or damages somebody else they are in contact with (Table 16.1).

The first thing a client usually notices is their own reaction which is manifested by a strong emotional reaction or sudden behavioural change (**C**). Having identified this, the event or situation (**A**) apparently causing this is clarified. Only then is the link between the thoughts and beliefs (**B**) and the reaction explored. Disputing the thoughts and beliefs (**D**) takes the form of establishing that either they are not logical, empirical or self-helping. However justified, logical and true the negative thoughts or beliefs may be, they probably do not help. Another likelihood is exaggeration; for example: 'I can't go on without him'; 'Losing this job is the end of the world'; 'Everybody hates me', etc. The term 'awfulizing' is often applied to this. It may be possible to then change the belief or thought to something less emotive, such as: 'I shall probably find it very hard to go on without him, but will find a way in time' (**E**). This mechanism will then reduce the emotional reaction a little. So if originally in column (**C**) there was anxiety, guilt or anger, it could then be reduced having worked through **D** and **E**, in column (**F**) to concern, regret or annoyance, and the same reduction would apply to the extreme behavioural reactions (Ellis *et al.*, 1997).

This technique seems cumbersome to start with, but with practice is extremely effective and relatively swift to apply. Many of the author's more logical clients prefer it to any other method, as they can really see for themselves exactly how it works. It incorporates the ideas of the clients building up self-acceptance rather than self-esteem, which is much more vulnerable to the opinions of others and the effects of life events.

Multimodal approach

This method, introduced about 20 years ago (Lazarus, 1989), is a way of providing a holistic assessment framework. For each section of this a

Table 16.1 Rational emotive behaviour therapy – the ABC model

A	B	C
Activating Event or Situation	Beliefs or Thoughts	Consequences, Behaviour, Strong Emotion(s)
D	E	F
Disputing (B)	Effective approach used to change (B)	Formulation of less acute responses

suitable modality can then be chosen to try to combat that particular strand of stress reaction. For this method, questions are asked to establish Behaviour (**B**), Affect (**A**), Sensation (**S**), Imagery (**I**), Cognition (**C**), Interpersonal functioning (**I**), Drugs/Health/Biology (**D**) – **BASIC ID** (acronym). This builds up a structural profile of the client and how they see themselves functioning on all these levels, with a scoring system of 1–10. This helps to prioritize the areas needing working on and to select which modalities of therapy to introduce first (Palmer and Dryden, 1995). The idea is to use the higher scoring positive aspects to build up the weaker ones, incorporating chosen appropriate techniques.

Stress mapping

Sometimes, particularly when dealing with workplace stress, it is useful to work out exactly how patterns of stress interact. Stress mapping is a clear, graphic way of doing this (Palmer, 1990). A scoring system of 1–10 is used to record the degree of stress, and arrows are used to show the direction of stress between employees. At the centre of all of it is the client, but they need to recognize that they may cause stress to others who may also be under stress from somebody else.

Physical exercise

Many people find that exercise is a good form of stress relief and relaxation. Some clients prefer a tough workout in a gym, or similar intense exercise, getting a feeling of well-being subsequently, partly as a result of endorphin release. Others prefer a more leisurely approach. However, some very highly competitive sports, e.g. squash, may increase stress reactions and certainly could be hazardous to anyone already in a highly-stressed state who is also mainly sedentary in their occupation.

Case study

A very high-powered businessman, aged 56, had had relatively recent heart bypass surgery. The first operation had caused serious complications and a second one had been necessary in close proximity to the first. The result of all this, 6 months later, was a man who was – mainly for psychological rather than physical reasons – largely housebound. He felt too depressed and unmotivated to do anything at all and just sat all day brooding. He also was dyspnoeic (breathless), despite the fact that the second operation was a success and no physical reasons were identified for this distressing problem.

During the **assessment** visit he was obviously very low in mood and spoke minimally and appeared very cynical about any techniques working. He was also breathless on exertion and found it difficult to make eye contact. His chest expansion remained fairly good laterally. He could do diaphragmatic expansion when he concentrated, but his tendency was to breathe most of all apically – rather short, sudden breaths both in and out. He could not motivate himself to (a) do his favourite hobby – woodwork, for which he had a well-equipped workshop in part of the garage, (b) walk his dog, (c) socialize, (d) drive – concentration too poor, and (e) help about the house – something he previously was always 'too busy' to do anyway.

All this was putting a strain on his relationship with his wife. He hated her being the main breadwinner and, although he clung to his house rather than going out, he was experiencing a trapped feeling.

Treatment – initially he was taught **breathing techniques**, (a) to help him deal with his anxiety and (b) to minimize the hyperventilation. Despite his obvious resistance to any intervention, he was normally a compliant person and was always conscientious in applying what he was taught.

He was surprised at the slight improvement he felt. Other techniques were worked through in the following order – relaxation, negative thought changing, problem-solving – which was more a sharing of ideas as he had taught this to management trainees in the past – rational emotive behavioural therapy and then gradual exposure to (a) exercise, (b) going out, and (c) socializing. Once he found that this all began to improve things, his anxiety and depression gradually lifted and he was able to go out and started his woodwork again. At the end of his 6 sessions he stated: 'Now I get the idea – it is a bit like having a tool-kit and I can select and mix the tools as I wish, depending on my needs at the time'. The author could not have put it better herself!

Conclusion

This chapter is a kind of 'whistle-stop tour' of stress counselling and management techniques. A great deal can be achieved by clients building up their own personal 'tool-kit' of these interventions and mixing and matching them as they find most effective. When life feels like a constant battle, much energy is wasted trying to force oneself through it all. Conservation of the precious positive life force is important, as is the dispersing of negative energy which can build up and feel at times quite overwhelming and defeating. Balancing out all the pressures and preventing them becoming stressors is part

of the lifetime's learning curve that everyone needs to follow in order to function at their optimum level.

References

Burns, D. (1989) *The Feeling Good Handbook*. Malden: Plume Books.

Dryden, W. and Gordon, J. (1990) *What is Rational Emotive Therapy?* Loughton, Essex, UK: Gale Centre Publications.

Ellis, A., Gordon, J., Neenam, M. and Palmer, S. (1997) *Stress Counselling: A Rational Emotive Behavioural Approach*. London: Cassell.

Jacobson, E. (1938) *Progressive Relaxation*. Chicago: University of Chicago Press.

Lazarus, A.A. (1989) *The Practice of Multimodal Therapy*. Baltimore, MD: John Hopkins University Press.

Marks, I.M. (1978) *Living with Fear*. New York: McGraw-Hill.

Palmer, S. (1990) Stress mapping: a visual technique to aid counselling or training. *Employee Counselling Today*, 2(2), 9–12.

Palmer, S. (1992) *Stress Management – A Course Reader*. London: Centre for Stress Management.

Palmer, S. (1998) 'Stress', BBC Radio 4 programme.

Palmer, S. and Dryden, W. (1995) *Counselling for Stress Problems*. London: Sage.

Seaton, L. (1995) Hyperventilation Leaflet (tel. 0161-929-8101).

17 Qigong and Taichi in physical therapy

Sara Mokone

Introduction

Experience demonstrates that the practice of Qigong and Taichi enables practitioners to enhance their healing skills, as well as their own health and vitality. This chapter will be looking into the origins and practice of Qigong and Taichi. This approach to therapy recognizes the connection between body, mind and feelings. The slow graceful, low impact exercises of Qigong and Taichi are ideal for building coordination and postural awareness and of value as part of therapy. It is said that Qigong cultivates energy through regular practice and development of the experience of the energy. According to one teacher 'Qi and Qigong must be experienced rather than defined' (Dong and Esser, 1990). To give an analogy, a strawberry cannot be known from a dictionary definition – it has to be tasted to experience what a strawberry is.

What is Qigong?

Qigong (pronounced chee goong) is also spelt Chikung, or chigong. The word can be divided into two parts, Qi and Gong. **Qi** (written as Ch'i or chi) means air, breath of life or vital essence. Qi refers to the principle of change and flux in the universe. Qi is known by different names in other cultures. It is the quantum field in modern physics, and known as Prana or Shakti in India. In this chapter, Qi will be used to describe 'biological energy' in all its forms. **Gong** means work, to develop skill and competence. Qigong literally means working to cultivate biological energy. It is the Chinese method of health practice for harnessing this biological energy, based primarily on a system of physical training for preventive and therapeutic health care. It is a form of psychosomatic self-training that enables the practitioner to achieve mental and physical well-being (Dong and Esser, 1990). To achieve this aim, practitioners are required to undertake a series of actions. These include movements involving muscle coordination, with breathing exercises and mental concentration. The object of the approach is to:

● calm the mind
● promote good health
● prolong a healthy life
● cure disease
● develop physical strength and prowess.

Qigong is a mind–body approach to health, widely used in China for its 'anti-ageing' effect (Watkins, 1997). As longevity is increasing, it is important that physical and mental health are supported. Other factors which may interfere with the achievement of this end, relate to the person's lifestyle. Environmental, economic and social stress factors in society can lead to imbalances which affect mental attitude. These include, balance of rest, work, and nutrition (Government Health Document, 1998).

The aim is to achieve balance in all aspects of life – through the use of this practice. Qigong is accessible to people of all ages and abilities, and different styles can be performed sitting, lying down or standing. Health benefit can be achieved with a short period of daily practice.

Origins of Qigong

Qigong is one of the branches of Traditional Chinese Medicine, which includes acupuncture and moxibustion, herbal remedies, massage or tuina (Dong and Esser, 1990).

Lao-tzu, a philosopher who wrote the *Dao De Jing* 5000 years ago and is thought of as the originator of Taoism, described breathing methods to gather Qi at Dantian (the sea of Qi below the navel) and so protect the essence of a person's strength. Forms of the movements described are still used in both medical and fitness fields today, for the promotion of tranquillity enhanced by relaxation of the sympathetic and stimulation of the parasympathetic nervous activity (Takahashi and Brown, 1986).

Qigong's modern history dates back to the 1950s, when research institutes were established to investigate 'All forms of traditional Chinese medicine, which were being integrated into the health system in China after the establishment of the Peoples' Republic of China in 1949' (Eisenberg and Wright, 1983). Acupuncture has achieved widespread recognition in the West but it is only in the past 20 years that awareness of the medical benefits of Qigong has grown.

How does Qigong work?

The principles are simple and yet profound. Bioelectrical energy flows through the body constantly. The goal of an individual studying Qigong is to learn to sense the energy, develop it and control it. This takes a lifetime to master, even though learning the basic principles may only take a few moments. The further the student progresses, further subtleties are perceived, and the understanding broadens. The subtle energies circulate throughout the entire body in energy channels, known as meridians. Blockages in these meridians may cause physical or emotional problems.

Modern neurophysiological research shows that physical functions are directly influenced by a person's mental state (Pert, 1997). Therefore, it follows that if the mind can be harmonized then the autonomic nervous system will function more efficiently. For instance, the emotions can change the chemical balance in the tissues, through the action of neuropeptides. Anger causes release of neurochemicals, which effect the white cells and diminish the activity of T-Lymphocytes. Visualization of peaceful mental images may electrically activate the pituitary and pineal glands to release hormones, which stimulate the parasympathetic nervous system and lead to relaxation.

Qi is a concept or a function rather than a substance that can be measured. Qigong is thought to work through the autonomic nervous system and act as a regulating influence on the homeostatic mechanisms of the body (Figure 17.1).

How the body functions

Energy is fed by:

- food
- air
- water
- light
- sound
- sensory stimulation.

Blood and body fluids travel through the body, giving nutrition and removing waste. Western medicine can, by various methods, measure the input and output of these fluids. However, energy in itself is more difficult to define and measure:

> Although the subtle energies which the Chinese refer to as Qi are hard to measure there is indirect evidence for some type of electromagnetic energy circuit which involves the meridians and acupuncture points. (Gerber, 1996)

Physiology

Some of the changes taking place in the body continuously include renewal of bone, and

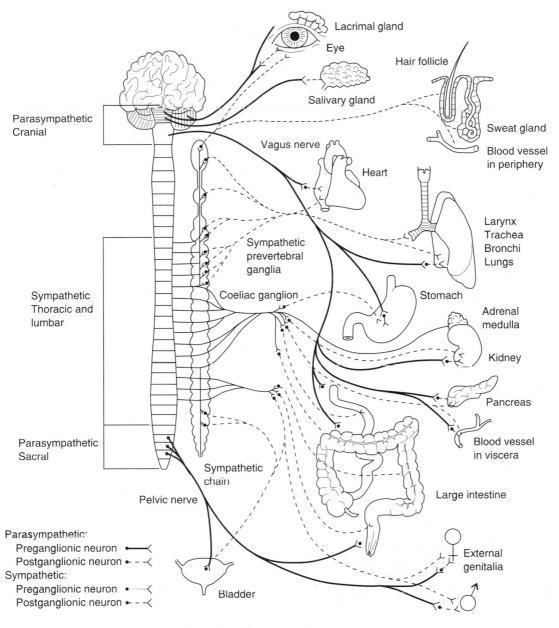

Figure 17.1 The autonomic nervous system

activity of the phagocytes and mast cells. Research into osteoporosis shows that the bony base of the body renews itself completely every 7 years (Dixon and Woolf, 1989). So, as you sit and read this chapter, there are vital forces at work in your body all the time. Physiotherapy aims to promote the body's natural processes, and abilities to heal by speeding up the effects of phagocytosis and mast cell action. This can be enhanced by the Qigong effect on 'vitality' which underpins the body's ability to regenerate and grow.

Forms of Qigong

'One river, many tributaries' – there are a number of different forms of Qigong:

- Medical
- Fitness training
- Martial arts
- Combined Daoyin – massage which awakens the energy channels
- Spontaneous movement
- Meditation
- Healing – Sending sound and electromagnetic waves from the hands with the intention of directing energy to heal someone else; the latter form requires specialized training and practice.

Qigong is therefore an umbrella category, covering a wide range of ways of building vitality that can include activities like walking and dancing (Figure 17.2) (MacRitchie, 1993).

Basic principles, and elements

All forms are based on common principles and elements. Whether Qigong is practised as a martial art, a form of fitness training or for medical purposes the principles are to combine movement, relaxation and breathing with meditation and visualization:

- Motor control
- Postural awareness

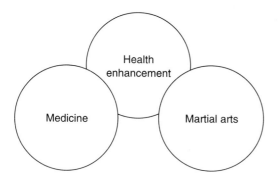

Figure 17.2 Different forms of Qigong

- Relaxation
- Breath control
- Visualization – a very important element of Qigong
- Mental control or meditation.

Motor control. This includes all muscle types – voluntary skeletal muscles, and smooth or (so-called) involuntary muscles, such as Cardiac muscles – which work continuously.

Postural awareness. This is developed as the person practises sitting, standing and lying. In all of these, attention is paid to the alignment of the body in space, in relation to the earth's gravitational field and the position of the spinal segments. The effects are on all the surrounding tissues, connective tissues, including cartilage, tendons, joints, and nerves to the organs at each spinal segment (Dr Shen Hongxun, 1995).

Relaxation or a 'soong' (the mandarin word for relaxation) *attitude.* This is one of the goals to be attained by the frequent practice of Qigong. Achieving a calm mind eliminates stress factors (Eisenberg and Wright, 1986). The training of autogenic responses is another way of achieving this, as is the Mitchell method of physiological relaxation (Mitchell, 1987).

Breath control. Through the practice of slow, controlled movements awareness of breathing increases, and the body naturally gains a more rhythmic slower and deeper range of breathing. Not all schools concentrate on breath control, because some individuals may find difficulties in changing their breathing patterns. Rather, slower and deeper breath control is an outcome from the slow, gentle movements learned. Other forms allow the practitioner to 'breathe like a baby' – a reverse breathing which is more like panting. Observation of this is needed. (See other texts in the recommended reading list, or find a teacher who teaches this method.) (Cohen, 1997)

Visualization. The ability to release the right brain, through visualization and direct the thoughts at where breath goes – so sending healing thoughts to different body parts: 'Where the thoughts go, there goes Qi – and where Qi goes healing follows' (Cohen, 1997): the creative release of right brain activity.

Meditation (usually associated with spiritual practices). Learning to clear all thoughts from the mind. A skill which comes with practice. Students are encouraged to practice to improve their exam results outcomes.

Energy will flow through the line of least resistance, termed wuwei. This is a further element of Qigong, based on doing less rather than making the effort to do more, thus promoting generative and nutritive effects. Regular practice leads to gaining relaxation of the flight-and-fight muscles via neurochemical pathways.

Methods

- Practise slow, controlled movements
- Maintain static postures, simultaneously directing the flow of Qi and blood through the tissues, by the development of breath control
- The flow of Qi in the meridian channels is stimulated by movement and massage. According to Traditional Chinese Medicine (TCM) these meridian channels are those which are stimulated with acupuncture. Areas of lower electrical conductivity indicate points called energy gates, where the body can be more easily stimulated by visualization, stretch, touch, pressure, massage or needles (Figure 17.3).

Summary

The aim of practising Qigong is to cultivate personal energy. By the above mechanisms, the body is enabled to produce energy-storing effects while reducing wasted energy consumption and increasing energy accumulation. This is achieved by cleansing the meridian pathways and collaterals, and regulating the homeostatic mechanisms (MacRitchie, 1993).

The benefits of practising Qigong can be shared between those practising together. Teachers of Taichi and Qigong prefer to teach groups, who are encouraged to practise together, because of the transfer of healing energy within the group. The facilitation of a group dynamic

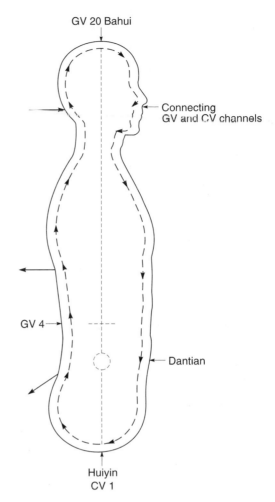

Figure 17.3 Key energy gates on the Du and Conception vessel channels, around the middle of the body. Mental concentration at these points promotes the flow of blood and Qi (Wang Yifang, 1992)

may have to do with the particular healing energy of the group leader.

What is Taichi?

Taichi is one of the many forms of working with Qi – a form of Qigong. The symbol Taichi means the 'supreme ultimate' – the Yin-Yang symbol of balance and harmony. Taichi was developed as a martial art for self-defence. It is an immensely popular form of Qigong for those seeking fitness, and has both internal and external aspects. Taichi is referred to as a form of 'moving meditation'. Slow controlled movement, are combined with breath and intention, utilizing the key elements of Qigong as mentioned above. The external form, developed as a martial art, moves with the energy in the cosmos and the environment. Neidan, the internal medical form of internal exercises, is for improving the flow of vital energy through the internal organs and pathways within the body.

> Taichi aims at stress reduction, improved flexibility and better body awareness.
> The continued practice acts as a challenge to learning self-development. The Taoist philosophy itself is attractive. The Taoist society offers social aspects and the opportunity to help one another, so learning a philosophy of selfless sharing.
> (Baker, 1997)

The practise of Taichi involves more formal sequences of movements known as forms – popularized as the Long and Short Yang school forms. Other forms of Qigong are easier to learn and practice.

Research into the effects of Qigong and Taichi

A number of studies describe the use of specific Qigong exercises as being successful in treating the following conditions: hypertension, diabetes, coronary artery diseases, kidney disorders, peripheral vascular diseases, tuberculosis, cancer, arthritis, neurasthenia and a host of other chronic maladies (Eisenberg and Wright, 1986). Other health areas influenced and improved by the practice of Qigong include general mobility, joint movements in rheumatoid arthritis, reductions of falls in the elderly, reductions in mood disturbance-tension; depression; anger. Outcome measures employed include quality of life indices. Physiological studies have shown some of the effects, such as the lowering of blood pressure and slowing the respiratory and pulse rate (Sancier, 1996).

The positive effects in lowering blood pressure is shown in a follow-up report on 242 hypertensives over 30 years (Benor, 1993; Wong Chongxing *et al.*, 1993). This longitudinal study of the effects of Qigong on preventing stroke and alleviating the cerebrocardiovascular risk factors concluded that Qigong plays a major role in improving self-regulation and alleviating the multiple cerebrovascular risk factors. Here the method of using Qigong was to achieve a calm mind, smooth breathing and a relaxed body, practised mainly in sitting, as self-healing (Benor, 1993). A review of research studies indicates that Qigong exercises can benefit health and that emitted Qi can produce significant changes in different kinds of living systems, including plants and animals (Sancier and Hu, 1991).

Experiments measuring electromagnetic fields radiating from a Qigong Master have been documented by Chinese researchers (Dong and Esser, 1990). Some Chinese scientists believe that healing with a Qigong Master's external Qi is from infrared heat waves. The power of this radiation is much lower than that used in 'diathermy' which is measured in watts. The strength of these emissions is in microwatts (Figure 17.4) (Li Yingbo, 1985).

The interaction of energy between participants in a group can be verified experimentally (Dong and Esser, 1990). Mention has been made of the benefits obtained from practising Qigong and Taichi in group settings.

Research into Qigong for stress at work

A study of the (acute) effects of the practice of Qigong suggests that 'Qigong training as a stress-coping method affects and plays a role in hormonal regulation related to the maintenance of homeostasis' (Ryu and Lee *et al.*, 1995). In this study, 20 healthy men and women of an average age of 28 who practised Qigong, had their blood levels measured. Endogenous opioid peptides, beta-endorphin and stress hormones such as ACTH and cortisol were measured before, during and after Qigong practice. The levels of endorphins was raised and the ACTH lowered. There was no effect on cortisol levels. This seems to indicate an effect on the immune system, and increase in pain-relieving hormones.

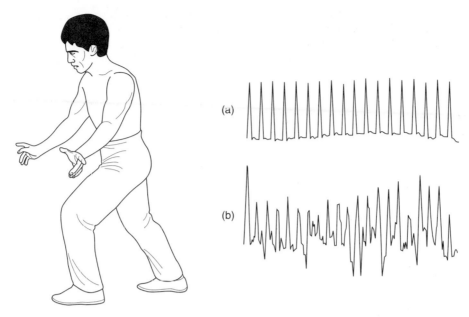

Figure 17.4 Pulse waves between the hands of a Qigong Master: (a) taken before his Qigong exercise; (b) taken when he was practising Qigong

Cortisol levels are increased by being alarmed or stressed (Figure 17.5), and diminished at rest.

An interesting study was directed to investigate the benefits of Qigong training in reducing stress at work (Skoglund, 1998). This paper measured some of the physiological changes following a 2-week period of Qigong training. A comparison was made between a control group and Qigong group of adult computer operators (Skoglund, 1998). Immediate responses to the effects of practising Qigong were measured and long-term effects were measured over a 5-week period. Skoglund's findings showed that the Qigong training reduced the heart rate and the noradrenaline excretion, thus indicating a reduced activity in the sympathetic nervous system. There was also a reduction of spinal backache symptoms among the Qigong group. Her conclusions were that the preliminary results of the pilot study indicate that Qigong exercises reduce stress related to computerized work environments. Further investigation, using a control group engaged in some other form of stress reduction activity or exercise, is needed to confirm the results.

Exercise training effects

There is a field of study in Western universities known as psychoneuroimmunology (PNI). This is a growing area that studies how psychological factors, mediated by neuroendocrine agents, can affect the immune system. New physiological knowledge has been acquired on the mechanisms internally by which the neuro-transmitters 'communicate' between systems (see Appendix at the end of this chapter).

One study showed the potential of exercise intervention in coping with mental stress:

> Exercise has been associated with decreased levels of mild to moderate depression and anxiety, which are symptoms of failure to cope with mental stress. (Morgan, 1987)

Vigorous exercise is now believed to be effective in treatment for at least some mental health problems. Further research on the relationship of exercise to the immune system has shown that in general, moderate physical exercise enhances immunity while intense exercise is immunosuppressive (La Perriere *et al.*, 1994).

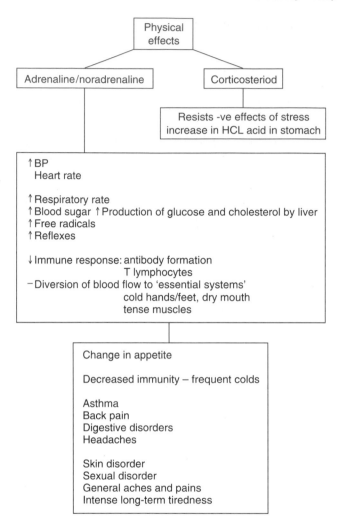

Figure 17.5 Effects of stress

The article concludes that exercise has been associated with improved mental health and well-being. Exercise training modulates endogenous opiates and stress hormones. Moderate exercise enhances immunity with the possibility of lowering the risk of some infections.

Prevention of falls in older people

The above effects of exercise are illustrated in the results of research in the USA into the applications of Taichi for the prevention of falls in older people. The Taichi exercises augment the exercise effects through the use of both mental concentration and relaxation of tension, which are thought to benefit emotional states. Lai and colleagues (in Davis, 1997), showed that elderly Taichi exercisers showed a significant improvement in VO_2 (oxygen) uptake as compared to an age-matched control group of sedentary individuals (Davis, 1997).

In a further study the stress reduction effects of Taichi quan exercises was measured by heart rate, blood pressure and urinary catecholamines, and salivary cortisol levels. A comparison was made with matched groups of brisk walkers, meditators and quiet readers. The groups doing moderate exercise had similar outcome in heart rate, blood pressure and urinary catecholamines. However, in addition the Taichi group expressed feelings of lowered anxiety states and enhancement of 'vigor' (Jin, 1992).

An American study comparing two groups, to test the effects of computerized balance training and Taichi on postural stability (Wolf *et al.*, 1996, 1997), showed a statistically significant decrease in the number of falls among older participants in a Taichi exercise group. Taichi was found to gain success by promoting confidence and reducing the fear of falling. This may be because of the natural practice outside of controlled laboratory conditions.

In further studies conducted at Department of Rehabilitation Medicine, School of Medicine, Emory University, Atlanta, Georgia, USA (on the benefits of Taichi practice by older people), the data suggest that when mental as well as physical control is perceived to be enhanced, older persons' motivation to continue exercising also increases, with a generalized sense of improvement in overall well-being (Kutner *et al.*, 1997).

Comparison of Taichi and Qigong with other forms of exercise

Qigong works from inside out, with the intention of moving energy in the body, unlike most other forms of exercise which work on developing strength, suppleness and stamina. Taichi and Qigong combine Mind intention, and Relaxation of tension with active exercise, therefore having a profound affect on the autonomic nervous system. Yoga is another exercise form which shares these characteristics.

Practitioners interviewed find Qigong simpler to teach than Taichi. Some forms of Taichi are like a choreographed dance, and follow a long form. Even the short form requires disciplined use of a set of movements. With Qigong it is possible to use different exercises at different times, according to which is appropriate. This widens its applications, so it can be used more easily for the particular condition or effect required, for example in situations where people have physical disabilities and cannot stand to practice. Qigong is the base, and can be used for training particular systems.

Introduction to methods of working with Qi

The first stages are to sink the weight, intention and centre of gravity into the legs and soles of the feet. The practitioner visualizes connecting with the centre of gravity of the earth. This helps to centre the body and move thinking from the head down into Dantian, the psychic centre which is three fingers' breadth below the navel (Dong and Esser, 1993). Each body organ has an emotional side – we are used to ideas like 'tightness in the throat', to indicate fear, or 'butterflies in the stomach' – to indicate nervousness, or 'have a heart', meaning to be kind. Therefore, we are used to linking emotions, organs and intention.

Outcome measures

How can one define feelings of 'vigour' and 'energy'? A subjective feeling of well-being. After some months of practice signs can be observed in the skin tone and performance levels. Measures can be made of changes in speed of completing tasks and levels of concentration.

As learning is experiential, it may benefit the reader to participate in the following exercise.

Qigong posture

1. Sit on the edge of your chair with your head balance above your base. Imagine a golden chord attached to the centre of your crown, gently elevating your head.
2. The centre of your crown is directly above the midpoint of your perineum, a point in Chinese medicine known as Huiyin (the greatest yin). The top of your crown is known as Bahui (the greatest yang) – meeting a thousand pathways.
3. Your feet need to be shoulders' width apart, and firmly positioned on the ground.
4. Breathe out, tightening your stomach muscles on the exhalation.

5. Imagine your breath going down to your toes, as you breathe out. Stretch and release your fingers and toes to promote clearing toxins from your system.
6. At the end of the out-breath, let go of your stomach muscles so that air fills your abdomen without effort.

Continue with three to four long breaths on the first occasion, then let your breathing become more natural. This is a process of Qigong – you have participated in a Qigong exercise. It is advisable to follow a routine when practising. Begin with warm-ups then the form, and then a closing ceremony.

Clinical indications

Clinical applications depend on the extent of training of the individual therapist. The author applies Qigong as an integral part of the whole package of therapeutic techniques, of physiotherapy and acupuncture, integrated within the therapy sessions.

1. Self-preparation of the therapist – clearing and self-cleansing and maintaining personal fitness. The intention of the individual therapist may augment the treatment.
2. Relaxation of the patient before and during acupuncture treatments, in order to improve the effectiveness of the therapy.
3. For specific conditions – to alleviate balance problems, and postural awareness for example, hemiplegia, one side weakness, Parkinson's or complex neurological conditions. Reduce blood pressure, repetitive strain injuries, reduction of stress.
4. Group dynamics – as a warm up exercise before commencing meetings. This helps to improve concentration. Benefits neuromuscular facilitation groups.

These indications are reflected in the literature (Cohen, 1996). Various models of Qigong are used, based on studies with many teachers both in China, the UK and Canada. For example Liu Xiao Ming and Yuan Li Ren, Michael Tse, Dr Stephen Aung. Use is made of an approach called *Qinetics* devised by Lydia Wong (1995).

Relaxation technique

This relaxation Qigong technique was taught to the author by a doctor of Traditional Chinese Medicine from Beijing School of TCM. She based her work on Dr Liu's work from Shanghai Qigong Institute (Liu Xiao Ming and Yuan Li Ren, 1993). This method can be practised lying, sitting or standing, keeping the tongue raised against the upper hard palate, and the eyes slightly drooping. Again the concentration is on the Dantian–Qihai point three fingers below the navel. A three route relaxation is used to clear stray thoughts from the mind. Suggest that the person visualize water flowing over the body:

1. Down the front, from eyes to toes.
2. From the top of the head (Bahui point) over the neck, shoulders, down both arms and out of the finger tips.
3. The Third route is from the top of the head down the back, waist, thighs, calves and the soles of the feet exiting via the toes.

This method can be included with all acupuncture treatments. It can be taught for self-use, between treatments, especially for overcoming sleeplessness.

Cleansing and clearing (tuning in)

The Taoist approach to Qigong aims to enhance physical and mental life, connecting the person to their environment (Guo, 1994). Therapists will be better grounded, and more available for treating others if they work on clearing any toxins from their own system first. One method is by bouncing on the heels on the spot for a minute while doing deep breathing exercises, then shaking hands and feet to open all the circulatory channels.

This preparation is usually done before any strenuous exercises routine – and is commonly taught to athletes in training. Theoretically this provides the opportunity of enhancing performance by achieving a more helpful attitude and intention. It may benefit a health practitioner, to learn to clear the channels and rid the body of any toxins before beginning to work. This requires consciousness, and intention to move blood, fluids and 'energy' around the body. This point of view has been corroborated by other physiotherapists who use Qigong as part of their work.

Precautions and contraindications

Always study with suitably qualified teachers, and have someone to refer to when developing the skills.

The standard precautions relating to physical activity apply:

- Do not practice immediately after a meal, or when very tired.
- Take care to maintain a warm and protected environment. According to the TCM explanation, illness results from external causes such as cold, wind, damp and storms – or from excessive overwork, or from a deficiency or internal disease. Other internal causes of disease are the 'internal devils' – emotions and attitudes. They do apply in modern society. Therefore, do not practise outside in the cold. The desire is to be able to develop a 'Qigong attitude' of mental calm. In such a mental state, the body may be quite vulnerable to cold and damp. This is particularly so for static and 'standing like a tree' postures. Early morning is a time that traditionally in China, thousands of older people are seen exercising, but frequently by doing limbering up exercises first.
- Active Qigong is not recommended during an infection. The circulation of blood in the tissues may spread infection further. Resting methods may be used.
- During menstruation women must take the precaution of not visualizing the flow of energy below the waist as this may increase blood flow. Certain movements, such as straining downwards or hold low postures are contraindicated. This precaution applies for pregnant women as well.
- A very important precaution is to study Qigong in stages – not attempting to advance too quickly (Aung, 1994). In the fast pace of Western Society, this may seem very conservative, however, it is important to prevent adverse effects. There are many different forms, and for safety a

choice can be made to do basic training first before moving on to more advanced forms of visualizing the movement of energy for healing others.

Adverse reactions

If attention is paid to precautions there should not be adverse effects when practising Qigong. However, there are studies in China of adverse mental effects resulting from practising too long or using too much intention to direct the flow of Qi inappropriately. This may result in either physical or emotional illnesses (Cohen, 1997). However, it is still possible to practise other forms of Qigong.

Qigong has been a closed field to the West until recently, but in Traditional China was practised in some form by many professions to enhance their mental prowess and art, these included calligraphers, poets and theatre artists, as well as monks who taught their students, within a very rigid system. Now there are hospitals which use Qigong as the main means of treatment, by Qigong Masters, and regular daily personal practice by the patients.

Finding a teacher who is well versed in the practice of Qigong can be difficult. There are international institutions and accredited training packages. For this reason, Taichi teachers are much easier to find, and within the class, the elements of Qigong will be recognized.

Further case histories

A small study has been conducted by the author, as part of research for this chapter. Thirty-five physiotherapists who use Qigong, either for self-healing or for patient treatments have been contacted by postal questionnaire. One conclusion reached is a recognition of the importance of treating yourself for the sake of the wellness of the patient. As one practitioner put it: 'you need to recharge your own batteries, so that you do not run into empty while working – and do not get drained of charge by the work that you do.' The study was presented at the World Confederation of Physical Therapy (WCPT) Congress 1999, in Japan.

Case history 1

An 88-year-old man with Parkinson's, cervical and lumbar spondylosis. Treatments are aimed at improving balance and well-being; increasing joint range of movement and decreasing pain.

Therapy included acupuncture, muscle balancing exercises as well as postural advice. He does a number of exercises modelled on Qigong postures, and postural awareness. He has been taught slow controlled movements for transferring his weight from leg to leg, with knees bent and to visualize sinking concentration down to his feet, while counting his breaths out. A grounding exercise.

The outcome has been that he has been able to keep walking safely to the local shops, and maintain a reasonable upright posture. He has lost the shuffling gait and rigidity which are classical signs of the condition.

He depends on taking aldopa in the form of sinemet tablets regularly. This requires liaison with the neurology consultant to vary the times and amounts of sinemet.

The combination of the exercise programme with medication has allowed for the best outcome. Other symptoms which have responded are: improved continence, less constipation, better swallowing and speech.

Treatments are regular – a monthly monitoring visit now, but at times, weekly visits if some crisis affects him.

The following is a case history received from a therapist working with learning disabilities in a community setting.

Case history 2

A 30-year-old lady with a learning disability has impaired vision and spina bifida. She uses a wheelchair. Her symptoms are poor lung capacity and poor mobility in her shoulders. Day Centre and Residential Centre staff requested advice on managing her chronic respiratory difficulties. She has needed continuous medical prescriptions for repeated chest infection. Copious sputum has been produced on waking every day for years.

Action: The physiotherapist introduced sound therapy especially for lungs with the 'SSSSS' sound made while arms are elevated on making the sound. The staff were requested to

reinforce these sounds and movements and shown how to perform this activity with the client at least 3 times daily.

Outcome: One month later her chest symptoms had been alleviated and sputum was cleared. Two years later, she reported that she still remembers and has not had a recurrence of chest infections.

Explanation: This uses the six healing sounds approach, from the Taoist school of Qigong. Each of the body organs is said to resonate with a particular sound, performed with particular arm and body movements. The sound for the lungs is like the word Sir ('r' silent), while the arms are elevated as high above the head as possible (Chia, 1986).

The application of Qigong and Taichi for special health needs is being developed through the Taichi Society, which has its headquarters in the UK in Colchester, Essex. At a treatment centre in Toronto, Canada, Dawn Baker, a physiotherapist from England, is appointed as coordinator of health care. They are conducting studies evaluating treatments for chronic health problems, including MS, strokes and other illnesses affecting older people.

Summary

This chapter has described in brief the relationship of Taichi to Qigong and how one is a part of the other. An explanation of the way these techniques affect body physiology when practised has been given and supporting research evidence has been cited. The relative ease of inclusion of Taichi and Qigong in an exercise programme for clients and for practitioners has been addressed.

Mention is made of the need to find suitably qualified teachers and to be aware of the precautions in preventing adverse reactions when working with this form of moving energy in the body.

Universities may consider further research into the applications of this holistic approach to health and well-being.

Appendix (reproduced with permission from a *Guardian* interview with neuroscientist Candice Pert, 1998)

Why the body and mind are inseparable, by Eileen Fursland

Candice Pert is Professor of Physiology and Biophysics at Georgetown University Medical Centre in Washington DC. She is at the heart of the scientific establishment yet she has come up with a scientific rationale for alternative and complementary therapies. She has, she believes, found the link between the mind and the body – the biomolecular basis that could explain everything from psychosomatic illnesses to why so many people swear by meditation, acupuncture, massage and similar therapies. 'Your emotions run every system of your body, from your intestines to your immune system' she says. 'Complementary therapies recognize the importance of the emotions, they do not ignore them. They recognize that people are full humans spirits with feelings and thoughts, which is so often left out by high-tech conventional medicine.'

Pert was a 26-year-old research student in 1972, when she discovered the opiate receptor – the sensing molecule on the surface of a brain cell which can pick up a message carried by opiates such as morphine or heroin. She found herself at the epicentre of psychoneuroimmunology – the study of the body's 'information substances' and their receptors. These substances include hormones such as oestrogen, neurotransmitters such as serotonin, and other chemical communicators called peptides.

The story of this research is told in her book 'Molecules of Emotion: Why we feel the way We feel', Scribner, New York, 1997.

The tiny changes which these information substances bring about at the level of the cells can add up to changes in our physiology, behaviour, physical activity and mood, making them, she believes the 'molecules of emotion'.

Pert and her colleagues have already shown that endorphins, the body's natural opiates, are released by exercise as part of the 'runner's high'. 'Endorphins are sexy, people love them' she explains. 'But there are at least 200 different chemicals that are probably just as important.'

Her research showed that the information substances are produced not only by the brain, but by other parts of the body as well. In her view, the mind – in the form of the 'molecules of emotion', the neuropeptides, can 'wander' through the body and the blood and the cerebrospinal fluid. This in turn leads the immune system and the endocrine system to communicate with and influence each other, thus explaining why our thoughts and emotions can affect our health. Body and mind she says are one the same thing.

'I am critical of the over-use of drugs, particularly antidepressants.' You can, she insists, learn to release more of the natural substances through exercise, sex and thought – to induce your own 'high'. 'It's an interesting theory that what you believe comes true' she says.

Complementary Therapies do not get the recognition they deserve. 'A study at Stanford University showed that when people with cancer got together in groups to express themselves emotionally, those people survived twice as long. If a new drug had somebody living twice as long, that would be front page news.'

References

Aung, S. (1994) A brief introduction to the theory and practice of Qigong. *Am. J. Acupunct.*, **22**(4), 335–48.

Baker, D. (1997) Personal communication. Taoist Taichi Centre, Toronto, Canada.

Benor, D. (1993) *Healing Research*, Vol. 1. Oxfordshire: Helix Editions.

Chia, M. (1986) *Chi Self-Massage – The Taoist Way to Rejuvenation Healing*. Huntington, NY: Tao Books.

Cohen, K. (1996) *The Way of Qigong – The Art and Science of Chinese Energy Healing*. London: Bantam Books.

Davis, C. (ed.) (1997) *Complementary Therapies in Rehabilitation*. NJ: Slack.

Dixon, A. and Woolf, A. (1989) *Avoiding Osteoporosis*. London: Macdonald Optima.

Dong, P. and Esser, A. (1993) *Chi Gong: The ancient Chinese way to health*. New York: Marlow.

Eisenberg, D. with Wright, T.L. (1983) *Encounters with Qi – Exploring Chinese Medicine*. London: Jonathan Cape.

Gerber, R. (1996) *Vibrational Medicine – New Choices of Healing Ourselves*, 2nd edn. Santa Fe, NM: Bear.

Government Health Document (1998) Green Paper, *A Healthier Nation*.

Guo, B. (1994) Introducing Qi Gong: turn back the clock and rejuvenate. *J. Complementary Med.*, **45** (May), 14–17.

Jahnke, R. (1997) *The Healer Within*. San Francisco: Harper.

Jin, P. (1992) Efficacy of Tai Chi, brisk walking meditation and reading in reducing mental and emotional stress. *J. Pschosom. Res.*, **36**, 361–70.

Kutner, N.G., Barnhart, H., Wolf, S.L., McNeely, E. and Xu, T. (1997) Self-report benefits of Tai Chi practice by older adults. *J. Gerontol. B. Psychol. Sci. Soc. Sci.*, **52**(5), 242–46.

La Perriere, A. *et al.* (1994) Exercise and psychoneuro-immunology. *J. Am. Coll. Sports Med.* **26**(2), 182–90.

Li Yingbo (1985) *The Wonders of Qigong* (compiled by China Sports magazine). Wayfarer.

Liu Xiao Ming and Yuan Li Ren (1993) Traditional Chinese Methods of Health Preservation. *J. Chinese Med.*, no. 41, January, summary.

MacRitchie, J. (1993) *Chi Kung – Cultivating Personal Energy. Health Essentials*. Shaftesbury: Elements Books.

Mitchell, L. (1987) *Simple Relaxation*. London: John Murray.

Morgan, G. (1987) *Exercise and Mental Health*. New York: Hemisphere Publishing.

Pert, C. (1997) *Molecules of Emotion: Why We Feel the Way We Feel*. New York: Scribner.

Ryu, H., Lee, H. *et al.* (1995) Acute effect of Qigong training on stress hormonal levels in man. *Am. J. Chinese Med.*, **XX1V**(2), 193–98.

Sancier, K.M. (1996) Medical applications of Qigong. *Altern. Therapies*, **2**(1), 40–6.

Sancier, K.M. and Hu, B.K. (1991) Medical applications of qigong and emitted qi on humans animals, cell cultures and plants: a review of selected scientific research. *Am. J. Acupunc.*, **19**(4), 367–77.

Skoglund, L. (1998) The use of Qigong as a method of reducing stress amongst computer operators. Are stress levels and/or psychosomatic symptoms influenced by Qigong training? MSc paper Karoliinska Institute, Sweden.

Takahashi, M. and Brown, S. (1986) *Qigong for Health*. Tokyo: Japan Publication.

Wang Yifang (compiled) (1992) *Illustration of Channel Points for Acupuncture, Moxibustion and Qigong*. Changsa, People's Republic of China: Human Science and Technology Press.

Watkins, A. (ed.) (1997) Successful ageing. In *Mind–Body Medicine. A Clinician's Guide to Psychoneuroimmunology*. London: Churchill Livingstone.

Wolf, S. *et al.* (1996) The ancient Taichi exercises effective in preventing fall in the elderly population. Emory University. A Study Sponsored by NIA (National Institute of Ageing). *J. Trad. Eastern Health Fit.*, Qi journal.

Wolf, S. *et al.* (1997) The effect of Tai Chi Quan and computerised balance training on postural stability in older subjects. *Phys. Ther.*, **77**(4), 371–81.

Wong Chongxing *et al.* (1993) The effects of Qigong on preventing stroke and alleviating the multiple cerebro-cardiovascular risk factors – a follow-up report on 242 hypertensive cases in 30 years. (Paper presented at the Second World Conference for Academic Exchange of Medical Qigong, September. Quoted in Eisenberg and Wright (1986).)

Wong, L. (1995) *Qinetics* (book and video) available from 14 Howsclose, Uxbridge UB8 2AS.

Recommended reading

Beinfield, H. L. and Korngold, E. (1991) *Between Heaven and Earth*. New York: Ballantine Books.

Bensousan, A. (1991) *The Vital Meridian*. London: Churchill Livingstone.

Cen Yue Fang (ed.) (1996) *Chinese Qigong Essentials*. Beijing, People's Republic of China: New World Press.

Ellis, N. (1994) *Acupuncture in Clinical Practice: A Guide for Health Professionals*, Therapy in Practice Series. London: Chapman and Hall.

Guo, B. (1996) Applying the method of emptying the mind whilst filling the abdomen to enhance the effect of acupuncture in clinical practice. *J. Chinese Med.*, **45**, 14–17.

Hall, J. with Jacobs, R. (1992) *The Wise Woman – a Natural Approach to the Menopause*. Shaftesbury: Element Books.

Hongxun, S. (1995) *BUQI Chinese Healing and Self-healing*. Ghent: Buqi Institute.

Housheng, L. (1994) *300 Questions in Qigong Exercises*. Guangzhou, People's Republic of China: Guangdong Science and Technology Press.

Jwing-Ming, Y. (1995) *Chinese Qigong Massage*. Massachusetts: YMAA Publication Centre.

McKenzie, E. (1999) *Chi Kung: Cultivating Personal Energy*. London: Hamlyn.

Patterson, C. (1996) Measuring outcomes in primary care: a patient generated measure, MYMOP compared with the SF-36 health survey. *Br. Med. J.*, **312**, 1016–1020.

Quinn, K. (1991) *Chi Kung – Reclaim your Power*. London: Thorsons.

Tse, M. (1995) Balancing Qigong for your back. *Qi Magazine*. February/March.

Tse, M. (1998) *Qigong for Health and Vitality*. London: Piatkus.

Sifu Wong Kiew Kit (1996) *Chi Kung for Health and Vitality: A Practical Approach to the Art of Chi Kung*. London: Gaia.

18 Aromatherapy

Tessa Campbell and Elisabeth Jones

Introduction

This chapter on aromatherapy will hopefully give some insight into why, when treating patients, physiotherapy and aromatherapy combine well together. In many respects aromatherapy allows physiotherapists to return to their roots by renewing the art of healing through touch, with massage being the main means of application. Physiotherapists have always been good at treating physical problems, and by incorporating aromatherapy into the skill base it is hoped to increase the scope of treatment to also cover mental, emotional and possibly spiritual factors. In addition, the efficacy of treatment may be improved by applying those essential oils which are indicated by the physical symptoms. Since it is now accepted that there is a strong link between the mind and the body, it must be of benefit to the patient to try to treat all the factors affecting them, not just one. This impacts on the initial assessment of a patient, in that it must be holistic in nature and cover all aspects of their health and lifestyle. This is extremely important, as physical problems with the body are rarely found in isolation, but as part of the larger picture of that person as a whole. Aromatherapy has been observed to be of most use in chronic conditions and stress-related problems, both of which are areas of great interest to physiotherapists.

Conventional medicine and complementary therapies should not be seen as an either/or situation, but as a melding of knowledge for the greater good of the patient. By combining the best from natural and synthetic sources, medicine can continue to be increasingly effective, and physiotherapists are in a very good position to lead the way in combining conventional medicine with the complementary therapies in order that patients receive the best possible treatment.

What is aromatherapy?

Aromatherapy is the treatment of the human organism, either internally or externally, by the application of essential oils of aromatic plants.

Physiotherapists using aromatherapy apply the oils externally, whereas an aromatologist would be more likely to treat using internal applications. This latter type of treatment is not common in Britain, but is used more on the Continent by qualified practitioners. This chapter will look solely at the external application of essential oils.

Historical background

The history of aromatherapy is very much associated with that of herbal medicine, and can be traced as far back as 3000 BC. Many of the ancient civilizations, the Chinese, Egyptians, Jews, Greeks and Romans, made their own contributions to the art, using aromatics both for medicinal and for beautifying purposes. Around AD 1000, Avicena improved on the basic distillation process of extraction of oils, and wrote books on the properties of plants. In the sixteenth century Paracelsus came up with 'The Doctrine of Signatures' in which he associated various plants with particular diseases, e.g. lungwort leaves, which resembled the shape of the lungs, would be used for the treatment of chest complaints. Then in the seventeenth century Nicholas Culpeper combined astrology with herbalism, and wrote his famous work *The Complete Herbal*. As more books were written, and particularly once they appeared in English rather than Latin, knowledge of herbs and oils was opened up to the general public.

Interest in herbalism began to wane in the eighteenth and nineteenth centuries with the advent of synthetic drugs, and remained in the wings until the early part of the twentieth century when the work of the French Chemist René Gattefosse led to the advent of the term 'Aromatherapie'. He wrote many articles on the medicinal qualities of herbal oils, particularly for the treatment of skin cancer, gangrene, burns and chronic wounds. This work was carried on by another Frenchman, Dr Jean Valnet, who, during World War II, treated war wounds with essential oils. Madame Maury, a Swiss biochemist researching the therapeutic use of essential oils at the same time as Valnet, decided to use massage with pure essential oils as a treatment.

By the late 1970s, Michelene Arcier, William Arnold-Taylor, Elisabeth Jones, Eve Taylor and Robert Tisserand were leading the field in the training and development of aromatherapy. In the 1980s, a number of therapists felt it was important that there should be an independent representative body for the profession of aromatherapy. Thus the International Federation of Aromatherapists (IFA) was formed in Britain in 1985. Since its inception, IFA branches have also been set up in Australia, Holland and Japan. Another major organization was founded in Britain in 1990, the International Society of Professional Aromatherapists (ISPA). Its international membership represents such countries as Australia, Singapore and the Republic of Ireland. Both the IFA and ISPA are self-regulating and democratically elected bodies which liaise with similar national bodies in the formulation of recognized training standards.

In 1991, the Aromatherapy Organisations Council (AOC) was set up as an umbrella group for several aromatherapy associations. Both the IFA and the ISPA belong to the AOC, and it is the governing body for the aromatherapy profession in the UK. Its aims are:

1. To unify the profession through bringing together its various organizations.
2. To establish common standards of training, and to ensure that all organizations registered with the Council provide appropriate standards of professional practice and conduct for their members.
3. To act as a public watchdog.
4. To provide a collective voice for all organizations within aromatherapy, through which to initiate and sustain political dialogue with government, civil and medical bodies, in order to enhance the best interests of professional aromatherapy.
5. To offer a mediation and arbitration service in any disputes involving aromatherapy organizations.
6. To initiate, support or sponsor research into aromatherapy.

In 1995, a massage special interest group (ACPIM) was set up under the auspices of the Chartered Society of Physiotherapy, and this incorporates a subgroup for those physiotherapists using aromatherapy. The aims of this group are to provide a forum for discussion of ideas, to keep abreast of current research, and to keep members aware of the ongoing work to standardize training.

Anyone wishing to train in aromatherapy should apply to the AOC for a list of approved colleges.

Research into aromatherapy

Physiotherapists have always been taught to question what they are doing and why, so it is only natural that they want to know why aromatherapy appears to work. Unfortunately, however, science is only just beginning to unravel the mysteries and complexities of essential oils, so we do not have all the answers yet.

As Andrew Vickers (1996) says: 'There is a dearth of good quality clinical research investigating aromatherapy as typically used by practitioners.' This is beginning to change and physiotherapists with their specialist knowledge should be in the forefront of this research. In the meantime, the relevance of the single case study should not be ignored.

There are two main areas of research, the studies carried out in the clinical setting and the basic research into the oils carried out in the laboratory. The latter is a long process, in some cases taking up to 3 years to fully analyse the effects of two oils.

Examples of laboratory experiments on oils are the study by Carson and Riley (1995) which showed the antimicrobial activity of the major components of the essential oil of *Melaleuca alternifolia* (Tea-tree oil), and another by Larrondo *et al.* (1995) which showed the antimicrobial activity of *Lavandula officinalis* (Lavender), *Melissa officinalis* (Melissa) and *Rosmarinus officinalis* (Rosemary).

Clinically-based experiments have shown that:

- 5% Tea-tree oil gel is an effective treatment for mild acne (Bassett *et al.*, 1990).
- Different species of Lavender will yield oils with different therapeutic effects (Buckle, 1993).
- Peppermint oil in ethanol solution, massaged into the forehead, is an effective treatment for tension-type headaches (Gobel *et al.*, 1996).
- Lavender oil has a sedative effect on elderly patients, and helps promote sleep (Hudson, 1996).

This is just a small sample of the data available, but the relevance to the Health Services can be appreciated; for instance, some hospitals are using Lavender oil to aid sleep, in care of the elderly wards, instead of sleeping pills.

Research has also been done into the effects of massage with essential oils, in various health settings, such as

- The use of foot massage with neroli on post-cardiac surgery patients in intensive care was found to help psychologically with patients' recovery (Stevenson, 1994).

- Massage with essential oils was found to be beneficial to the well-being of cancer patients (Corner *et al.*, 1995).
- Citrus fragrance, which comforts through stimulation of the olfactory system, was applied to 12 depressive patients and the results indicated that the doses of anti-depressants necessary for the treatment of depression could be markedly reduced. The citrus fragrance normalized neuroendocrine hormone levels and the immune function (Komori *et al.*, 1995).

More in-depth information on research can be obtained from the Research Council for Complementary Medicine.

What are essential oils?

The term 'essential oil' may be defined as referring to an odorous, volatile product obtained by a physical process from a natural source of a single species, which corresponds to the source in both name and colour (Williams, 1989). The 'natural source' can be one of many parts of a plant or tree, e.g. bark, seeds, flowers, twigs, berries, fruits, leaves, rhizomes or roots.

The 'physical process' most commonly used to extract essential oils from their parent plants is distillation. In steam distillation, the plant material and water are heated together in a vessel called a 'still'. As the oils are released from the plant material, they rise up in the vessel along with the steam, pass into a condensing coil and start to cool. This leads into a collecting vessel where the oil and water mixture is cooled further, and then separated.

There are various other methods of extraction, including dry distillation, expression, solvent extraction and maceration.

When using a natural substance on the body it *must* be pure and unadulterated, so it is very important that it comes from 'one species'. Even within one species there will be variations in the chemical make-up due to differences in growing conditions, i.e. soil type, altitude, rainfall, sunshine and the time of year it is harvested. It therefore follows that essential oils must be purchased from a knowledgeable and reputable source.

Chemical make-up

Gas chromatography shows that one essential oil can consist of hundreds of different compounds and these can be divided up into hydrocarbons, oxygenated compounds and trace elements.

Hydrocarbons.   The main hydrocarbons found in essential oils are monoterpenes and sesquiterpenes and very occasionally diterpenes: monoterpenes have 10 carbon atoms; sesquiterpenes have 15 carbon atoms; and diterpenes have 20 carbon atoms. The carbon atoms are linked to hydrogen atoms in chains.

Oxygenated compounds.   These are classified into different types according to their chemical structure. There are alcohols, aldehydes, esters, ketones, lactones, phenols and oxides. These compounds, when used in isolation, act on the body in differing ways, and some of them can be quite irritating to the body, e.g. phenols can be a skin and mucous membrane irritant.

Trace elements.   These may contain sulphur or nitrogen, and may be skin irritants.

The different constituents contribute to the perfume of the essential oil, dependent on various factors – the proportion of the constituent, its volatility and quality, and the strength of its odour. It is thought that the constituent parts of the oils can have differing effects on the body, e.g. the terpenes can be antiseptic and bactericidal, alcohols can be antiviral, and aldehydes, anti-inflammatory and sedative. The therapeutic outcome, though, is not directly related to the perceived effects of the constituents found in the oils, as seen in this quote from Dr Maria Lis-Balchin:

> It is wrong to group essential oil
> components of similar chemistry e.g.
> ketones, aldehydes etc. together and allocate
> biological properties to these groups. With
> few exceptions, similar components can
> influence the action of different essential oils
> in different ways. (Lis-Balchin *et al.*, 1995)

In aromatherapy we believe that it is important to use the whole oil, as we do not yet know how all the individual constituents interact with one another and affect the therapeutic outcome. We do know that the proportion of any one constituent is not relative to its effect, so it may be present in a small amount but have a major influence on the overall odour or therapeutic effect of that oil. We also know that the interaction of the constituents of an oil has the ability to counteract irritating effects of individual constituents, e.g. Lavender oil contains an oxide 1,8 cineole which, on its own, is a skin irritant, but Lavender in total is considered to be a safe oil. This is known as the **quenching effect**.

Precautions

There are four possible adverse reactions to essential oils:

- *Toxicity.* This is commonly called poisoning, and is dose dependent, i.e. the greater the dose the higher the risk. If the guidelines for choosing oils and percentage of essential oils are followed, this should not be a problem. The constituents of which to be most aware are phenols and ketones.
- *Irritation.* This falls into two sections, irritation of the skin and irritation of the mucous membranes. The constituents which cause the main problems are the phenols, e.g. thymol, carvacrol and eugenol, which can cause inflammation of the skin or the mucous membranes.
- *Sensitization.* This is when an essential oil causes an allergic reaction, so is very much an individual problem. Only a small amount is needed to have an effect, so this reaction is not dose dependent.
- *Photosensitization.* This is a pigmentation of skin which is exposed to ultraviolet light, natural or otherwise, after the application of certain oils. These are mainly Expressed Citrus Oils, like Lemon (*Citrus limonium*) and Bergamot (*Citrus bergamia*). Photosensitization can be avoided by using Distilled Lemon (*Citrus limonium*) Oil, or Bergapteneless Bergamot (*Citrus bergamia*) which is labelled Bergamot (FCF).

There are also some specific conditions where extra care must be taken when selecting the oils:

- **Pregnancy.** Avoid the strongly emmenagogic oils (i.e. those oils which promote menstruation) such as Basil (*Ocimum basilicum*), Hyssop (*Hyssopus officinalis*), Juniper (*Juniperus communis*), Marjoram (*Origanum marjorana*), Myrrh (*Commiphora myrrha*), Thyme (*Thymus vulgaris*) and Sage (*Salvia officinalis*). This is purely precautionary as there is, to date, no evidence that these oils are abortifacient in the dosages that are used by a professional aromatherapist.

- **Epilepsy.** Oils to be avoided because they may precipitate a seizure in certain circumstances are Hyssop (*Hyssopus officinalis*), Rosemary (*Rosmarinus officinalis*), Sweet Fennel (*Foeniculum vulgare*) and Sage (*Salvia officinalis*). Oils which may be helpful in epilepsy are Roman Chamomile (*Anthemis nobilis*), Lavender (*Lavandula augustifolia*) and Ylang Ylang (*Cananga odorata*). This information comes from the British Epilepsy Association and is based on the research of Betts (1993).

- **Blood pressure.** Oils to be avoided in high blood pressure are Mandarin (*Citrus reticulata*), Rosemary (*Rosmarinus officinalis*), Sage (*Salvia officinalis*) and Thyme (*Thymus vulgaris*). Oils to be avoided in low blood pressure are Clary Sage (*Salvia sclarea*), Lavender (*Lavandula augustifolia*), Lemon (*Citrus limonium*), Marjoram (*Origanum marjorana*), Melissa (*Melissa officinalis*), Rosemary (*Rosmarinus officinalis*) and Ylang Ylang (*Cananga odorata*). Hyssop (*Hyssopus officinalis*), Rosemary (*Rosmarinus officinalis*) and possibly Ylang Ylang (*Cananga odorata*) are thought to be able to balance blood pressure.

Commonly used oils

Following is a list of 21 oils which have been found to be useful when used in conjunction with physiotherapy, but this is only a small proportion of the oils that are available to an aromatherapist:

1. **Basil** (*Ocimum basilicum*). Refreshing and tonic effect.
2. **Benzoin** (*Styrax benzoin*). Warming, calming and soothing to the skin.
3. **Bergamot** (*Citrus bergamia*). Refreshing, relaxing and uplifts the spirit.
4. **Chamomile Roman** (*Anthemis nobilis*). Soothing for physical and mental states.
5. **Coriander** (*Coriandrum sativum*). Uplifting and reviving.
6. **Eucalyptus** (*Eucalyptus globulus*). Refreshing, stimulating and good for respiration.
7. **Geranium** (*Pelargonium graveolens*). Refreshing, good for all skin types, particularly oily skin.
8. **Ginger** (*Zingiber officinale*). Warming, drying and helps aches and pains.
9. **Juniper** (*Juniperus communis*). Refreshing, astringent and good for fluid retention.
10. **Lavender** (*Lavandula augustifolia*). Restores and balances mind and body, excellent for skin problems and is very versatile.
11. **Lemon** (*Citrus limonium*). Astringent, refreshing and stimulating.
12. **Marjoram, Sweet** (*Origanum marjorana*). Warming, relaxing and good for muscle rubs.
13. **Melissa** (*Melissa officinalis*). Uplifts the spirit, soothes the mind and is good for respiratory conditions.
14. **Patchouli** (*Pergostemon patchouli*). Soothing, relaxing oil, which decongests oily skin.
15. **Peppermint** (*Mentha piperata*). For digestive and nervous upsets, and cools the skin.
16. **Black Pepper** (*Piper nigrum*). Stimulates circulation, reduces muscular aches and pains, aids digestion and respiration, and is aphrodisiac.
17. **Pine** (*Pinus sylvestris*). Antiseptic and refreshing.
18. **Rosemary** (*Rosmarinus officinalis*). Refreshing, invigorating and clears congestion.
19. **Sandalwood** (*Santalum album*). Calms and soothes, balances secretions of the skin, and is sensual.
20. **Tea Tree** (*Melaleuca alternifolia*). Powerful antiseptic and fungicide, therefore used for infections of all kinds.
21. **Ylang Ylang** (*Cananga odorata*). Uplifting, soothing, sensual and good for the skin.

Oil profiles

Aromatherapy oils can be classified according to their smell, i.e. citrus, floral, herbal, musky, spicy and woody. Below is an in-depth profile of six oils, one from each of these categories. The therapeutic uses of these oils are based on empirical evidence.

Glossary of terms

Antiphlogistic – reduces inflammation and vasoconstricts.
Carminative – eases bowel pain and expels wind.
Emmenagogue – promotes menstruation.
Febrifuge – reduces fever.
Rubifacient – stimulates circulation.
Vulnerary – heals sores and wounds.

Citrus – Bergamot (*Citrus bergamia*) Rutaceae

Extracted by expression from the peel of the nearly new fruit.

Traditional uses

Digestive	Antispasmodic/Carminative/ Digestive Colic, flatulence, indigestion.
Nervous	Analgesic/Antidepressant/ Sedative Anxiety, depression, nervous tension, headaches.
Respiratory	Antiseptic/Febrifuge Infections, fevers.
Genito-urinary	Antiseptic For infections.
Skin/Hair	Antiseptic/Astringent/ Vulnerary Acne, oily skin and hair, ulcers, wounds.

General effects. Refreshing, relaxing and uplifts the spirit.

Main constituents. Limonene, linalyl acetate, linalool.

Caution. Avoid using before or after ultraviolet light treatment or sunbathing.

Floral – Geranium (*Pelargonium graveolens*) Geraniaceae

Extracted by distillation of the green leaves.

Traditional uses

Circulation	Haemostatic Helps to arrest bleeding.
Digestive	Antispasmodic/Digestive Diarrhoea, gastroenteritis.
Nervous	Analgesic/Antidepressant/ Sedative Neuralgia, depression, anxiety.
Genito-urinary	Antiseptic/Diuretic Infections, fluid retention.
Skin/hair	Antiphlogistic/Antiseptic/ Vulnerary Dry skin and hair, inflamed skin, bruises, burns, dry eczema, wounds, ulcers, decongests.

General effects. Refreshing, decongestant in skin care, good for all skin types, particularly oily skin.

Main constituents. Citronellol, geraniol.

Caution. Can have irritating effect on hyper-sensitive skin.

Herbal – Marjoram, Sweet (*Origanum marjorana*) Labiatae

Extracted by distillation of flowers and leaves.

Traditional uses

Circulation	Hypotensor Lowers blood pressure.
Digestion	Antispasmodic/Digestive Colic, indigestion.
Muscles	Analgesic Muscle aches and pains.
Nervous	Analgesic/Sedative Anxiety, hysteria, insomnia, migraines, nervous tension.
Respiratory	Antiseptic/Antispasmodic Colds, sinusitis.

Genito-urinary Diuretic/Emmenagogue
Fluid retention, painful
periods, leucorrhoea.

General effects. Warming, relaxing, good for muscle rubs.

Main constituents. Geranyl acetate, pinene, sabinene, terpineol, terpinenol-4.

Caution. Avoid in pregnancy.

Musky – Patchouli (*Pergostemon patchouli*) Labiateae

Extracted by distillation of dried young leaves.

Traditional uses

Nervous Antidepressant/Aphrodisiac/
Sedative
Counters depression, anxiety
and nervous tension,
stimulates sexual desire.
Urinary Diuretic
Fluid retention.
Skin Antiseptic/Astringent/
Vulnerary/Decongestant
Acne, oily skin and wounds.

General effects. Soothing, relaxing oil, good for decongesting oily skins. Fixative in perfumery.

Main constituents. Benzaldehyde eugenol.

Spicy – Black Pepper (*Piper nigrum*) Piperaceae

Extracted by distillation of the dried, nearly ripe fruit.

Traditional uses

Circulation Rubifacient/Febrifuge
Circulatory stimulant, reduces
fevers.
Digestive Antispasmodic/Carminative/
Laxative
Gastroenteritis, flatulence,
appetite loss.
Muscles Analgesic/Rubifacient
Muscle aches and pains.

Nervous Aphrodisiac/Stimulant
Stimulates sexual desire,
for debility.
Respiratory Antiseptic/Antispasmodic
Coughs.
Urinary Diuretic
Fluid retention.

General effects. Stimulates circulation, reduces muscular aches and pains, helps digestion and respiration, and is aphrodisiac.

Main constituents. Caryophyllene, phellandrene.

Woody – Sandalwood (*Santalum album*) Santalaceae

Extracted by distillation of the heartwood of the tree.

Traditional uses

Digestive Antiseptic/Antispasmodic/
Carminative
Colic, diarrhoea, gastritis,
flatulence.
Nervous Aphrodisiac/Antidepressant/
Sedative
Stimulates sexual desire,
depression, anxiety, nervous
tension.
Respiratory Antiseptic, Antispasmodic/
Expectorant
Bronchitis, catarrh, coughs,
colds, laryngitis.
Genito-urinary Antiseptic/Diuretic/
Emmenagogue
Genito-urinary infections,
fluid retention.
Skin/hair Antiphlogistic/Antiseptic/
Astringent/Vulnerary
Acne, oily and dry skin and
hair – balances secretions,
counters inflammation and
sensitivity.

General effects. It calms and soothes, balances secretions of skin, sensual.

Main constituents. Santalol.

Assessment (as taught at the Elisabeth Jones Natural Therapy Centre)

Having studied the essential oils, it is now time to look at the patients. As mentioned earlier, in an aromatherapy assessment it is necessary to look at the patients holistically. The assessment is broken down into three main sections, and will take approximately half an hour to complete, preferably taking place in warm congenial surroundings, which helps the patient to relax.

1. **Verbal.** Notes should be taken on past medical history, medication and present problems. Also note lifestyle and family circumstances which have a bearing on the physical problems. Ask about their mental state, e.g. any problems with depression, anxiety, stress, etc., and ascertain the patient's personality type.

2. **Visual**

   and

3. **Tactile.** These elements of the assessment are carried out in tandem. Observe spinal alignment, both in standing and sitting, and note skin colour and texture. Check movement between the superficial and deeper layers of fascia, assess circulation through the back, and test for pain or discomfort between the facet joints of the spine. Palpate the abdomen for pain or tenderness, while observing the face for signs of tension or anxiety. Note the facial skin type, colour and texture. Palpate any painful areas using standard physiotherapy techniques. Finally palpate the various reflex areas of the feet as in reflexology, and question the patient on any areas which show up as tender or have altered 'feel' or sensation. This helps to jog the patient's memory about problems which may not have come up previously in the assessment, as well as reinforcing information already given.

Check for contraindications (see next section) and obtain the patient's permission to contact their GP if there are any queries about their medical condition. Do not hesitate to contact the doctor if there is any uncertainty as to the advisability of carrying out the treatment. The patient must sign the form accepting responsibility for the aromatherapy treatment.

Lastly, ask the patient about their odour preferences, i.e. do they like floral, citrus, herbal, spicy, musky or woody smells, as it is important that they like the smell of their treatment oil. The assessment is now complete and the physiotherapist has a much better idea of 'who' he/she is treating and 'why', and can now concentrate on the 'how'.

Contraindications

If you are using massage as the means of applying essential oils to the body, the contraindications to massage would be applicable, i.e. *do not massage if*:

- the client is running a temperature, unless under orders from the medical practitioner
- there is recent scarring, unless under orders from the medical practitioner
- there is an open wound, infection, bites, or rash of unknown origin
- there is an inadequate blood supply, or haemorrhage is occurring
- there is acute inflammation
- there is acneic skin
- there are internal organ disorders
- there is active bone growth, i.e. recent fracture, myositis ossificans or periostitis
- the patient is pregnant – not over the abdomen.

Precautions should be taken if there is or are:

- varicose veins – do not apply pressure over them
- malignant disease – first obtain consent from the consultant
- heart disease – avoid massaging the anterior chest wall and neck area, and take care over the reflex areas between the shoulder blades
- diabetes – beware of poor circulation
- rheumatoid arthritis – in the advanced case, beware of collagenous weakening

- steroid treatment – long-term treatment can cause the skin to become thin, so pressure must be very much lighter (Holey and Cook, 1997).

With particular reference to aromatherapy massage, there are a number of other precautions:

- essential oils *must* be diluted in a vegetable carrier oil to enable the oils to be absorbed through the skin – mineral oil does not offer this facility
- the percentage of essential oil to carrier oil should not exceed 5%, and is normally 0.5–2%
- rubifacient oils should not be applied to vasodilated skin
- the 'Precautions' section (see earlier) for each oil must be observed
- advise the patient not to sunbathe or have ultraviolet light treatment on the same day as their massage
- if in any doubt about a client's medical condition, check with their GP or consultant
- essential oils are flammable – keep away from naked flames
- reduce concentration of essential oils by 50% when treating babies, young children, the elderly and heavily medicated patients
- if essential oils accidentally get into an eye, wash out with distilled water.

Blending of oils

Now the fun begins – the client's history has been taken, their problems ascertained and an individual blend of oils is now to be made up. Why blend the oils? It is believed that the essential oils work together **synergistically,** i.e. the overall effect is greater than the sum of the individual effects, so blending creates a more powerful tool.

The perfumery business has studied the different rates at which essential oils evaporate, and classed them accordingly. Oils which evaporate quickly are called Top Notes and these are the most volatile and tend to be the first smell that can be detected in a blend. Then there are the Middle Notes, which are less volatile and tend to relate to bodily functions. The least volatile are the Base Notes and these oils also act as fixatives, i.e. they help to slow down the evaporation of the Top Notes, fixing them in the blend for longer. Table 18.1 gives the 'Note' classification of the 21 oils listed earlier.

Having decided on the desired therapeutic outcome, choose several oils which are most likely to achieve this, then find a basic three which provide a Top, Middle and Base Note. For example, a patient presents with chronic backache, constipation and dry skin. The choice of oils can be made from:

- *Chronic backache* – Benzoin, Chamomile, Coriander, Eucalyptus, Ginger, Juniper, Lavender, Lemon, Marjoram, Peppermint, Black Pepper, and Rosemary.
- *Constipation* – Ginger.
- *Dry skin* – Benzoin, Chamomile, Geranium, Sandalwood, Ylang Ylang.

The blend could include Benzoin (Base), Chamomile (Middle), Ginger (Top).

Table 18.1 Classification of oils into Top, Middle and Base Notes

Top Notes	Middle Notes	Base Notes
Basil	Chamomile	Benzoin
Bergamot	Geranium	Patchouli
Coriander	Juniper	Sandalwood
Eucalyptus	Marjoram	
Ginger	Melissa	
Lavender	Black Pepper	
Lemon	Pine	
Peppermint	Rosemary	
Tea Tree	Ylang Ylang	

Carrier oils

Having decided on the essential oils, the carrier oil must now be chosen. As previously mentioned, it must be vegetable oil as this will be absorbed through the skin. The main vegetable oils used are: Sweet Almond, Apricot Kernel, Avocado, Grapeseed, Jojoba, Peach Kernel, Safflower, Sunflower and Wheatgerm oil. These may be mixed or used on their own. The range of vegetable oils is constantly increasing, with some now thought to help the therapeutic outcome, e.g. Hypericum oil is thought to be anti-inflammatory, and Calendula to soothe and relieve skin rashes.

Basic formula for an oil blend

There can be anything from one to five essential oils in a blend with a carrier oil, but it is usual to have three, as this should be sufficient to cover most problems. If too many different essences are added, the subtlety of the smell can be lost. Formula:

0.5–2% essential oil to 30 ml carrier oil
(3–12 drops)

So, with reference to the previous example the blend could be:

3 drops Benzoin, 2 drops Chamomile and
3 drops Ginger in 30 ml Sweet Almond oil

Once this formula has been made up, treatment can begin.

Application of oils

Sufficient oil is applied to the hands of the therapist, and then applied to the patient. In aromatherapy massage, three techniques are used – Swedish, neuromuscular and Shiatsu. The **Swedish massage** provides the initial relaxation and gentle influence on circulation and lymphatic drainage, then the **neuromuscular massage** achieves a more dynamic effect on the musculature through deep kneadings, while stimulating the nervous system. The **Shiatsu massage** is given to influence the lines of energy flowing through the meridians of the body and clear any blockages through pressure on the Tsubo or acupuncture points (see Chapter 15). The overall result is to relax the patient, both physically and mentally, to improve the circulation and lymphatic drainage, help remove metabolites and toxins from the body, calm the nervous system, and normalize meridian energy flow. From a physiotherapy point of view this provides a very good base from which to start other manual therapy techniques such as mobilizations, manual traction and 'nags and snags' (joint mobilizing technique).

A full body massage may take up to 1.5 hours, so smaller areas are often treated due to time constraints, e.g. hand, foot, or neck, back and shoulders. Massage is not the only way in which essential oils can be applied; the other methods are given below.

Basic formulae for other applications

- **Baths**. 6–10 drops of essential oils diluted in either 20 ml milk or unperfumed bath gel, and added to the water once the bath has been drawn. Agitate the water to aid dispersal. This is a useful means of applying sedative oils particularly to enhance relaxation.
- **Foot baths**. 6–8 drops of essential oils diluted in 20 ml milk or unperfumed bath gel, and added to a large basin of water. This is very useful for those late afternoon outpatients with foot problems. Add, for example, some Lemon oil or Tea Tree oil to a foot bath half-full of warm water and leave feet to soak for 10 minutes, explaining that this is part of the treatment! On the other hand, after a long clinical day, a foot bath with Peppermint oil added provides blissful relief for aching feet. Variations on this would be hand and sitz (hip) baths.
- **Vaporizers**. 3–4 drops of essential oils added to warm water in an oil burner or aromatic diffuser. This can be used to create a calm mood in a room to help stressed or agitated patients. Equally, it is useful to vaporize antiseptic oils to help counteract airborne infections. For safety in the hospital situation, it is better to use a diffuser.

- **Steam inhalations.** 6–10 drops essential oils in 2 pints steaming water. Again, in the ward situation, check up on any safety regulations before carrying out this type of treatment.
  Oils for sinusitis and colds – Eucalyptus, Peppermint, Rosemary.
  Oils for expectorant effect – Bergamot, Eucalyptus.
  Oils for antispasmodic effect – Sandalwood, Lavender.
- **Compresses.** 1–6 drops of one or more essential oils to 100 ml hot or cold water. The compresses can be used to help reduce swelling, reduce fever or soothe pain.
- **Tissue.** 2–3 drops essential oils put onto a tissue. This can then be sniffed by the patient as and when they want. This is the simplest and quickest way to administer essential oils, and can be used to influence the mental state of a patient, due to the direct route to the limbic system.
- **Lotions and creams.** Essential oils can be added to unperfumed, hypoallergenic base lotions or creams in the same proportions as for an oil, i.e. 0.5–2% (3–12 drops essential oil to 30 ml lotion or cream). This can be an effective means of applying the oils between treatments when an oil carrier would not be appropriate.

Absorption of essential oils

There are three routes by which essential oils enter the body: by absorption through the skin; by inhalation; and by olfaction.

1. **Absorption.** When essential oils are diluted in a vegetable oil or in water, as in massage, baths and compresses, the oils are absorbed by the skin and enter the circulation, and thus travel to the muscles, joints and body systems.

When the essential oils are breathed in through the nose there are two pathways that have a combined action – inhalation and olfaction:

2. **Inhalation.** This is where the oils are absorbed through the mucous membrane of the nose and thus into the circulation, and transported as above.
3. **Olfaction.** Here the essential oils trigger electrochemical signals in the smell receptor cells of the olfactory centre, which are then transmitted by the olfactory nerve to the limbic system, where they can trigger memories and emotions. These messages are then sent to the brain and body systems, stimulating the release of sedative, stimulating or euphoric neurochemicals.

Storage of oils

Essential oils are volatile substances which will react with oxygen, causing changes in the chemical composition and therefore the effect on the body. In order to cut oxidation down to a minimum, great care must be taken to store the oils correctly. This means:

- buying oils from a reputable dealer who will ensure that they arrive in good condition, marked with 'use by' dates
- storing oils in a cool, dark place, preferably the fridge, in dark-coloured glass bottles
- observing the 'use by' dates
- mixing blends in dark-coloured bottles, and ensuring that patients store their blends for home use in the fridge, not on the bathroom window sill!
- labelling blends for home use with clear instructions, and marking 'For External Use Only'.

Home care advice to patients

For the patient to gain maximum benefit from aromatherapy, advice should be given where necessary, on lifestyle problems affecting their condition, for example:

1. *Stress.* Discuss measures to reduce stress levels, including the use of relaxing oil blends to put in the bath.

2. *Diet*. All patients must drink plenty of water after aromatherapy massage, to help flush the toxins out of the system. Encourage patients to eat and drink healthily.
3. *Sleep problems*. If necessary, make up oils to be put on a tissue, which can be placed inside the pillowcase at night to aid sleep.
4. *Posture* and *gait* re-education.
5. *Exercises*, either specific or for general fitness.

The advice given should relate to problems highlighted during the assessment, with referral to other professionals where necessary.

Figure 18.1 provides a schematic overview summarizing the factors that combine to make aromatherapy an effective treatment.

The clinical setting

It is very exciting for the authors to hear about the different ways in which physiotherapists are using aromatherapy in their everyday practice. Many have been involved in planning the introduction of complementary therapies into the NHS by sitting on steering committees and presenting a case for the inclusion of this very valid treatment modality for their patients. A strong point could be made that physiotherapists should oversee a modality so closely linked to their primary core skill of massage. Here, for example, are the main areas where aromatherapy is being used to good effect, both in the NHS and in private practice: Ante-

and postnatal; musculoskeletal problems; palliative care; paediatrics; elderly care; learning disabilities; mental health; stress management; and care of the carers.

- **Ante- and postnatal.** Aromatherapy is being used in preparation classes for mothers, in labour wards and in classes in baby massage, the latter helping mothers to bond with their babies, and giving them a strategy for coping with a screaming infant, for example, with colic. Safe oils such as Chamomile and Lavender would be used.
- **Musculoskeletal problems.** The main benefit of aromatherapy in this area is relaxation of muscle tension and spasm, which helps to relieve pain, and thus allows more thorough examination and treatment of the affected part. It is also used to counteract emotional stress which could exacerbate the condition.
- **Palliative care.** Complementary therapies are well accepted in this area of work, and aromatherapy in particular has been found to help with nausea (Mandarin), loss of appetite (Peppermint and Ginger), general emotional support (Grapefruit, Elemi, Myrrh and Frankincense) and oedema (Juniper and Fennel).
- **Paediatrics.** Children react well to aromatherapy, and it is a useful tool in gaining a child's confidence and trust, reassuring them that not all hospital treatments have to hurt.

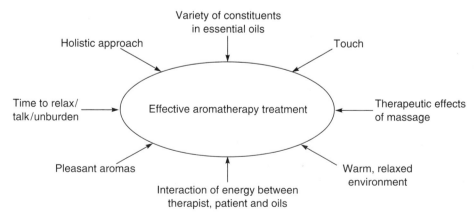

Figure 18.1 Factors which make aromatherapy an effective treatment

- **Elderly care**. For these people, the very human act of touching in a caring way can have a quite dynamic effect on their lives in hospital, and a simple hand or foot massage can have many benefits both physically and mentally. Aromatherapy can also be of benefit in the treatment of constipation, using abdominal massage with oils such as Orange and Black Pepper to bring relief.
- **Learning disabilities**. The use of 'smell' and 'touch' with this group provides another route for learning, and can also help in the formation of relationships. Some oils have also been shown to aid the learning process, e.g. Peppermint and Rosemary.
- **Mental health**. Aromatherapy is another tool that can be used to combat stress in these patients, both as a self-help technique and one that is administered. It is also a pleasurable experience, giving relaxation and a non-threatening touch situation. Useful oils include Frankincense, Neroli and Chamomile.
- **Stress management**. There is no better treatment for stress than aromatherapy. Patients really appreciate the time and space to fully relax, once they have learnt how to make that time available, and that they deserve it! Self-administration of the oils at home, e.g. in the bath, gives another way of taking control of their lives.
- **Care of the carers**. This is a very valid use of aromatherapy. Whether the carers are hospital staff or family members, it is important that they are nurtured and cared for, so that they in turn can do their job happily. Some physiotherapists are organizing support group sessions in hospices for carers, and in hospitals for staff. With the present awareness of high stress levels among health workers, it would be an interesting study to monitor how aromatherapy could relieve stress-related illness in staff.

This is a brief overview of the ways in which aromatherapy is, and can be, used in health settings, and is the object of ongoing research which will be of increasing benefit for those who anticipate practising in this field.

Typical comments the authors have received from physiotherapists using aromatherapy are:

I use aromatherapy as another tool, e.g. alongside mobilizations, ultrasound, and exercises in the treatment management.

I find it a very useful modality of treatment in conjunction with other physiotherapy techniques.

When I have the opportunity to use aromatherapy with the children I find it relaxes them in preparation for passive movements and stretchings. It seems to calm the fear of painful movement.

I was surprised how often I decided to use essential oils in a varied caseload of patients.

Some physiotherapists commented on the very positive response of their patients to aromatherapy, with many patients expressing a feeling of well-being after treatment, which helped them to cope more positively with their physical problems.

Many physiotherapists adapt their technique to suit (a) the needs of the patient, (b) the time available, and (c) the treatment location. Applications other than massage are used when appropriate, often as self-help strategies and part of the home care routine.

The empirical evidence behind the therapeutic uses of essential oils is backed up by the results obtained by those applying them, and physiotherapists have found that, for example:

- Lavender does help relieve pain, stress and insomnia.
- Eucalyptus/rosemary/marjoram blended helps orthopaedic/musculoskeletal problems.
- Roman chamomile is good when used with children.
- Mandarin helps nausea after chemotherapy.
- Neroli helps depressed patients.
- Lavender oil helps in the treatment of burns patients.

Case histories

Here are three case histories which illustrate the effective use of aromatherapy in physiotherapy.

Case history 1

Mrs A, a middle-aged lady, came to the clinic 2 years ago with a number of problems, revealed during consultation. She was thin, highly strung and had considerable pain in her right shoulder and neck, radiating into the head, causing repeated headaches. She also had irritable bowel syndrome. She was waking 2–3 times a night and showed signs of tiredness and anxiety. During the consultation it transpired that, due to her husband's redundancy, she had been left the sole breadwinner for the family.

It was obvious that she was under great stress, so on her first visit she received $1\frac{1}{2}$ hours of aromatherapy massage using a blend of Lavender/Chamomile/Sandalwood in Grapeseed oil. The massage routine included manual traction and passive movements to the neck, and also scalp massage, all of which helped her neck/shoulder/head pains, and increased her range of movement. She was visibly more relaxed after this first treatment.

When she returned 2 weeks later she reported that her sleep pattern had improved, though she still woke at least once at night. Her neck, shoulder and head pain had improved for 1 week. It was decided to include Marjoram in the blend, and this was used for subsequent treatments and for home care. She then had hourly treatments once a week, and after 3 weeks there had been great progress. The headaches had diminished, she was sleeping well, the irritable bowel syndrome was much improved and she had only a few tender areas on palpation of her right neck and shoulder.

By the sixth treatment she was feeling very well. Subsequently she attended the clinic once a month. Her husband was re-employed after 9 months, and she now comes for 'top-up' treatments 4 times a year.

Case history 2

Mrs W had been aware of pain in both sacroiliac joints and right hip for about 6 months. She was middle-aged, menopausal and on HRT. Her medical history included a bladder repair and a history of headaches. She had moved house recently and her work included a lot of heavy lifting and standing. On examination she presented with kyphosis and scoliosis in the thoracic spine, poor mobility between the superficial and deep fascia over the back area, and sluggish circulation in the lumbosacral area. There was no pain between the facet joints, but the right hip exhibited some signs of casular tightening.

Her first treatment was a neck/back/shoulder massage with a blend of Ginger/Juniper/Orange oils in Grapeseed oil carrier, followed by exercises to improve abdominal postural tone and discussion of postural pitfalls to avoid. The home care strategy was to massage her oil blend into painful areas at night, and to do her exercises.

Mrs W returned 3 weeks later having done her exercises and increased the contraction time for her abdominal muscles. The pain had decreased, so the same treatment was repeated and the exercises progressed.

At the third treatment the oils were changed to also help the menopausal symptoms: Vetivert/Chamomile/Fennel/Geranium in Grapeseed oil. The scoliosis had now gone but the kyphosis was still marked, so the manipulative procedure of 'nags' was applied to the lower thoracic spine to increase range of movement.

Mrs W was seen 1 month later, by which time her back problems were much better but the right hip was still aching and the menopausal symptoms were still present. The oils were changed to Benzoin/Geranium/Marjoram/Lavender in Grapeseed oil carrier and deep kneadings applied over the right buttock. Postural tone around the pelvis was now good, so more active hip and back exercises were taught. This treatment relieved Mrs W's symptoms and she then continued with a maintenance plan of 1 treatment per month for 3 months. During this time she had cystitis, for which a blend of Benzoin/Niaouli/Lavender was made which she added to her bath, and this helped to ease the discomfort. Mrs W was discharged with a blend of Peppermint oil in Sweet Almond oil (10% solution) to apply to her forehead should a headache start.

Case history 3

This client was an 11-year-old boy with cerebral palsy due to injury at birth. He was a difficult baby, with feeding and sleeping problems. He was now being cared for by his grandmother. Physically, he was a spastic quadriplegic with increased tone in all four limbs, and abnormal patterns of movement in his entire body. He was totally dependent on others for all his needs, and had great difficulty trying to learn to move due to the abnormal reflexes and postural responses present. Stimulation of his back caused him to thrust into extension, with his head pushed back and mouth open, and in order to prevent this his hips had to be bent to less than 90 degrees, which broke the spastic pattern and allowed him to relax. These factors had a bearing on his positioning for massage. His sight was poor, but he could hear well and differentiate between voices. He also suffered from epilepsy which was fairly well controlled by drugs. Due to the imbalance of muscle tone, he had acquired a deformity of the hips known as the 'windswept' position, which the orthopaedic surgeon decided to try and correct, in order to improve sitting position, hygiene and to prevent spinal problems. After complicated surgery, he was in plaster for 11 weeks, but unfortunately the operation did not work due to the strong pull of the muscles and the slow healing rate of the bones. He was in a great deal of pain and did not like being moved, as the operation site was still very tender.

It was decided to use aromatherapy with this child, for several reasons. First, to try to reduce the muscle spasms and spasticity to make movement easier and prevent further deformity, and secondly, to help calm his fear and nervousness enough for him to allow movement of his hips, knees and pelvis. Lastly, he needed help to obtain a good night's sleep.

For the first treatment a blend of Chamomile/Marjoram/Sandalwood in Sweet Almond oil was chosen to calm his fears and relax his muscles. The massage was done with the client lying on the floor on a thick quilt, with a pillow under his hips and towels to aid positioning. He was quite relaxed and enjoyed his massage and accepted passive movements of his legs afterwards. His grandmother reported that he was relaxed for the rest of the day and she was advised to put Lavender oil in his bath and on a tissue inside his pillowcase at night to help him sleep.

The broken sleep was still a problem, so the oils were changed for the second treatment and Petitgrain used instead of the Chamomile. The patient was very tired and tight and unwilling to move which made positioning him difficult. Once the massage started he began to relax, and fell asleep. After the massage his legs were stretched without complaint. He slept for 4 hours after massage and woke refreshed and happy. His grandmother was given a massage oil containing Chamomile, Marjoram and Sandalwood for home use.

The little boy was quite tense before the third treatment, so Petitgrain/Sandalwood/Ylang Ylang were blended in Sweet Almond oil to help him relax. His tolerance and range of movement were tested before and after treatment and there was a marked improvement. The same oils were used for the next session, but he did not relax as quickly, and abduction made him cry. He also had a small fit, and slept for a while afterwards, possibly as a result of this.

At the last session his grandmother reported that his sleeping was better. His legs and feet were rather cold so Black Pepper was used instead of the Petitgrain, to try and boost his circulation. He relaxed extremely well, his feet warmed up, and his grandmother noted the improved colour. The massage enabled him to sit and he accepted his physiotherapy well.

It was very clear that aromatherapy massage relaxed this boy in preparation for his physiotherapy treatment, and it was hoped that time and a suitable location could be found to carry on with this approach once he returned to school.

Conclusion

The needs of the patient are paramount, so it is incumbent on physiotherapists to seek out and use the best possible treatments, whether they are orthodox or complementary. When aromatherapy is integrated within physiotherapy it provides a complementary approach which is therapeutically effective for many patients. Future clinical trial research will help to clarify which combination of factors is most effective in different conditions, but present knowledge already provides a firm basis on which to incorporate aromatherapy within physiotherapy.

Acknowledgements

Our thanks go to everyone who has contributed to this chapter on aromatherapy. We are indebted to Vera Atlas, Nancy Bell, Chris Callaghan, Michelle Connell, Anne Dewhurst, Geoff Farrell, Christine McCue, Jessica Strachan, Chris Sutton and Sarah Varman.

References

Bassett, I.B., Pannowitz, D.L. and Barnetson, R.S. (1990) A comparative study of tea tree oil versus benzoylperoxide in the treatment of acne. *Med. J. Australia*, **153**, 455–58.

Betts, T. (1993) Sniffing the breeze. *Epilepsy Today*, **5**.

Buckle, J. (1993) Aromatherapy: does it matter which lavender oil is used? *Nurs. Times*, **89**, 32–35.

Carson, C.F. and Riley, T.V. (1995) Antimicrobial activity of the major components of the essential oil of *Melaleuca alternifolia J. Appl. Bacteriol.*, **78**, 264–69.

Corner, J., Cawley, N. and Hildebrand, S. (1995) An evaluation of the use of massage and essential oils on the wellbeing of cancer patients. *Int. J. Palliat. Nurs.*, **1**, 67–73.

Gobel, H., Fresenius, J., Heinze, A. *et al.* (1996) Effectiveness of *Oleum menthae piperitae* and paracetamol in therapy of headache of the tension type. *Nervenarzt*, **67**, 672–81.

Holey, E. and Cook, E. (1997) Pathological Principles. In *Therapeutic Massage*. London: W. B. Saunders, pp. 63–64.

Hudson, R. (1996) The value of lavender for rest and activity in the elderly patient. *Complement. Ther. Med.*, **4**, *52–57*.

Komori, T., Fujiwara, R., Tanida, M. *et al.* (1995) Effects of citrus fragrance on the immune function and depressive states. *Neuroimmunomodulation*, **2**, 174–80.

Larrondo, J.V., Agut, M. and Calvo Torras, M.A. (1995) Antimicrobial activity of essences from labiates. *Microbios*, **82**, 171–72.

Lis-Balchin, M. (1995) Essential Oil Components. In *The Chemistry and Bioactivity of Essential Oils*. East Horsley: Amberwood, p. 26.

Stevenson, C. (1994) The psycho physiological effects of aromatherapy massage following cardiac surgery. *Complement. Ther. Med.*, **2**, 27–35.

Vickers, A. (1996) Research on Aromatherapy. In *Massage and Aromatherapy. A Guide for Health Professionals*. Cheltenham: Stanley Thornes, p. 167.

Williams, D. (1989) Lecture 1. In *Lecture Notes on Essential Oils*. London: Eve Taylor, p. 7.

Recommended reading

Battaglia, S. (1995) *The Complete Guide to Aromatherapy*. The Perfect Potion (Aust) Pty Ltd.

Holey, E. and Book, E. (1997) *Therapeutic Massage*. London: W. B. Saunders.

Hollis, M. (1998) *Massage for Therapists*, 2nd edn. Oxford: Blackwell Scientific.

Price, S. and Price, L. (1995) *Aromatherapy for Health Professionals*. Edinburgh: Churchill Livingstone.

Research Council for Complementary Medicine (1998) *Essential Oils*, 3rd edn, A Resource Pack.

Tisserand, R. and Balacs, T. (1995) *Essential Oil Safety, A Guide for Health Care Professionals*. Edinburgh: Churchill Livingstone.

Vickers, A. (1996) *Massage and Aromatherapy. A Guide for Health Professionals*. Cheltenham: Stanley Thornes.

Flower essences

Ann Childs

Rationale

Consider the paradigm of health not as a static absence of symptoms, an almost unachievable Utopia, but as a dynamic continuum of being able to respond to life's challenges with a positive attitude, thereby maintaining some measure of personal control and giving some inner understanding to the process of personal response and personal responsibility.

Flower essences act as catalysts, enabling us to respond, at a more unconscious level, the observable changes being acknowledged at a conscious level. Dr Edward Bach, the founder of the therapy of flower essences, recognized that patients with a positive outlook and a will to get well were able to fight illness and recover more quickly than those who had become fearful, depressed, resentful or given up hope. He progressively based his treatment on each individual's temperament rather than the disease alone (Howard, 1998).

Conceptual framework

Vibrational medicine incorporates substances, usually essences or tinctures, which contain high-frequency subtle energies, capable of therapeutically altering the delicate human energy field. Each flower essence has an individual pattern of frequencies (signature), imprinted on and stored in water, similar to homoeopathy. Flower essences directly address the emotions, personality and mental attitude of the person, without

necessarily taking into account the physical manifestations of disease. It is not *what* is happening to the person, but *how* they are responding to the given situation, illness, etc., which is of importance. The specific flower essence energy field resonating alongside the disturbed energy field of a person brings this about. The result is a harmonic pattern at a specific frequency. This harmonic pattern will resonate through the whole energy system, having a therapeutic effect at all levels, including the physical. After the person has finished taking the remedies, the positive changes tend to be maintained as a result of behavioural and attitudinal changes. However, other issues may become apparent, as health and life is an ongoing process.

Type remedies correspond to potentials/imbalances, which are part of the personality's character structure. **Helping remedies** assist the personality to re-harmonize acute but temporary states of mind which are not part of the overall character.

For a comparison of flower essences, allopathic, herbal and homoeopathic medicine, Kaminski and Katz (1996) provides an in-depth discussion. It becomes easier to say what flower essences *are not* rather than what they *are*! Bach suggests that the apparent negative aspects of the personality are caused by a separation of the person from their 'higher selves'. The remedies flood the system with the corresponding positive attributes, thereby 'washing away' the negative aspects, which are there primarily to give guidance to personal development. This enables transformation of behaviour, thought processes and attitudes, thereby meeting the challenges of life.

It is interesting to note Bach's philosophy of enhancing the underlying, if often obscured, inherent positive qualities of each individual personality.

Origins of Bach flower remedies

In the 1920s, Bach was a highly successful and eminent physician, London University lecturer and Chief Bacteriologist to the London Homoeopathic Hospital. He owned a large Harley Street consulting practice, his own research laboratories (providing training for many doctors worldwide), published discoveries in both general medicine and homoeopathy (many of which are still in use today), and continued non-paid work with low-income groups.

He was always searching for an ultimate, simple remedy, which would heal at the deepest level without causing harm to the person, nor requiring anything to be destroyed or altered in its production. To achieve this he gave up his medical practices in 1930 and devoted the last 6 years of his life to studying plants.

The discovery of the profound and powerful attributes of the living flower heads on the human psyche came about by Bach intentionally experiencing a specific negative emotional state. He would then intuitively seek out a flower in its natural habitat, which neutralized his symptoms, consequently achieving a corresponding positive state of mind.

Fifty years prior to current psychoneuroimmunological research, Bach had correctly intuited that different emotional and personality factors contribute towards a general predisposition to illness.

Production

The flower heads are carefully harvested in the early morning at the peak of their bloom. The entire surface of spring water, in a glass dish, is covered with the flower heads and left outside in sunlight. The sun's rays potentize the water with the 'living' energy of the flowers, thereby leaving an electromagnetic imprint on the water. A small amount of natural seepage also occurs. However, Bach was meticulous to use non-harmful plants. This 'primary' essence (often referred to as a 'mother' essence) is diluted down to a 'stock' essence, which is available commercially in most health stores. At both these levels the essences are preserved in brandy.

Application

Generally, 4 drops are taken from the purchased stock bottle and diluted in 30 ml of spring water and preserved by 5 ml of brandy to form the dosage bottle, lasting approximately 3 weeks. Alternatively, 2 drops from the stock bottle can be diluted in a glass of water and drunk throughout the day. For best effect, essences are taken orally, under similar conditions to other homoeopathic remedies. However, remedies may also be used in a cream base and applied externally to the skin, in compresses or added to bath water.

Owing to the low potency and absence of harmful side-effects, the essences are deemed safe to use with all persons including babies, during pregnancy, and in frail and debilitating conditions.

Remedy descriptions

Bach identified 38 different remedies pertaining to 38 specific states of mind which he maintained covered all our serendipitous emotions and soul qualities. These are listed in leaflets available with the remedies. Further information can be found in the References.

The 'Bach' essence **Rescue Remedy** is the most widely-used flower remedy for broad-based first aid involving shock or trauma at any level. It is actually a combination of 5 separate flower essences consisting of:

- *Star of Bethlehem* – to neutralize energy depletion after any form of trauma and shock at all levels.
- *Rock Rose* – to address the state of terror, panic and 'frozen with fear' feeling.
- *Clematis* – to help the sense of numbness, any tendency to faint, and bring someone into the here and now.

- *Impatiens* – eases irritability and excessive, impatient reactions. Brings inner peace, releasing body tension.
- *Cherry Plumb* – relates to the fear of losing control of both the mind and emotions and 'breaking down' in every sense. Helps to regain composure.

There are countless numbers of empirical cases where rescue remedy (RR) has quite literally rescued people and animals from severe shock by activating their own physiological support systems to function appropriately, thereby neutralizing the effects of shock and, on many occasions, relieving pain and a whole gamut of mental distress. The following are some of the examples taken from personal use of RR or direct observation:

- acute tenderness and sensitivity over wounds and surgical scars respond particularly well to external application of RR cream
- before and during childbirth, dentistry, exams and panic attacks
- a cynical farmer tried RR on his newborn lambs and discovered a significant increase in survival rates; he has continued to use it at lambing time
- wild animals and birds in distress.

Cram (1998) uses a broad conceptual framework of stress profiling (psychophysiological procedure to study the emotional reactivity of the body) by incorporating multi-site surface electromyographic (sEMG) recordings at the paraspinal sites of the Chakras (energy centres). From this study, empirical data suggests that the five-flower RR reduces stress by specifically working at the level of the throat (C4) and heart Chakra (T6). Cram interprets the metaphysical influences of RR as appearing to assist us in letting go of our attachments and desires, while promoting a sense of calmness.

Selection process

To quote Bach: 'Take no notice of the disease, think only of the outlook of the one in distress'. Bach intended the selection of essences for each individual to be a simple process, relying on

perception, observation and keen, sensitive, listening skills. Self-selection is convenient yet requires a degree of self-awareness and honesty. A therapist or counsellor would help to identify the issue using attentive listening. Having a deep knowledge of psychology is not required; however, the use of flower essences alongside psychotherapy is supportive, enhances insight and helps to move the process forward.

If the choice of remedy is unclear, communication difficult or time short, the specific essence for that moment in time may be identified by muscle testing. Diagnostic vibrational testing techniques result in a more perceptive and effective choice of essence when used within the context of a therapeutic relationship.

To clarify the rational underpinning the choice of remedy, several are highlighted in the following two case histories. Descriptions of essences are, by necessity, brief, but in reality are more complex.

Superficially, people may appear to present with similar symptoms, in similar circumstances, but on further questioning it is apparent that the feelings underneath are very different. Conversely, the symptoms may be totally different, yet the underlying feelings can be identical. Therefore, there is not a Bach Flower Remedy for grief because we all respond differently to grief. The following are two case histories of people in the early stages of bereavement. They presented with low motivation, tiredness, confusion of thought, lack of interest, poor concentration and headaches.

Case history 1: Cath

Cath was an immensely sensitive and maternal person. While on a family car outing her two teenage daughters died in a horrific traffic accident, Cath sustained a fractured wrist and musculoskeletal injuries and her husband sustained no major physical injuries. During the first few weeks, Cath used *Star of Bethlehem* for shock, *Rock Rose* for terror, panic and nightmares and *Sweet Chestnut* for extreme mental anguish and despair. Drops were taken whenever needed (almost hourly). After these initial few weeks Cath's mind would constantly return to the events of the accident, reliving every moment both day and night. Although part of the grieving process, this was causing great distress. *White Chestnut* helped to alleviate the continuous cycle of unwanted thoughts, allowing a better quality of sleep. Headaches also ceased. Several weeks later the prescription changed to *Pine* and *Willow*. The *Pine* works on the guilt and self-reproach (she felt guilty, even though she wasn't, again part of the natural grieving process) and *Willow* for her justified bitterness and resentment.

After several months, Cath mentioned how she experienced difficulty sitting or travelling in a car owing to the specific fear relating to her accident. Within a week of taking *Mimulus* and using emotional stress release this was no longer a problem. By this time Cath was unmotivated, spending most of her time absorbed in her memories and not able to focus or adjust to life. *Honeysuckle* helped her to let go of the past while still providing a living relationship to it. By increasing her awareness of the present she was enabled to look towards the future. At a later stage *Walnut* was helpful in the transitional stages from home to work, with *Larch* giving the self-confidence required.

Throughout this difficult time Cath was receiving physiotherapy for the orthopaedic problems sustained in the accident. This facilitated the introduction and maintenance of the Bach Remedies. Simultaneously, she was supported by friendship from her local community and family. During this most traumatic year, Cath did not require medication for sleep problems, mood control or anxiety. In the subsequent years she achieved readjustment levels beyond any thought possible under the tragic circumstances.

Case history 2: Richard

Richard is 70 years old and has initially coped well with the loss of his wife after her long illness, but is becoming tired, demotivated and has difficulty making decisions. His lack of interest, enthusiasm, motivation, tiredness and resignation to enduring a lonely future points towards *Wild Rose* remedy. Decision-making becomes a priority problem having lost the driving force and directive of his wife who made most of the major decisions. This compounds his tiredness. *Scleranthus* helps with decisiveness and clarity of life direction, resulting in a sense of inner balance. Within a month of taking the remedies, Richard had renewed energy, increased motivation and became more socially outgoing. This enabled him to learn new life skills, such as cooking and shopping, which helped gain his confidence in his own decision-making. Further interests ensued including painting, pottery and dancing.

Application to physiotherapy practice

The external application of drops of essences onto the skin, essences combined with a carrier cream, essences in water soaked in a compress or the commercially made all-purpose rescue remedy cream, provide ease of implementation for physiotherapists. For the treatment of recent tissue trauma, inflammatory joint conditions and soft tissue injuries, anecdotal evidence and the author's experience have observed a decrease in the inflammatory response, decreased local pain and improved function, in a matter of minutes. This amelioration of symptoms enhances further soft tissue mobilization. The improvement is further enhanced with self-application.

There is a legal difficulty in who can prescribe products that are to be consumed internally, but advice can be given and clients can purchase their own flower essences over the counter. Within a good communicating NHS network, some doctors will prescribe the remedies after consultation with the therapist.

Mimulus is an extremely useful remedy in health care and hospital settings. It relates to specific fears, e.g. fear of surgery, injections, pain, death, darkness or even hospitals. 'Mimulus' types tend to be hypersensitive to their surroundings and over-careful in convalescence, slowing down rehabilitation. Reluctance to move a joint for fear of pain can be helped by using this remedy added to massage cream.

Compatibility with other therapies

Bach flower essences are deemed to be totally safe and without side-effects. If an unsuitable remedy is chosen, there is no effect, i.e. there is no resonance with the disharmony. If the correct remedy is chosen, changes happen slowly, gently and appropriately. The essences are compatible with all other therapies and medication. Combined with counselling or any psychotherapeutic work, the flower essences enhance and consolidate the therapeutic process, especially when combined with individualized and appropriate affirmations. For example, for someone learning assertiveness skills and taking the essence *Centaury*, an appropriate affirmation would be 'I value my strength of will'. When involved with any treatment intervention involving people exhibiting severe mental health problems, communication at a multidisciplinary and medical level is of the utmost importance to achieve maximum benefit and to monitor changes. As with other homoeopathic remedies, strong medication and certain aromatherapy oils may neutralize the effectiveness of essences.

Other varieties of flower essences

Edward Bach was unequivocally the originator of flower essences and maintained that his 38 essences covered all essential soul qualities. Nora Weeks, his immediate confidante and successor, promised to ensure that Bach's work 'remained complete, unpretentious and straightforward'. Since that time a basic continuity and unbroken link has existed between the successive curators at the Bach flower centre, 'Mount Vernon', in Wallingford, Oxfordshire. Bach himself wrote, 1 month before his death: 'Attempted distortion is a far greater weapon than attempted destruction. . . . '

Currently there are many flower essence centres. Some specialize in the Bach essences, whereas others have developed their own individual essences in response to the changing social, spiritual, psychic, personal and ecological challenges of this time. The Flower Essence Society (FES) promotes and encourages an ongoing research programme of controlled clinical studies, detecting, analysing and interpreting the presence of subtle energy forces within the plant. Data is recorded from practitioners worldwide. At present over 70 FES remedies are available, while many others are in the process of testing.

One of the FES products is the North American *Yarrow Special Formula*, originally developed in response to the Chernobyl nuclear plant disaster in 1986. This essence is reported to strengthen the etheric body against radiation. It has been developed for uses related to video display units, terminals, radiation therapy, geopathic stress and other invasive electromagnetic fields.

Vita Fons II (formerly *Vita Flora*) is made from a combination of living wild flowers to produce one essence. It is described as improving the interface between the subtle energy systems, thereby improving the quality of energy absorbed through the Chakras. Its users make many medical claims. Although based upon a complex philosophy, having one product which helps everything eliminates the need for choice and may be locally applied by the external application of Vita Fons cream, oil or talc. For the therapist tentatively setting out to use flower essences, rather than choose different remedies for each specific condition, Rescue Remedy or Via Fons II would be applicable.

References

Cram, J. (1998) Flower essences and stress profiling: a matter of head and heart. *Research Web Site of Flower Essence Society* (http://www.flowersociety.org/Cram-FFF.html).

Howard, J. (1998) Bach Flower Remedies: a personal commentary on the work of Dr Edward Bach. *Complement. Ther. Nurs. Midwif.*, 4, 148–49.

Kaminski, P. and Katz, R. (1996) *Flower Essence Repertory*. Nevada City, CA: Flower Essence Society.

Recommended reading

Bach, E. (1931, reprint 1987) *Heal Thyself. An Explanation of the Real Cause and Cure of Disease.* Saffron Walden: C.W. Daniel.

Cunningham, D. (1992) *Flower Remedies Handbook*. New York: Sterling.

MacPherson, H. (1989) *Affirmations for the Bach Flower Remedies*. York: Chien Clinic, 13 St. Saviour's Place, YO1 2PJ.

Scheffer, M. (1990) *Bach Flower Therapy*. Wellingborough: Thorsons.

20 ElectroCrystal therapy

Trish Niblock and Kirsty Petre

Introduction

ElectroCrystal therapy was developed by Harry Oldfield in 1988. It is based on a system of pulsed high-frequency current and electro-magnetic induction. In essence, it consists of the application to the body of a tube filled with crystals in a saline solution through which is passed a pulsed high-frequency current which brings about healing changes in the body by normalizing tissue frequencies through induction and resonance.

Background

Initially, Oldfield was interested in Kirlian photography, developed by the Russian researcher Semyon Kirlian. Kirlian studied the electrical discharges emitted by living bodies as recorded by electrophotography. This is based upon observations of a phenomenon known as the 'corona discharge'. Electrically-grounded objects in high-frequency electrical fields characteristically demonstrate spark discharges between the object and the electrode generating field. The term 'corona discharge' arises from the observation of discharge patterns around circular objects, where the spark pattern along the edge of the object resembles the outer corona of the sun during an eclipse. This can be captured on photographic film.

Oldfield first came across Kirlian photography in a magazine article some time in 1976, which showed a Kirlian photograph of a leaf and described how to make the apparatus that took the photograph. At that time he was a science teacher and also ran a school science club. The making of Kirlian apparatus became a project for the club, which soon produced its own Kirlian photographs. Following on from this came another project inspired and funded by Colonel McCausland to examine Kirlian photographic differences between whole foods and processed foods. There were obvious differences between these foods, in that the corona patterns of the processed food were weaker and in some cases non-existent. These results were presented to a meeting of the Health Education Council and caused interested discussion. At the end of the meeting, Glen Rein, a young American biochemist working with cancer cells and tissues, suggested that Oldfield should start examining tissue samples with Kirlian photography. This was the beginning of a long and fruitful friendship. During the course of their work they showed that Kirlian photography was able to diagnose carcinogenic tissues in their early stages, in that the corona discharge pattern was far greater than that of normal cells, probably indicating that the energy of these cells is out of control.

Their wide range of experiments included Kirlian photographs of human subjects, including Rein himself. Occasionally, Rein's handprints would show little or no energy for no apparent reason until the connection was traced to his work with radioactive tracers which severely affected his energy levels. This was interesting and useful as a diagnostic tool, but

Oldfield began to wonder whether this knowledge could be used to treat conditions in situations where energy was out of balance. He worked with electromagnetic fields for some time, trying to find a technique for normalizing distorted energy fields. At about this time he was introduced to the concept of crystal healing – a technique that had been used in ancient times and in which interest was reviving – so he began to use crystals with his electromagnetic work.

In his early days of research into Kirlian photography, Oldfield noticed that an object energized in the Kirlian field gave off radio waves and an audible sound. He decided that there must be information in both sound and radio frequencies as well as light. In order to measure this information he lowered the voltage and increased the frequency so that he could send a three-dimensional signal over the whole body and scan the energy field in decibel levels both on the surface and away from the body. These signals can be picked up by a simple soundmeter, which has the advantage that it can be used with procedures which do not involve touching the patient. This lessens the possibility of artefacts which can arise with the Kirlian photographic method. This is the method, known as the Electro Scanning Method (ESM) which is generally used by practitioners.

A further development of Oldfield's diagnostic methods is Polycontrast Interface Photography or the PIP scan. The great advantage of this method is that it is in real time. Light waves impinging on the force field around the body create an interference pattern which can be picked up and recorded on video. When playing back this video through a computer with sophisticated software, this pattern can be interpreted and printed out in colour. In this way, current energy flows, distortions and energy configuration points can be seen and compared. These printouts can be kept as records and are more readily understood by patients than the readings of the ESM scan. PIP scans can be performed very quickly, thus having the great advantage of offering immediate proof of the results of a treatment, as they can be taken before and after treatment.

'Energy configuration points' is the name Oldfield gave to seven vortices which he noticed appeared regularly down the central line of the body. Subsequently he discovered to his surprise that these corresponded to the energy centres known universally as the Chakras (see Chapter 4). There are seven major Chakras, each of which spins at its own specific frequency, the slowest being the Base Chakra and the highest the Crown Chakra. Chakras are thought to draw in energy from the universal energy field which is then stepped down to the frequencies of the physical body which they affect through the nerve plexuses and the endocrine glands. Table 20.1 gives the relationships which are known to exist in Ayurvedic medicine. Some authorities use different associations of Chakras and organs, depending on whether they are using systems derived from the East or the West.

Oldfield has observed the Chakras and colours on the PIP system. He has found that green crystals are very effective in the solar plexus region and crystals with a yellow ray are very effective in the Heart Chakra zone, so that electrodes containing crystals of these rays may be used specifically on these Chakras. In practice, the electrodes most often used contain a mixture of crystals which have proved to be most generally effective. Oldfield theorizes that this seeming 'reversal' of 'classical' colours

Table 20.1 The Chakras and their relationships

Chakra	Nerve plexus	Endocrine	Colour
Base	Sacrococcygeal	Gonads	Red
Splenic	Sacral	Pancreas	Orange
Solar Plexus	Solar plexus	Adrenals	Green
Heart	Cardiac plexus	Thymus	Yellow
Throat	Cervical ganglia	Thyroid	Blue
Brow	Hypothalamus	Pituitary	Violet
Crown	Cerebral cortex	Pineal	White

could be due to the fact that modern man has to cope with a polluted environment and green (balance) is needed in the area of the solar plexus and its associated organs of cleansing and elimination. Each Chakra represents a band of frequencies, knowledge of which is essential in the use of ElectroCrystal therapy.

Crystals have played a crucial role in a variety of modern discoveries. For instance, the piezo-electric effect whereby mechanical distortion creates a surface electrical potential and the application of a potential difference creates mechanical distortion that can be used to pro-duce a spark. A ruby crystal, for example, was used in the first laser. Crystals can convert poten-tial difference frequencies into acoustic frequen-cies, as in ultrasound machines, and there are many other well-known uses of both natural and artificially produced crystals. Because the molecules which form a crystal are arranged in an identically ordered lattice array, it is in perfect energy balance. Therefore, energy going in to the crystal must be balanced by an equal amount of energy leaving the crystal. For example, in the piezoelectric effect mentioned above, mechanical energy applied as pressure causes the emission of an equal amount of light and electrical energy in the form of a spark. In ElectroCrystal therapy, this perfect energy balance is enhanced with pulsed high-frequency currents through crystals in order to affect vibrations of cells and organs in the body.

Each crystal vibrates at a known frequency according to its size and type. Knowing the fre-quency of particular crystals enables Electro-Crystal therapists to use appropriate crystals or crystal mix in order to stimulate, tranquillize or balance vibrational frequencies of organs and energy centres which have become disturbed. Oldfield states that most mineral specimens can be electrically activated, especially the quartz crystal lattice (Oldfield and Coghill, 1988). There is no doubt in Oldfield's mind that crys-tals, gemstones and many other minerals have intrinsic healing properties.

The characteristics of stones come in three main groups:

- stimulators, e.g. garnets, rubies
- balancers, e.g. emeralds, jade
- tranquillizers, e.g. amethyst, sapphire.

There is also a fourth group which Oldfield calls amplifiers. These are first and foremost quartz crystals which greatly increase the effectiveness of the healing aspects of minerals. The effects of these crystals themselves can be greatly increased by pulsed high-frequency electricity because of the harmonics they generate. This method Oldfield called ElectroCrystal therapy.

There is a clear relationship between the way ElectroCrystal therapy and homoeopathy have a balancing effect on the health of the individual. George Vithoulkas (1985) explained homoe-opathy in electromagnetic terms as follows:

Electromagnetic fields are characterized by the phenomenon of vibration. As electrons race around atomic nuclei, they first move in one direction then another, as viewed by an external observer. This oscillation back and forth occurs at a specific frequency which is determined by the type of subatomic particle and its level of energy. For our purposes however the significant point is that everything exists in a state of vibration, and every electromagnetic field is characterized by vibration rates (or frequencies) which can be measured. The human organism is no exception. To grossly oversimplify a highly complex situation, one can visualize an individual human being as existing at a particular vibrational frequency which may change dynamically every second depending on the mental state of the person, internal or external stresses, illness, etc. The electromagnetic field is very likely the 'vital force' that Hahnemann referred to.

Once a morbific stimulus has affected the electromagnetic field of a person, things may progress in two ways. If the person's constitutional state is strong and the harmful stimulus weak, the electromagnetic field changes vibration rate only slightly and only for a short time. The individual is not aware that anything has happened at all. But if the stimulus is powerful enough to overwhelm the vital force, the electromagnetic field undergoes a greater change in vibration rate, and effects are eventually felt by the individual. . . . The symptoms of a disease are nothing but reactions trying to rid the organism of harmful influences which are merely the material manifestations of earlier disturbances on a dynamic electromagnetic level. . . . As all substances possess characteristic electromagnetic fields the task of the homoeopath is to find that substance whose vibration rates most closely matches that of the patient during illness. . . .

When the vibration rates are matched, a phenomenon occurs which is very well known to physicists and engineers as resonance. This results in an increase of the patient's electromagnetic field at precisely the frequency needed to bring about a cure.

Theoretical basis of ElectroCrystal therapy

ElectroCrystal therapy works on the same principle as homoeopathy, in that disturbances in the electromagnetic level are corrected by applying a vibration frequency which resonates with that of the patient.

The electromagnetic spectrum covers a vast range of frequencies. Within this spectrum there are frequency bands that human organs are tuned into. Frequency windows that are most important for ElectroCrystal therapy are those of the energy centres of the body or Chakras which extend from 1 Hz to 45 kHz. They are covered by the pulse repetition rates, named A to D on the ElectroCrystal generator. Within these pulses are higher frequency components that contribute to the wave shape. The most effective healing response is obtained when the frequency or pulse repetition rate is matched to that of the Chakra or organ to be treated. As in homoeopathy, to achieve the maximum effect the 'remedy', i.e. the appropriate frequency, must be applied in the correct potency. In ElectroCrystal therapy potency means amplitude of signal rated 0 to 10 on the generator. Therefore, the treatment choice must include both frequency and amplitude of signal. (In the case notes shown below, where treatment is given as D10, for example, both the frequency and the amplitude of signal are high and the effect will be stimulating. Conversely A0 will be tranquillizing.)

Diagnosis and therapy

The ElectroCrystal generator was the first machine developed by Oldfield for the use of vibrational frequencies in the treatment of dis-ease, but he did not stop there. As both light and sound also form part of the healing spectrum, he has extended the range of treatment options by adding equipment to stimulate crystals through the use of pulsed light. This is known as the OptoCrystal Therapy Unit in which the crystal or crystals are stimulated by high-intensity, red-light-emitting diodes pulsed as in the ElectroCrystal generator. This unit can be more focused as the red light from the diode is passed through the crystal in a small applicator and therefore may succeed where the ElectroCrystal generator has failed. They are often used in conjunction, e.g. the Opto-Crystal therapy unit may be used on a high-frequency high-amplitude setting over the thymus to stimulate the immune system, while the ElectroCrystal generator is used on a tranquillizing setting to reduce an inflammatory condition elsewhere in the body. Equipment is also being developed to use sound directly as a healing medium.

The electroscanning method is a three-dimensional detection system and is used as follows: a glass electrode filled with crystals in saline solution is attached to the ElectroCrystal generator. The patient holds the electrode in his/her hand and stands upright in a relaxed manner. A soundmeter tests the reference field to discover magnitude and phase shifting which the generator sends into and around the patient. The field itself is pulsed from the generator into the electrode. A secondary field effect is set up in the subject by induction. The field can be tuned to a control spot on the subject by a frequency-tuning system.

To obtain a control reading an area is chosen on the body which is free from past or present injury, indicated by a '0' decibel reading on the meter. The field is tuned to the baseline reading for this patient. It is important to check the consistency of this reading by selecting another control area on the subject. Both areas should be of the same amplitude and in phase with one another. Readings on the seven major Chakras and on any areas of the body causing concern are then taken. Where the amplitude is close to and in phase with the control reading, this area is regarded as normal. Where there are noticeable changes, these may be due to some clinical abnormality. Changes may range from 1 to 2 db to 10 or more. For instance, a patient suffering from an inflammatory condition or a tumour gives a high reading over the affected area, and at the same time there could be a low reading over the thymus (immune system). These readings are recorded on a chart and treatment planned accordingly.

In taking this scan it is important that the patient remove all jewellery and metal objects and should not be standing near any metallic object. Since the scanner used is a soundmeter, the treatment room should be quiet. Adjustments are made for readings over clothes, hair or on skin, depending on whether the control areas chosen were clothed or on bare skin. Adjustments must also be made where areas under examination lie over postoperative pins or plates.

Treatment is given using either the Electro-Crystal generator or the OptoCrystal therapy unit, or a combination as required. Both these units are battery operated for safety and portability; the generator battery is rechargeable and supplied with a charger. Two controls alter the wave frequency and amplitude and there is a further control on the generator for fine tuning of amplitude as necessary. Electrodes consist of either glass or flexible plastic filled with crystals in a saline solution which are applied to the area to be treated and held in place using Velcro straps. It has been found that in most cases best results are achieved by treating both the affected area and the relevant Chakra, according to the scan readings.

Example of a scan reading and treatment

The patient presented with symptoms of chronic intestinal problems. She had had bowel surgery and her gall bladder had also been removed. She now suffered from a rectal prolapse, fluid retention and lower back pain. Scan tuned in at C6 80 on control points (both ear lobes, which had not been pierced), and the major

Chakras were then scanned to determine their levels of energy.

The readings showed as follows:

Crown	−3
Brow	−1
Throat	−4 (extremely low – holding back on expression of feelings? Thyroid tests clinically normal – low basal temperature)
Heart	−2
Solar Plexus	−1
Splenic	−2
Base (front)	−3
Base (back)	−2

This patient showed depression of function in all her major Chakra areas and complained of feeling run down with severe tiredness and lethargy. Treatment consisted of stimulating frequencies beginning with the Chakras with the worst distortion, i.e. Crown, Throat, Splenic and Base Chakras. This patient was assessed and treated during a training session and it was not possible to follow her progress, but treatment would be expected to have continued over at least 8 sessions.

Case histories

Case histories 1 and 2 were kindly provided by Pauline Tyndale-Biscoe, Registered Homoeopath, Allergist and ElectroCrystal therapist, while case history 3 was from one of the authors (T.N.).

Case history 1

Five years ago Pauline's husband fell 32 feet (10 m) and broke the talus bone in his right ankle. He made a good recovery but was warned of the likelihood of necrosis in the affected ankle. Recently he started feeling pains in his right ankle from time to time. These became more frequent and intense. As the ankle benefited from exercise, Pauline thought it might need some energy put into it. The reading of −1 and −2 at the back of the affected ankle confirmed her theory. Before treatment, the right ankle was particularly painful. Four sites at the back of the ankle were treated with a ruby diode on D10 for 10 minutes each with the OptoCrystal therapy unit. Immediately after treatment her husband could walk without pain. There was no recurrence of the pain up to the time of writing (1 month following the treatment).

Case history 2

Alan aged 13 was a top swimmer. He fell, damaging his left shoulder, which caused much pain at any motion, even writing. An X-ray showed that the top of the scapula was jagged. He was told he would have to stop all sport and take painkillers to enable him to do his school work. The shoulder read −5. It was treated with D10 for 10 minutes on the Opto-Crystal therapy unit with a ruby diode, which increased the pain. This was followed with an amethyst rod on the clinical unit for an hour, which eased the pain. Over the next 3 weeks Alan was treated every 3 days with a combination of D9 and A10, D8 and A9, D10 and A8 and D10 and A9. Slowly, the time needed with the amethyst was reduced to 20 minutes. Then the treatments were spaced out gradually, until once a week was enough. Two months after the treatment there was no pain. The patient returned for another X-ray which showed that the bone was completely healed. Alan returned to competitive swimming and went on to win many titles.

Case history 3

Barbara was a very active housewife and mother, secretary and keen organic gardener. After redecorating her home by herself she began to suffer from bilateral carpal tunnel syndrome. Her hands were puffy and painful. She found she could do very little without acute pain. The orthopaedic consultant advised surgery to both wrists at once. Her scan showed that her Throat Chakra was at a high, +4, and her wrists were off the scale at +10. Treatment was C0 to the Throat Chakra and A10 to both arms. Her wrists received an alternating treatment of C0 and A10. On the next day her wrists read +6, but the Throat Chakra was still

high at +4. On the third day her Throat Chakra read +3 and her wrists remained at +6, but felt much better. She then felt able to go away on holiday. When she was seen later on in the year her readings were Throat Chakra +2 and her wrists were +3. She reported back to the surgeon that she would not be having any surgery, and has not suffered from any recurrences.

Research notes (from Dr Muriel Mackay, Homoeopath, Naturopath and Reflexologist)

Knowing how very important it is for the health of the whole body that the colon, in particular the ileocaecal valve, functions well, I have been doing some research into using ElectroCrystal therapy on this site. If the valve is not working properly, digestive and many other problems are caused. I find that by using A3 on site to relax and reduce spasm of the ileocaecal valve, alternating with D10 to stimulate its function, many improvements in health are achieved. (More detailed notes on this research have been sent to Harry Oldfield.)

(Contribution to *ElectroCrystal Therapy Newsletter*, December 1992)

Conclusion

ElectroCrystal therapy is an useful adjunct to physiotherapy treatment. It provides a simple mechanical method of assessing and balancing a patient's subtle energy field. It is therefore a practical step in the metamorphosis of a traditional physical therapy into a more holistic and truly complementary therapy. It can be applied during the course of other treatments. Once the measurements have been taken and the energy needs assessed, the electrodes can be applied and left *in situ* while other treatments such as massage, mobilization of joints are used, or when hot or cold packs are being deployed.

References

Oldfield, H. and Coghill, R. (1988) *The Dark Side of the Brain*. Shaftesbury: Element Books.

Vithoulkas, G. (1985) *Homeopathy – Medicine of the New Man*. Wellingborough: Thorsons.

Recommended reading

Bonewitz, R. (1983) *Cosmic Crystals*. London: Aquarian Press.

Collins, J. (1991) *Life Forces*. London: New English Library.

Gerber, R. (1996) *Vibrational Medicine*, 2nd edn. Santa Fe, CA: Bear.

Simpson, L. (1997) *The Book of Crystal Healing*. London: Gaia Books.

Solomon, J. and Solomon, G. (1998) *Harry Oldfield's Invisible Universe*. London: Thorsons.

21 Using the sensory environment as therapy

Ann M. Davies

Introduction

For everyone their eyes, ears, nose, mouth and skin are their points of sensory contact with the world. The sensory input changes and each neurological system perceives the change in the surroundings and this leads to a corresponding alteration physically and emotionally. Everyone is personally aware how they are changed in the physical and mental state by their surroundings and how sensory stimulation affects their well-being and balance. It alters them physically, as well as their mood and mental balance. Most people find it very hard to completely relax in a bright red room with red light, Shostakovich playing loudly and Rosemary oil burning! Conversely it is difficult to remain completely alert in a soothing blue room, Enya music gently playing and Lavender oil burning.

How can physiotherapists use the sensory environment to balance their clients and help them to heal themselves and to achieve their maximum potential? How can surroundings be altered to achieve this? How can the sensory input of colour, light, sound, smell, spatial awareness and texture be altered? How will this affect the human body and mind? These are the questions that will be answered in this chapter.

Sensory environments can be used as a sensory environment for an individual or group, with only general aims in mind, e.g. stimulation or relaxation. Alternatively, they may be designed for an individual or group to achieve specific changes and the changes monitored, e.g. reduction in muscle tone or reduction in blood pressure. The environment may be chosen personally by the client, but sometimes for specific results the environment would be chosen by the therapist. The therapy may be task orientated, enabling, or used as directed therapy.

History of sensory stimulation for healing

Sensory input has been used to heal since ancient times. The Egyptians had healing temples of light and sound, such as at Thebes and Karnak, where the colours were produced by passing sunlight through crystals. Almost all religions use the combination of colour, sound and smell to alter the physical/mental/spiritual state of the people participating.

The Christian church has traditionally used different symbolic colours for ceremonial clothing and this is combined with specific energy frequencies of sound in church music and specific smells using incense to produce the exact sensory input required for any particular ceremony. Each ceremony produces a different effect on the participants. Light was also used for healing in bygone times in some churches, and people receiving the healing were laid in specific recesses so that the sunlight passing through the stained glass windows fell on them, producing the colours required.

Man has always used sensory input to change himself, whether it be in the home, clothes, religion or healing. This is not a new science but a very ancient one. Although science recognizes the effects of cosmic, gamma, X-rays, ultraviolet, microwaves, shortwaves, infrared and longwaves on human physical bodies, there still exists controversy over whether the visible portion of the spectrum also affects bodies physically. The non-visible portions of the spectrum frequently have deleterious effects on health. Is it not possible that the rainbow of visible light that has nourished all life since the beginnings of time is here to enhance health as well as life?

Electrotherapy uses microwaves, shortwaves, longwaves, ultrasound, ultraviolet and infrared. Doctors use X-rays and gamma rays to both diagnose and treat, but, for some strange reason, light and sound wave frequencies are rarely used. The visible light spectrum runs from 400 to 700 nm, which is through the colours of the rainbow from violet to red. Sound waves cover the audible frequency between 20 Hz and about 15 kHz (babies to 20 kHz).

Research is now being undertaken, mostly in the USA, which is addressing this lack of knowledge of the effects of visible light on the human body.

Snoezlen as therapeutic environments

The word 'Snoezlen' is a contraction of two Dutch words equivalent to 'sniffing and dozing'. The word suggests a relaxing atmosphere. Developed in 1975 by Ad Verheul at the Hartenburg Centre in the Netherlands, to help improve the quality of life for people with learning disabilities, the concept has been extended and used in elderly care, paediatrics, pain control and obstetrics.

Snoezlen consists of pleasurable sensory experiences generated in an atmosphere of trust and relaxation. The sensory experiences stimulate the primary senses without the need for intellectual activity. The senses stimulated can include sight, hearing, touch, smell and taste.

Sensory rooms are usually set aside and kept for this particular purpose. However, the principles can be adapted to any particular room/ area and can even be extended to a small area of a larger room or department, although this would of necessity consist of simpler and easily dismantled and transported equipment. Small areas can also be set up at home.

The Snoezlen room

Typically a purpose-built Snoezlen room set aside for this particular use only, and therefore permanent, will be constructed as follows. It would be a completely white room, with the windows covered to enhance concentration and to cut out external stimuli. Frequently the room will use plastic-covered padded white foam mattresses throughout, which increases the comfort and insulation of the unit. These also make it easier to clean. The room needs some kind of ventilation and heating system to maintain a steady comfortable temperature. If physically disabled clients are to use the room, some kind of hoisting system needs to be built into the original plans.

Within the blank unit is installed equipment that can be operated by the therapist or the client. Special on–off switches are available that are easy to operate and stimulating in colour, shape and texture. There are numerous pieces of apparatus that can be installed, ranging from simple home-made equipment to expensive purchased items, depending on the permanence of the unit and the amount of money available. Such equipment should include a source of music and tapes covering a wide spectrum of music from stimulating to relaxing; a method of burning oils (not an open-lit candle oil burner which can be dangerous) and a collection of selected oils; a range of objects for their tactile and textural differences; and a method of altering light and colour. Included may be coloured light bulbs, rotating mirror balls, projectors to produce changing colours and images, and pulsating (not flashing) lights that will not induce epileptic fits. Anyone photosensitive should not be subjected to changing light, but constant light should be used. Focal points of light might include fibreoptics, bubble tubes, spotlights and light tubes. Tactile experiences might include different textures and shapes where clients can explore them, and also vibrations through massage mattresses or vibrating tubes.

A wide range of pillows, cushions and foam shapes should be available.

All the above can be centred in one room or spread out into different rooms and areas, each area having a specific purpose, e.g. Relaxing Room. Sound Room, Touch Corridor, Adventure Room. Sometimes hydrotherapy pools can be included in the overall plan. If the equipment is all in one room it is essential that an objective is agreed for the session and only the appropriate pieces of apparatus are used. Not every item of equipment in the room should be switched on at the same time. It should be decided whether the session is to be stimulating or relaxing, and if the client will be passive or expected to participate.

As well as white rooms which reflect light and where the colour in the room can be changed, black rooms can be used. These are rooms draped in black curtains, again a blank canvas upon which the sensory environment can be altered. These rooms are particularly good for sound rhythms and visual tracking. They are also excellent for deep relaxation and concentration. If only one room is available, the basic white room can have black curtains which can be put away; therefore, one room serves as white or black.

The sensory environment

Most people have some abilities with most senses – even those who are deaf or blind quite often have the ability to feel vibrations, can tell the difference between light and dark colours, feel different shapes and textures, and perceive sounds and rhythms, although they may not always be able to communicate what they are perceiving.

Again, before the session commences, a particular objective needs to be set and if there is a group with conflicting needs it may only be possible to have a very general treatment which could be classified relaxing or stimulating. For specific treatments the session will probably need to be one to one and individually planned:

- For *sight* stimulation, use bubble tubes and fibreoptics, alter the colour of the light, rotate the light colours, alter the shapes and angles, use pictures on the wall that do not require understanding. For some treatments, basic colour changes are enough. For specific results, a single overall colour should be used.
- For *hearing* stimulation, apart from relaxing or stimulating, the music pitch, tone and rhythm should be varied in a simple way, with a variety of sounds and silence. Musical instruments and sound beams can also be used for active participation.
- The *smell* chosen for a session should fit into the overall aims of the session.
- *Taste* is very difficult to fit into a multi-sensory session and is usually a specialist activity undertaken on its own.
- *Movement* is encouraged if there are powerful stimulators, e.g. lights that can be switched on/off, different textures to explore or a sound beam utilized.

With even a small amount of equipment in a small area of a large department/room the therapist can achieve significant results. The rationale behind some of the above treatments is explained further, with particular emphasis on how it can be used in physiotherapy sessions.

Visual stimulation – light and colour therapy

All organisms, whether plant, animal or man, respond to light. Visible light has wavelengths of 400–700 nm and although humans are affected by radiation of many other wavelengths, they are unable to see it. Humans evolved under the light of the sun which reaches earth with its greatest strength in wavelengths 400–700 nm, the visible portion of the electromagnetic spectrum. These are the colours of the rainbow, with violet at 400 nm being the shortest ray, through to red, the longest at 700 nm. Through sensing these vibrationary rates, blind people can be trained to 'see' colours. Helen Keller describes this in her book, *The World I Live In* (Keller, 1933). These colours also produce specific visual sensations – red burns, orange warms, green is neutral, blue and violet are cool. Everyday expressions indicate most people's feelings about colour: 'in the pink', 'feeling blue', 'seeing red', 'under a black cloud', 'golden moments', 'silver lining'.

The eye has two separate functions. Light via the optic nerve to the occipital cortex enables humans to see. Light via a special layer of cells in the retina sends neural impulses to the hypothalamus. The hypothalamus is composed of two major zones. One zone controls the sympathetic nervous system and stimulates hormone production, while the other zone controls the parasympathetic nervous system and inhibits hormone production. As the body's major collecting centre for information concerning its well-being, the hypothalamus receives all external information picked up by sense organs and all internal signals from the autonomic nervous system as well as from the psyche. Its major functions include control of the autonomic nervous system, energy balance, fluid balance, heat regulation, sleep, circulation, breathing, growth, maturation, reproduction and emotional balance.

The pineal gland was thought to have no scientific purpose until recently, but mystics have always considered it to be very important and the 'seat of the soul', the third eye. The size of a pea, it has been discovered that its functions are vast. It acts as the body's light-meter, receiving light information (via the eyes and hypothalamus) and sending out hormonal messages that have a profound effect on the mind and body. Its activity, regulated by environmental light changes and the earth's electromagnetic field, is to transmit information to the body concerning the length of daylight. The pineal gland is highly active in human beings when young and is responsible for preventing the premature onset of puberty and development of sexual functions. Its light information synchronizes the body's functions relating to the external environment. The gland releases a powerful hormone, melatonin, in response to the body's biological clock, in turn controlled by light messages to the hypthalamus. Melatonin levels can change in response to very small amounts of light. Melatonin is found everywhere in the body and affects all the bodily functions. It is at its highest in the middle of the night and lowest during the day. Low levels of melatonin induce wakeful activity; high levels produce relaxation, inactivity and sleep.

How do specific wavelengths of visible light affect the human body?

From an extensive review of the research literature undertaken by Liberman on the physiological and psychological effects that light, both as a whole spectrum and across different frequencies, can have, a few examples have been taken to illustrate the therapeutic effectiveness of light (see references in Liberman, 1991).

Many enzymes and hormones are coloured and very sensitive to light. They frequently undergo molecular changes when stimulated by different colours that alter their original colours. These light-induced changes affect the power of these enzymes and hormones to cause dynamic reactions within the body. Martinek and Berezin (1979) found that some colours can stimulate certain bodily enzymes to be 500% more effective, and some colours can increase the rate of enzymic reactions, activate or deactivate certain enzymes and affect the movement of substances across cell membranes.

The use of colour as a therapeutic tool to treat hyperbilirubinaemia has now widespread acceptance, e.g. full spectrum visible light or blue light to break up bilirubin in the skin and tissues of neonatal babies. The relationship was originally noticed in the 1950s and was clinically confirmed by Lucey (1972). McDonald (1982) demonstrated that the same blue light was effective in reducing pain in people with arthritis. More recently, Anderson (1990) showed that red light is effective in the treatment of migraine headaches.

Alexander Schauss (1979) in Tacoma, Washington, has reported that aggressive, hostile and anxiety-ridden behaviour can be suppressed in minutes by exposure to a specific shade of pink. The sedating and muscle-relaxing effects of pink are now being tried for geriatric, adolescent and family therapy, prison reform and business. Even those suffering from colour blindness can be tranquillized by pink rooms. Schauss (1985) researched specially painted Baker Miller Pink holding cells in jails. A reduction of muscle strength happened in inmates in 2.7 seconds. Baker Miller Pink (bubble gum pink) therefore exerts a physical rather than psychological effect and it has been proved to calm nerves within muscles.

Legwold (1988), in a study at Texas University, found that the viewing of red light increased strength 13.5% in viewers and also elicited 5.8% more electrical activity in the arm muscles of viewers compared with other light conditions. This study also indicated that briefly looking at a red light ray may assist athletic performances requiring quick bursts of energy output.

Gerard (1958) studied the differential effects on psychophysiological functions of veiwing coloured lights. Gerard's results showed that red light increased blood pressure, increased respiratory movements, eyeblink frequency, and increased tension and excitement. Blue/white light decreased blood pressure, respiratory movements, eyeblink frequency, lessened anxiety and increased relaxation. Heart rate showed no difference under red or blue light.

Ertel (1978) discovered that the use of bright warm colours such as yellow and orange improved IQ and academic achievement of school-age children. Wohlfarth (1984a,b and 1985) substituted warm shades of light yellow and light blue wall paint in schools and there were lower disciplinary incidences, IQ was raised, there was less stress, children were quieter and there was less illness if full spectrum lighting was also added (Wohlfarth and Schutz, 1983).

Theo Gimbel at Hygeia Studios, has found that asthma, tension and insomnia are helped by the blue spectrum, and lethargy and lack of vitality by red, orange and yellow spectrums (Gimbel, 1980).

As can be deduced from all the above information, human beings react to visible light physically and mentally. All this modern research (and old, accepted knowledge) concerning light and colour has applications in physiotherapy treatments. The actual use of colour and light in specific treatments will be discussed later in this chapter.

Sound in therapy

Sounds and music can be used to convey emotions and feelings, but conversely it can be used to alter the emotional and physical states. As quoted by Martin (1997), Dr Francis Brannaf of Wilkes University in Pennsylvannia has shown that pleasant music increased levels of immunoglobulin A (IgA), thus boosting the immune system, and 'annoying sounds' decreased levels, thus making people more susceptible to all sorts of viral infections. There are a number of ways of using sound in the physiotherapy setting of learning disabilities:

1. As a background to set the scene mentally and physically. For relaxation gentle music (there are many excellent relaxing music tapes on the market) or if strong stimulation is required rousing music, with lots of changes and harsher sounds, should be used.

   Some animal and nature sounds are soothing, e.g. whales and dolphins, also gentle waves on the shore, whereas other natural sounds can be stimulating, e.g. storms, thunder, tigers.

   As well as soothing background music to induce relaxation, the music and general atmosphere can be used by the physiotherapist to reduce agitation and challenging behaviour, to decrease muscle spasm and to enable easier movement to take place.

   Gentle music can be used to accompany Taichi-type exercises where the movement is combined with breathing exercises and the movements flow gently one into the next. Adults with learning disabilities respond readily to Taichi-type exercises combined with relaxing flowing music.

2. Involvement in producing the music using various instruments including sound waves. Vibration and percussion instruments are particularly good and the client is encouraged to feel the different vibrations. Sound waves, where the movement of hands, arms, legs or feet in the wave will produce different notes depending on the movement, can be combined with the physiotherapy programme. Physiotherapy involvement in a music session can combine movements desirable from a therapeutic viewpoint with the production of the sound and music of the group.

3. Physioacoustic therapy is the use of low-frequency sound for the treatment of musculoskeletal, neurological and psychological disorders. It increases vascular circulation,

relaxes muscles and reduces pain. It has a wide application in stress-related symptoms, e.g. neuromuscular pains, headache, migraine, hypertension, insomnia, spasticity, brain injuries, strokes and also athletic injuries.

The usual method of application is a reclining chair housing a computer and six audio speakers. The computer creates and controls low-frequency sinusoidal sound waves which are broadcast through the speakers. Clients feel the sound as sympathetic resonance within muscles and other soft tissues (Lehihoinen, 1990).

The low-frequency sinusoidal sound is usually combined with specially selected music. The frequency range varies from 27 Hz to 113 Hz. Thus low-frequency sound comes from a specially designed computer. Any sound source (e.g. tape or CD) can be used to produce the musical effect.

Three sound parameters are important in the physioacoustic method (a) pulsation (b) scanning (c) direction.

- *Pulsation.* The low-frequency sound is varying in a certain, controlled time, sequence. The purpose of power pulsation is to prevent muscle contraction. Continuous stimulation commonly causes numbness and contraction. With the sound pulsating slowly, this effect can be avoided and relaxation obtained instead.
- *Scanning.* The computer causes the frequency to vary with a certain amplitude and speed. This is necessary to guarantee that each muscle is treated at its optimal frequency, i.e. the pitch at which the particular muscle responds naturally.
- *Direction.* Sound can be made to move from the lower parts of the body upwards or in the reverse direction. The ability to change direction appears to be beneficial in the treatment of certain stress-related symptoms such as psychosomatic pains and muscle tensions. Pulsation, scanning and direction together provide enormous possibilities in designing programmes to meet individual therapeutic needs. It is possible to make a change in programme, even in the middle of a session, when it

seems therapeutically appropriate. A typical treatment lasts 15–30 minutes. No special client preparation is required. The physioacoustic therapy is effective through clothes, casts and corrective braces. No significant adverse effects have been found, although some clients may experience nausea or vertigo during the first treatments. However, clients with confirmed or suspected cardiac problems, pregnant women and clients taking psychoactive medications should get approval from their doctors.

4. Using musical sounds to reinforce the movements required (see treatment section for further details).

Therapy using smell

As with colour and sound, people experience certain smells as pleasant, unpleasant, relaxing, stimulating, etc. Not everyone reacts to the same smell in the same way. Smells are stored and evoke reflex responses, depending on previous experience.

The therapist chooses a particular colour, sound, aroma, etc., because its vibration corresponds to something needed by the person seeking help. The easiest way to control the smell of an environment in a therapy or Snoezlen area is by using essential oils. Essential oils are obtained from plants, and plants were central to medicine and spiritual practices as far back as evidence is available. Previously, medicine and religion were linked (even in early Christianity), but today in most societies medicine and religion have become separated. However, the use of plants is still practised in religions, e.g. incense and anointing oils. The contents of the incense and anointing oils are very specific for a specific purpose in a specific ceremony.

The techniques and uses of aromatherapy are discussed in Chapter 18. Smell may be administered using massage via aromatherapy or it may be achieved through an oil burner. An essential oil diffuser is a small piece of electrical apparatus which uses an electric pump to propel minuscule droplets of essential oil into the air. They do not heat the oil, therefore there is no distortion of the aroma, and they can perfume a large space very quickly. There is some noise associated with them, however. The ceramic burners using a night-light candle are not suitable on health and safety grounds; instead an electric burner or ring burner for a light bulb should be used.

Physiotherapists should obviously know the medical background of any clients they are treating. Advice from a qualified aromatherapist must be sought, especially in certain fields, e.g. learning disabilities where a large percentage of clients have epilepsy, and certain oils that may precipitate an epileptic attack should not be used. These include Rosemary, Fennel, Hyssop, Camphor and Sage.

Very small amounts of oil must always be used. They should be very good oils that have not been adulterated, so that they are very pure. Below are a few of the combination of aromas that have been found useful with particular colours, sounds and specific physical and mental properties. Again it cannot be stated too often – all essential oils have physical and mental properties and some have side-effects and contraindications. Some are actually toxic. It is imperative that only oils suitable for a group or individual are used, taking into account their physical and mental history. Professional help must be sought.

Calming relaxing aromas

These would be used in combination with relaxing music and green, pink and blue rooms.

- **Lavender.** Excellent for relaxing, with no side-effects. Good for muscular aches and pains and arthritis.
- **Chamomile.** Again, no side-effects, good for relaxing, aches and pains after sport and for arthritis and rheumatism.
- **Orange.** Calmative, good for nervous tension and stress. Not suitable for babies.
- **Jasmine.** Ultrarelaxing but very expensive. Not to be used for babies or children.
- **Geranium.** Good for nervous tension, stress-related conditions, especially menopausal problems, and PMT. It is sedative and uplifting. Not to be used for babies.

- **Rose.** Again, extremely expensive but good for depression, insomnia, nervous tension and stress. Not to be used for young children.

Stimulating aromas

These would be used in conjunction with red, orange and yellow colours and stimulating music. Care needs to be taken, as a number of stimulating essential oils have contraindications. Stimulation with these oils should not take place in the evening as the client will not sleep.

- **Rosemary.** An excellent oil, stimulating and a tonic. Stimulating on mental and physical levels. Good for tiredness, migraine, muscular aches. *Caution:* Not to be used with babies and children, pregnant women, epileptics or clients with high blood pressure.
- **Peppermint.** Used for mental stimulation, and is refreshing and cooling. Not to be used with young children and babies.
- **Juniper.** Is both stimulating and relaxing and was used to purify air in hospitals. It is antiseptic and astringent, generally non-toxic, but can be slightly irritating. It must not be used in pregnancy (an abortifacient) or in kidney disease due to its nephrotoxic effect. Also not to be used for babies or children.
- **Lemongrass.** Toning and refreshing. Good for lack of interest, boredom and overwork. Not to be used with babies and children.
- **Eucalyptus.** Is a stimulant and is used for head clearing. Good for exhaustion and inability to concentrate. Not to be used for babies.
- **Cypress.** Tonic and astringent, good for sluggishness. Not for babies and young children.

The choice is personal and everyone will have their own favourites. If there are any oils the therapist does not personally like, they should be avoided, as they will be working in the environment. Some oils are never used because of toxicity, these include: Basil, Camphor, Clove,

Fennel, Hyssop, Marjoram, Sage, Thyme. Other oils are photosensitive and should be used with great care, e.g. Bergamot. Again, knowledge of the essential oils is critical when making choices for treatment.

Stimulation of other senses

The majority of sensory rooms use colour, sound, and smell, some also have tactile stimulation built into them, while taste is usually ignored. For some physiotherapy clients with learning disabilities, stimulation of the other senses can be an extremely useful adjunct to therapy. Sometimes the therapist may not want relaxation to be the aim, but stimulation and heightened involvement in the environment to encourage increased physical activity and awareness.

Tactile stimulation can be created by the use of different materials in the room, such as hangings, cushions, balls, mobiles or boards with different textures glued onto them (e.g. silk, carpet, wool, foam). Interspersed may be bell-pulls, chimes, rattles, etc., to encourage further exploration, again made up of different materials size and texture.

Vibration is a very useful tool and vibrating tubes, pads, mattresses and chairs are available commercially. Vibration can be used as a form of relaxation and massage, as in the mattress or chair, or it can be used as stimulation to encourage client participation. Vibration can also be used to focus the client so that therapy can take place; for example, many clients with poor concentration enjoy the vibrations of the massage mattress, and to feel and keep in contact with the sensation will quite happily lie prone or supine in one place for a period of time – something that they would not normally do. While the client is enjoying the mattress, the therapist can carry out his/her programme.

Use of taste stimulation is difficult to control in a sensory room and taste sessions are better when taken place separately with no other sensory input, where concentration is easier and where clients can be encouraged to physically reach out to take the taste and place it in the mouth. This activity usually takes place sitting at a table rather than in a sensory room. Fruit can be used for sweet, sour, different textures and exotic new flavours. Dips are useful and can include curry, chilli, spices, herbs, cheeses, etc. All that is needed is imagination by the therapist. Obviously when using food the client's medical background and feeding abilities need to be known.

Case histories

The examples of physiotherapy treatments using sensory stimulations, given below, are for clients with learning disabilities, although the principles would apply to many other areas of physiotherapy. From the previous information given, physiotherapists in many specialities could adapt the information for their particular field, e.g. neurology, obstectrics, palliative care, elderly care, mental health.

Case history 1

Mr A. Forty years old, challenging behaviour, severe learning disabilities, epilepsy, labile mood swings, recent cardiovascular accident resulting in hypertonic spasms.

Twenty minutes before the exercise session began the sensory room was used to relax, calm and stabilize the client. The colour of the room was pink and green, the oils used were Lavender and Chamomile. Music was played at low volume and consisted of a relaxation tape or soothing natural sounds of dolphins, waves or birds. As well as relaxation, the session reduced muscle tone (this was also encouraged by acupressure and Shiatsu massage of the limbs).

For the physiotherapy session, more visual stimulation was introduced including a projector to produce images on the walls, a bubble tube and the music slightly louder and more stimulating. This encouraged concentration and participation while still encouraging relaxation.

Case history 2

Mr B. Twenty-four years old, challenging behaviour, dyspraxia, generally hypotonic but with some hamstring contraction. Half an hour before physiotherapy, a session in the sensory room with either the psychologist or the physiotherapist took place.This was to produce relaxation. The client was allowed to talk at the beginning of the session, then encouraged to gradually become quiet and relaxed. Relaxing music, colours and smells were used. The client enjoyed visual stimulation of bubble tubes and fibreoptics, so these were allowed in moderation.

Mr B greatiy enjoyed music and chose the music for the exercise session, although the therapist encouraged him to choose music not too loud or too stimulating. Again he chose the colours and images; red was discouraged, although the client enjoyed that colour, because it was too stimulating and caused agitation. If the client insisted on loud music and red, then they were used, but a shorter than normal session was followed by a further session of relaxation. The exercise programme was undertaken using Taichi-type exercises which encourage flowing movements. The exercises were performed to the music.

Case history 3

Mr C. Severe learning disabilities, cerebral palsy. Recently became withdrawn, requires stimulation and encouragement to participate in his exercise programme.

The music was fairly loud using animal noises and rock music (which the client loves), and the smells used were stimulating. Colours were bright, alternating on the wall and directed onto a revolving mirror ball. Fibreoptics and bubble tubes were used with hand-operated on–off switches which the client was encouraged to control with his right hand. Tactile stimulation was used, as well as a vibrating tube. All the above stimulations were incorporated into his general exercise programme.

Case history 4

Mr D. Young male with cerebral palsy and learning disabilities, becoming more detached, sleeping long periods, harder to stimulate and arouse.

The following regime using sound was devised by the physiotherapist and occupational therapist and taped so that the carers could carry out the exercise programme daily. The physiotherapy exercise programme was reduced to five simple main movements. Each movement was analysed and a sound that represented and sounded like each movement was chosen.

The tape consisted of: (a) a jingle written especially for the client to wake and arouse him – after a while he became alert and waiting each time he heard 'his jingle'; (b) five musical sounds, with one exercise carried out by the client and his carer to each sound. Each sound was repeated 4 times.

1. One of the carer's hands on each of the client's wrist to assist movement. Arms out to side then into middle to accordion music – accordion out, arms out, accordion in, arms in.
2. Arms out to front then lower – accordion sounds.
3. Feet up and down to drum beats.
4. Knees bent in midline, gently rocking side to side using 'shushing' sound from brushes on drum.
5. Bend and straighten legs alternately. Chords up and down on electric organ, holding for a few seconds on top chord with legs bent.

After a few sessions the client not only anticipated the exercises, but carried on the exercises unprompted to the correct sounds.

Energy systems and environmental influence

How does the information given in this chapter relate to the Chakra and energy theories explained elsewhere in this book? The information given and experimental rationale have mostly related to the physical and mental solid-state processes and how thcy have been changed and measured. This is a Newtonian model, where the body is envisaged as a machine controlled by the brain and peripheral nervous system.

It is possible to look at this chapter's information in a completely different way. Just consider everything as energy. Einstein stated in his equation $E = mc^2$ that all living systems are energy. Living matter and human beings are networks of complex energy fields. Although the majority of biological researchers are still working from a Newtonian model of living systems, some researchers are now working on the Einsteinian concept of matter as energy, based upon the understanding that the molecular arrangement of the physical body is a complex network of energy fields.

How can the physical and mental changes occurring by altering the environment and senses be explained by the Einsteinian model? In the Einsteinian model, colour, light, sound and smells, etc., are all energies. Any energy system (the client) placed in these energy fields would react to them and subtle changes would occur in the client's energy system. These subtle changes introduced into the client's energy system could be used to balance, heal, alter mental states and produce physical changes within the body. Whether working in the Newtonian or the Einsteinian models, it is clear that the environment (light, colour, sound, smell, etc.) has a profound effect on each person's mental state and physical body. This has implications not only for physiotherapy treatments for clients, but in the surroundings that people are treated in, and the surroundings in everyday life.

Although this idea may appear very modern and these ideas are only just being introduced into mainstream medicine, the knowledge has been known and used for thousands of years.

References

Anderson, J. (1990) The effect of colour on the severity of migraine symptoms. *Brain/Mind Bulletin*, 15(4), 1.

Ertel (1978) *Kinder Farbstudien*. Munchen: Gesellschaft fur Rationale Psychologie.

Gerard, H. (1958) Differential effects of coloured lights on psychophysiological functions PhD Diss. University of California at Los Angeles.

Gimbel, T. (1980) *Healing Through Colour*. Saffron Walden: C.W. Daniel.

Keller, H. (1933) *The World I Live In*, 3rd edn. London: Methuen.

Legwold, G. (1988) Colour boosted energy – how lights affect muscle action. *American Health*, May, 10–12.

Lehihoinen, P. (1990) *Low Frequency Sound in Vibrational Medicine* (brochure). Norwich: Kirton Healthcare.

Liberman, J. (1991) *Light Medicine of the Future*. Santa Fe, NM: Bear.

Lucey, R. (1972) Neo-natal Jaundice and Phototherapy. *Pediatric Clinics of North America*, 19(4), 1–7.

Martin, P. (1997) Light relief. *Sunday Times Magazine*, 27 August, 34–42.

Martinek, G. and Berezin, L. (1979) Artificial light sensitive enzymatic systems as chemical amplifiers of weak light signals. *Photochemistry and Photobiology*, 29 March, 637–50.

McDonald, S.F. (1982) Effect of visible lightwaves on arthritis pain: a controlled study. *International Journal of Biosocial Research*, 3(2), 18–20.

Schauss, A.G. (1979) Tranquilizing effect of colour reduces aggressive behaviour and potential violence. *Journal of Orthomolecular Psychiatry*, 8(4), 218–21.

Schauss, A.G. (1985) The physiological effect of colour on the suppression of human aggression, research on Baker-Miller Pink. *International Journal of Biosocial Research*, 7(2), 55–64.

Wohlfarth, H. and Schultz, A. (1983) The effect of colour psychodynamic environment modification on sound levels in elementary schools. *The International Journal of Biosocial Research*, 5, 12–19.

Wohlfarth, H. (1984a) The effects of colour psychodynamic environmental modification on disciplinary incidences in elementary schools over one school year. A controlled study. *The International Journal of Biosocial Research*, 6(1), 44–53.

Wohlfarth, H. (1984b) The effects of colour psychodynamic environmental modification on absences due to illness in elementary schools. A controlled study. *The International Journal of Biosocial Research*, 6(1), 54–61.

Wohlfarth, H. (1985) The effects of colour psychodynamic environmental colour and lighting modification of elementary schools on blood pressure and mood. A controlled study. *The International Journal of Biosocial Research*, 7(1), 9–16.

Recommended reading

Allanach, J. (1997) *Colour Me Healing*. Shaftesbury: Element.

Ashby, M., Lindsay, W.R., Pitcaithly, D., Broxholme, S. and Geeken, N. (1995) Snoezlen – its effects on concentration and responsiveness in people with profound multiple handicaps. *Br. J. Occup. Ther.*, 58(7), 303–307.

Becker, R. (1991) *Cross Currents*. London: Bloomsbury.

Davis, P. (1991) *Subtle Aromatherapy*. Saffron Walden: C.W. Daniel.

Gerber, R. (1986) *Vibrational Medicine*, 2nd edn. Santa Fe, NM: Bear.

Haggar, L.E. and Hutchinson, R.B. (1991) Snoezlen – an approach to the provision of a leisure resource for people with profound and multiple handicaps. *Mental Handicap*, **19**, 51–55.

Kirton Litework (1995) Brochure. Norwich: Kirton Healthcare Group.

Lawless, J. (1992) *Encyclopaedia of Essential Oils*. Shaftesbury: Element Books.

Long, A.P. and Haig, L. (1992) How do clients benefit from Snoezlen? An exploratory study. *Br. J. Occup. Ther.*, **55**(3), 103–106.

McKenzie, C. (1995) Brightening the lives of elderly residents through Snoezlen. *Elderly Care*, **7**(5), 11–13.

Price, S. (1986) *Practical Aromatherapy*. Wellingborough: Thorsons.

Schofield, P. (1996) Sensory delights. *Nurs. Times*, **92**(5), 40–41.

Tisserand, R. (1988) *The Art of Aromatherapy*. Saffron Walden: C.W. Daniel.

Westwood, C. (1991) *Aromatherapy. A Guide for Home Use*. Christchurch: Kerbina Ltd.

White, J. (1997) Creating a Snoezlen effect in PICU. *Paed. Nurs.*, **97**(5), 20–21.

In the beginning and at the end

Part V

22 Complementary therapies for mother and baby

Fiona Mantle

Introduction

The emergence of complementary therapies during the last 20 years has been documented by Doyle (1993), noting specifically the increased use of homoeopathy, osteopathy, acupuncture, medical herbalism and aromatherapy. The Consumers Association, in a research paper published by the National Association of Health Authority Trusts (NAHAT, 1993), noted that one in four of its readers visited an alternative/complementary practitioner and that complementary therapies provide a significant second system in addition to conventional medicine (Fulder, 1996).

Fulder states that patients using complementary therapies come from all social classes (and not, as is popularly thought, from the wealthier middle classes), although there is some suggestion that economic grades A and B predominate. Sharma (1992) concludes from her survey of complementary therapy practitioners that the public are not fully aware of the range of conditions the various therapies can treat. Since the 1980s there has been an increasing integration of complementary therapies within mainstream health services, although, according to the NAHAT report, funding of complementary therapies is not generally considered a high priority in a system of finite resources. However, the British Medical Association report (BMA, 1993) went some way to acknowledge the benefits to patients and clients of complementary therapies and, more recently, HRH The Prince of Wales has given support to the report

Integrated Healthcare: A Way Forward for the Next Five Years? published by the Foundation for Integrated Medicine (1997).

Complementary therapies and modern midwifery (including the input from obstetric physiotherapists) sit comfortably together, since they share a philosophy of client empowerment, client choice and a holistic, non-interventionist approach. These tenets are enshrined in a report by the Department of Health (1993).

This chapter, which concentrates on the beginnings of life, will look at complementary therapies which obstetric physiotherapists can easily incorporate into their practice, both in the NHS and privately, and which will address common problems during labour and the first 3 months of the puerperium. Some of the therapies require specialist training, whereas others are available over the counter, and the use of these will depend on the physiotherapist's professional accountability.

Bach Flower Remedies

Physiotherapists who are interested in complementary therapies will no doubt have noticed the small dark bottles containing Bach Flower Remedies (BFR) in their local high street chemist or health food shop. BFR, along with homoeopathy, belong to the vitalist group of complementary therapies and were discovered and developed by Dr Edward Bach during the 1920s and 1930s. Bach's background was as a physician, homoeopath and pathologist who qualified as a doctor at University College Hospital in 1912. Bach was a disciple of Hahnemann and he was impressed by the gentle therapeutic approach of homoeopathy and its concentration on the patient, not the disease. From his own clinical observations Bach had come to a similar conclusion that it was just as important to address the patient's personality and presenting mood as it was to treat their physical condition. In spite of the value of homoeopathy, Bach had reservations about some of the substances which were used in its repertory of remedies and he wanted to develop a system of healing which was based solely on natural substances. The system Bach developed is highly flexible and the prescription is tailored to the individual and adjusted to their changing situation. This makes the system particularly valuable in childbirth, in which conditions are constantly changing and the mother's emotions are very near to the surface. Each flower essence is preserved in brandy and is taken as a few drops in a glass of water.

Premature labour

The onset of premature labour, which is defined as labour starting before 37 weeks' gestation, can be a profound shock to the parents, particularly if they have had a similar experience before. If the labour is very early there will be feelings of overwhelming fear and panic and the best flower remedy is Rescue Remedy. This is the most obvious choice since it is a composite remedy comprising of the five main remedies for this type of extreme situation. For the rising panic *Rock Rose* is indicated. Many people go into a state of denial when faced with impending tragedy, so *Rock Rose*, together with *Clematis*, will help to focus the mother into cooperating with the health professional in trying to save the baby, plus *Cherry Plum* to counter the fear of losing control. The remedy also contains *Star of Bethlehem* for the shock and *Impatiens* to help control the physical and mental tension and calm an agitated and irritable mind. Additional remedies which might be prescribed at this time might include *Red Chestnut* for the mother's fears for the baby and *Sweet Chestnut* for overwhelming despair, particularly if this has happened before. The remedy *Pine* is indicated

for the irrational feelings of guilt that some mothers have that somehow they have failed the baby, while *Crab Apple* will deal with the anger and disgust that she may feel that her body has let her down. While the baby is in the special care baby unit the mother and partner will benefit from *Red Chestnut* again, with *White Chestnut* for the worrying thoughts which will not go away.

Normal labour

During normal labour, BFR Rescue Remedy is the remedy of choice. Judy Howard of the Bach Centre in Brightwell recommends it in her book as almost the sole remedy (Howard, 1992) and having had twins herself has no reason to change her mind! For long and exhausting labour, *Olive* is indicated as well as *Walnut* for the transition stage.

Postnatal

In previous generations, the transition from working woman to full-time motherhood was a more protracted event. Most women gave up work on marrying and stayed at home, becoming acclimatized to a more housebound existence before having her first baby. Nowadays, the same transition can take only a few weeks and the consequential shock to the physical and emotional systems can be enormous. Rescue Remedy can be a great standby during labour, so it can be used to great effect immediately after birth, with the addition of *Walnut* which, with its properties of aiding transition, also helps to protect the mother from the influence of outside pressure and enable her to make up her own mind about her care and the care of her baby.

Unfortunately labour does not always go according to plan and some unanticipated medical intervention might be necessary. *Gentian* is indicated for the despondency which can occur if there is failure to progress as quickly as the mother might like and, if the labour does result in a caesarean section, *Pine* for the feelings of guilt which can often occur and leave the mother feeling angry and resentful in spite of having a lovely healthy baby. The new baby will also benefit from the remedies such as RR and *Walnut* at birth to aid transition from the womb to the outside world. *Impatiens* is for the irritable agitated baby, *Vervain* for the frustrated feeder, and *Clematis* for the sleepy, dreamy baby. As mother and baby get to know each other they will experience a range of emotions and the BFR can be a very useful catalyst to aid this process.

After childbirth, many mothers suffer from severe loss of confidence since babies have the habit of undermining the most organized mother and reducing her to tears of frustration, for which *Larch* and *Vervain* are indicated, along with *Elm* for the overwhelming responsibility that a new baby brings, much of which centres around feeding and sleeping. There is nothing worse than seeing other mothers apparently coping well, and *Holly* will help to regain a more balanced outlook.

Physiotherapists who are in contact with mother during the postnatal period will be alert to the signs of postnatal depression and often BFR can be used at the outset. *Gentian* has already been mentioned in relation to setbacks, but *Mustard* would be appropriate for the type of depression which descends without warning, as well as *Gorse* for feelings of helplessness.

Where paediatric physiotherapists will certainly be involved is if the baby is born handicapped. The parents will go through a bereavement in much the same way as for a stillborn baby or neonatal death, and *Star of Bethlehem* is the remedy for shock and bereavement. In addition, the parents who have been happily fantasizing about their baby for 9 months have to re-evaluate themselves and their own self-image. *Red Chestnut* is indicated for the concern for the baby's health and *Honeysuckle* to help them detach themselves from the baby they were expecting and to move on. For some parents the birth of an imperfect baby may be seen as a personal failure and they may feel guilty that something that they did may have caused this to happen, so *Pine* is indicated and, as some families will hide their sorrow behind a brave face, *Agrimony* will be the choice.

BFR are remedies which physiotherapists can incorporate into their care very easily. Training is offered at the Bach Centre in Oxfordshire, but Dr Bach himself declared that the remedies should be available to everyone whether medically trained or not so, technically, no training is required.

Aromatherapy and massage

Touch and massage have always been part of a physiotherapist's role and much of this section will be familiar. Massage, of course, is not one discrete therapy but one that can take many forms, ranging from soothing movements to the deep massage techniques used in Rolfing. Tiran (1996) suggests that in labour there is nothing intrinsically difficult about intuitive massage and that simple stroking will suffice in the absence of any knowledge of specific techniques.

Research into the effects of massage have unfortunately suffered from poor design and methodology, although a few randomized controlled trials have been conducted. However, Fulder (1997) suggests that the value of massage lies in its subjective effects. The studies cited are not directly related to maternity care, but demonstrate the physiological and psychological effects of massage in a variety of clinical situations. For example, Field *et al.* (1992), researching into the effects of massage on paediatric and adolescent psychiatric patients, assigned 72 subjects to either a group who watched a relaxing video, or a group who received massage. Sleep behaviour, activity rating and pulse rates were all measured. The results showed improvements in mood scores and a reduction in anxiety scores in the massage group compared with the video group. Overall, the massage group showed a greater improvement in sleep behaviour compared with the video group. Stevensen (1994) looked at three groups of post-cardiac patients who were either massaged with carrier oil, or essential oils, or had a short talk with the researcher. Results indicated that the psychological results in the massage groups, both with and without the essential oil, were each clinically and statistically significant compared with the 'talk' group.

A quick and effective way to reduce a person's anxiety by using massage might include massaging just one area of the body. Thomas (1989) demonstrated how a foot massage reduced the anxiety in a group of elderly patients, and this would seem a useful technique to teach partners to use during labour (particularly since many women in labour suffer from cold feet), as well as doing a back massage.

It is not only mothers who can benefit from massage therapy – premature babies have been shown to respond very well to touch. Porter (1996) has reviewed the history of neonatal care from the more 'hands-off' approach of the 1960s, when care centred around feeding and temperature control, through the minimal handling era to the more holistic present. Harlow's famous experiments with rhesus monkeys indicated that touch was as important as nutrients in normal development in infants, and this has been further demonstrated in infants. This has been further discussed by Russell (1993). Tactile/kinesthetic stimulation was given to pre-term babies weighing less than 1500 gm for 15 min, which included passive limb movements and gentle stroking. The results showed a significant increase in weight gain in the treatment group (Field *et al.*, 1986). In another study it was noted that babies who were suffering from the most complications gained most from the intervention (Scarfidi *et al.*, 1993).

Massaging babies is an integral part of mothering in many countries. In the UK it is becoming more popular and has developed into a formalized form of touch which mothers use already when anointing their baby's dry skin after a bath. The benefits of baby massage have been listed by McClure (1989) and include communication, improved sleep patterns, reduced anxiety and stress, promoting growth and development, and improved circulation and toned muscles. However, the concept of massage on babies and, subsequently, small children needs a few words of caution. Not all mothers feel that they can give the extra emotional input that this type of therapy involves, particularly those mothers who are emotionally deprived themselves, and professionals need to be aware of this, especially if the mother is suffering from postnatal depression. In addition, the issue of who does the massage will need to be addressed as the child gets older, as well as teaching the child who is allowed to touch them.

Aromatherapy refers to the therapeutic use of specially-prepared essential or aromatic oils. The oils can be found in different part of plants, including the flowers, leaves, seeds, wood, roots and bark. Chemists have found that essential oils interact with our bodies in three ways: pharmacologically, through chemical changes when oils enter the bloodstream and react with hormones and enzymes; physiologically, by producing an effect on the body such as sedation or stimulation; and psychologically, when the aroma of an oil is inhaled and we react to the smell.

Archaeologists have found evidence that, as far back as 3000 BC, people of the Indus valley knew how to distil oils and that other ancient civilizations were aware of their value. During the Middle Ages, oils were used to reduce the incidence of infection and it was noted that perfumers did not get the plague. In the 1950s, Dr Jean Valnet began using essential oils in his medical practice and their use is now part of mainstream medicine in France. Aromatherapy with massage or inhalation can be used for a wide range of conditions including skin conditions, infections, and as muscle relaxants, as well as a treatment for anxiety and depression.

The addition of aromatherapy oils to massage oil has been shown to enhance the therapeutic effect. Wilkinson (1995) used the essential oil *Roman Chamomile* in a massage and produced a greater reduction in anxiety levels than massage alone. One of the problems in the use of aromatherapy oils is the lack of consensus among aromatherapist regarding the therapeutic properties, dispensation and toxicity of essential oils. A look at a number of standard works shows a marked discrepancy in suggested use and safety in pregnancy. One example will illustrate this point. The oil *Bergamot* is suggested by Davis (1996) to be valuable in treating cystitis and depression, whereas Price (1993) fails to mention it in relation to either condition. Ryman (1989) states that it is good for infections, but does not mention it in relation to depression. More worryingly, Price (1991) does not indicate that *Peppermint* should not be used in pregnancy, whereas Tiran (1995) does. Tiran, who is a leading midwife/complementary therapy practitioner, lists a number of oils which should not be used in pregnancy. To ease the pain of labour, Tiran suggests the use of *Clary Sage*, *Jasmine*, *Lavender* and *Mandarin*. Of all these oils, perhaps the most useful is *Lavender*. It is a very safe oil and it has a wide range of application both during and after labour.

For physiotherapists who are not trained as aromatherapists, *Lavender*, *Chamomile* (which, unfortunately, is very expensive) and *Neroli* are three essential oils which they can use with confidence. *Lavender* has analgesic, antiseptic, antibacterial, antiviral and sedative properties, and it aids wound healing, although research undertaken by two midwives on healing of the perineum did not show a statistically significant difference in wound healing, but found that there was a marked reduction in perineal discomfort (Dale and Cornwell, 1994). *Neroli* is antidepressant and is excellent for relieving nervousness, tension and anxiety. The relaxing and sedative effects of *Lavender* and *Neroli* have recently been demonstrated by Buchbauer *et al.* (1991) and Jager *et al.* (1992).

Tiran (1996) describes the uses of essential oils in the treatment of specific conditions in maternity care. For labour she suggests a number of essential oils which can be used in various combinations, after taking into account the client's presenting symptoms and personal preferences which can change during the course of labour. She suggests that, for pain in labour, continuing with sacral massage is particularly soothing, and the use of essential oils of *Lavender* to promote contractions, *Clary Sage* for pain, and *Chamomile* for relaxation between contractions is beneficial. In addition, *Ylang Ylang* is particularly useful if the mother is getting stressed and emotional. The use of *Lavender* in perineal care has already been mentioned, but it is its antibacterial properties which are so valuable during the healing process and for healing bruises.

Many mothers lose their appetite after delivery (a problem encountered very frequently in health visiting), and poor maternal nutrition can prove a real obstacle in the establishment of breast feeding. In this instance, *Bergamot* is particularly good and is recommended by Davis (1996), who suggests that it is an appetite normalizer and is to be particularly recommended for its antidepressant qualities, as it is being regarded as 'uplifting'. For cracked or sore nipples, Stapleton (1995) recommends the application of a drop of *Geranium* oil added to 1 teaspoon of *Calendula* cream. Along with decreased appetite, constipation can be a problem during puerperium due to reduced appetite and the pain of perineal trauma, but can be aided by a gentle clockwise abdominal massage and the use of essential oils of *Orange nutmeg*, *Grapefruit*, and *Chamomile* (Tiran, 1996), while Davis (1996) suggests *Black Pepper* and *Fennel* (postnatal only).

To increase lactation, essential oils of *Lemon Grass* and *Jasmine* (also good for postnatal 'blues'), *Fennel* and *Dill* can be tried. It is important that the breasts are wiped clean before the baby is put to the breast.

The use of essential oils in the baby's massage oil can increase the tranquillizing effect of the massage to induce relaxation and sleep. Two oils which are useful and particularly safe for babies are *Chamomile* (known as the children's oil because of its gentleness and lack of toxicity) and *Lavender*. Davis cautions that the oils should never be added undiluted to the bath water, but mixed in a carrier oil first. One drop of *Lavender* oil can be put on a baby's sheet or sleep suit at night to help sleep from a few days old. Similarly, the addition of *Chamomile* to carrier oil, and massaged in a clockwise direction for 5 minutes, can do much to relieve colic.

Homoeopathy

Homoeopathy is a system of medicine based on the principle that 'like cures like'. Although Hahnemann is normally credited with the development of homoeopathy as a discipline, it was in fact Hippocrates, and later Paracelsus, who first developed the idea that an agent that can cause a disease might also be used to treat it, using the concept of '*similia similibus cretur*' – like cures like. However, it was Hahnemann who found that the more dilute the drug, the stronger the effect, and therefore he recommended that the remedies should be administered in the smallest possible doses – the concept of the 'minimum dose'. Germane to the development of a remedy is not only the dilution but also the succussion of the agent between dilutions. Remedies are made out of whole plants, minerals, salts and, in a variety of homoeopathy called isopathy, the offending agent. Homoeopathic remedies come in a variety of forms: tinctures, pilutes, granules or powders. The choice of remedy is dependent on a range of diagnostic criteria which includes: personality type, personal preferences, which covers such aspects as reactions to the weather, or time of day, and types of food enjoyed. Administration of the remedy is very flexible in terms of frequency and dosage and depends on the patient's individual situation. Of great relevance to homoeopathy is the concept of 'vital force' which is integral to the maintenance of bodily health. Homoeopathy has a long tradition of research in the empirical mode but has, more recently, been able to demonstrate its efficacy using randomized controlled trials.

The traditional form of defining homoeopathic efficacy has been the 'provings', which is the mechanism by which Hanneman identified the remedies. The word 'proving' comes from the German *'prufung'* meaning 'test', now known as the homoeopathic pathogenic trial (HPT). HPT involves the administration of the remedy under trial to a number of healthy individuals and noting their subsequent reactions. The remedy is then added to the homoeopathic repertory. The purpose of the proving of a homoeopathic remedy is to seek the character of a remedy and to test its qualities (Wieland, 1998). Each proving goes through a number of stages. Following the taking of a case history, the stages include:

- probability, confirmation that the same symptoms are experienced by more than one subject
- corroboration, where physiological effects are noted when the drug is taken in its raw state
- verification, when the substance is tried out on subjects
- characteristics – after lengthy verification it becomes characteristic for the remedy.

The validity of these provings has been critically assessed by Fisher (1998), who highlights issues around observer bias, lack of placebo control and no 'blinding' of the remedy. Elements of a minimum standard for provings has now been devised. In addition, because homoeopathy is such an individualized treatment, with success depending upon the accurate matching of remedy and patient, it makes more general research particularly difficult.

Dantas and Fisher (1998) undertook a review of homoeopathic provings published between 1945 and 1995, subjecting them to a critical examination of the reported effects, methodological rigor and reliability design outcomes, assessment and interpretation. The data collected was then submitted to a panel of practitioners for comment. Methodological quality was poor overall, clinical applications were not outstanding and details of volunteer selection were poor. In addition, it was concluded that it may not be appropriate to try out homoeopathic remedies on healthy volunteers. Research by Walach (1992) indicates that the more rigorous the methodology, the less symptoms were reported. The concept of provings has been fundamental to the concept of homoeopathy since its beginnings, but for other practitioners it is less applicable. All practitioners base their prescribing methods on their own clinical judgement.

There are a number of reviews of clinical trials of homoeopathy and two of these have been examined by Vincent and Furnham (1997). The main one, by Kleijnen *et al.* (1991), covered 107 controlled trials relating to a wide range of conditions. The standard of research design was often found to be poor, specifically citing low subject numbers of fewer than 25 subjects in the trial. However, overall, the results were positive in favour of the homoeopathic effect.

During labour, homoeopathic remedies can be administered very easily and do not affect any other medication which might need to be given. For a mother who is very anxious and fearful and with a tendency to panic, *Aconite* is the remedy of choice, and for the mother who is restless and anxious, with a fear of death which becomes worse during the night, *Arsenicum Album* is indicated. The remedy *Aconite* is derived from the herb *Aconitum napellus*, which is a deadly poison with a history of being used to poison arrow tips, hence the name from the Latin *'acon'* for dart. An excellent prophylactic for physical trauma and bruising is *Arnica*. This should be given as soon as labour starts to reduce bruising, and should continue to be taken postnatally. *Arnica* (which is also good for shock and fear) is derived from the herb *Arnica montana*, which was recommended by St Hildegard of Bingen

(1099–1179) as a valuable treatment for muscular aches and bruises and was commonly used among country people.

Hypericum is specific for the type of pain which results from a high number of nerve endings being cut and the consequent severe pain. It is derived from the herb *Hypericum perforatum* (St. John's wort), which has a long history of use in wound healing. Gerard, the sixteenth century herbalist, stated that 'it (hypericum) is a most precious remedy for deep wounds'. It follows that this remedy is particularly good for the pain of episiotomy. During labour, Lockie (1990) recommends *Coffea* for moderate or severe back pain, but with no signs of dilatation. *Coffea*, as the name suggests, is derived from the coffee bean and is a key remedy for insomnia. During labour it can be given in response to severe sensitivity to pain, since its main ingredient is caffeine, which has a long history of use as a stimulant and painkiller. If labour is prolonged due to malpresentation and the mother becoming very tired, chilly and distressed, *Pulsatilla* should be used. Sometimes referred to as a 'women's remedy', *Pulsatilla* does have a wider remit, but in labour is valuable for weepy, depressed mothers who need comfort and sympathy.

Homoeopathy is effective for a range of conditions during the postnatal period. Perineal discomfort will respond to *Arnica*, whereas difficulty in micturition might require *Aconite*. The loss of appetite which has been addressed under aromatherapy is subdivided into specific problems in homoeopathy. Lockie (1990) suggests the following variations in symptoms need to be taken into consideration. A craving for salt or fatty foods indicates *Natrum mur.*, a craving for sweets or sugary foods indicates *Lycopodium* and, for indigestion after fatty foods, *Pulsatilla*. For constipation, with resulting strain in trying to pass a stool, try *Nux*. For hard brown stools, *Bryonia*, and for mothers who are not only constipated but complain of feeling exhausted and irritable, *Sepia*. *Sepia* is also the remedy of choice for postnatal depression which presents itself as feelings of tiredness, irritability, loss of interest and feelings of indifference, particularly to loved ones: the mother who feels that she is unable to cope, is very weepy but resents help. *Sepia* is

itself a very interesting remedy. It is a potentized form of the 'ink' of the cuttlefish (*Sepia officinalis*) and the key to the remedy's effects lies in the behaviour of the cuttlefish itself, with its powers to change its hue with great speed into a variety of colours. This reflects the sudden mood changes for which *Sepia* is used as a remedy. The way the cuttlefish shoots away and hides reflects the depression of the *Sepia* subject who just wants to get away from it all.

Problems with breast feeding respond well to homoeopathic treatment, which has the added advantage of not coming through in the breast milk. If nursing is painful with a scanty milk supply and the mother is feeling low and weepy, *Pulsatilla* is the remedy of choice. If the nipples are too painful to nurse, making the mother irritable and intolerant of the pain, *Chamomilla* is indicated. This remedy is potentized from the camomile herb, which has a long history of medicinal use, being used for skin conditions, insomnia and as a gentle sedative.

Newborn babies often need the gentle care offered by homoeopathic medicine. On arrival, the baby may have some bruising of the scalp as a result of forceps delivery for which *Calendula* and *Arnica* are appropriate. Gemmell (1997) suggests giving the two remedies together. For soft tissue swelling which persists for more than a couple of days, *Calcarea Carbonica* or *Silica* is effective. For wind and colic, *Chamomilla* will help, particularly if the baby is better after passing a small amount of wind. For the more classic 'three months colic', *Pulsatilla* is advised, which is also useful later when the baby starts to teethe.

One question which is frequently asked, and an obstetric or paediatric physiotherapist may well be asked their opinion, is the often thorny problem of immunization. The Faculty of Homoeopathy is clear on this, in that they recommend orthodox immunization. Swayne (1998) states that the effectiveness of homoeopathic immunization is doubtful. Research by English (1987, 1992) on whooping cough was inconclusive, although Swayne suggests that homoeopathic treatment of the condition, should it arise, is a more satisfactory approach. The homoeopathic remedy *Apis* is of value if given at the time of immunization because of its action on burning, stinging pain when the skin is swollen and tender to touch. The remedy is potentized from the whole of the honey bee (including its sting!); however, it is recommended that this remedy is not given below 30c potency during pregnancy (c = centesimal and is a dilution of 1 part in 99 parts of water, so that 30c means that this process of dilution has been performed 30 times).

Hypnotherapy

Hypnotherapy is not a therapy in its own right, but a method of delivering a therapy more effectively. Hypnosis is usually described as a state of deep physical relaxation, with an alert mind producing slow alpha waves, and it is in this state that critical faculties are suspended and the subconscious mind accessed. The same state of altered consciousness is also found in meditation, relaxation and daydreaming. There is some debate as to whether there is in fact a separate distinguishable state of hypnosis, since no physiological differences have been identified. This has been clearly summarized by Heap (1996), who defines hypnosis as a two-way interaction between the subject and the hypnotist and is a complex psychological phenomenon. Hypnosis is therefore a condition which occurs quite naturally and everybody has at some time or other been hypnotized and indeed has hypnotized someone else – think of the way you daydream during unit meetings! Hypnotherapy is therefore the use of this daydreaming state for therapeutic purposes. Direct hypnosis is a very easy technique to learn and hypnosis is safe when used within the practitioner's professional scope of practice.

The value of hypnosis begins in the antenatal period, where it is of great value in the treatment of stress and anxiety by the use of post-hypnotic suggestions and guided imagery (Mantle, 1999). A conditioned response can be induced using hypnosis. Stein (1963) devised the clenched hand technique. This involves the subject identifying positive feelings of calm and relaxation, confidence and control and to experience them as strongly as possible, and to clench the fist of their preferred hand and to associate these feelings with this clenched fist. The procedure is then repeated using the non-preferred hand

and negative feelings. By clenching the appropriate fist, the client can then either 'throw away' the negative feelings or 'activate' the positive ones when confronted with a stressful situation. Other problems which respond well to hypnosis are what are referred to as the minor discomforts of pregnancy, which include constipation (Hartland, 1982), nausea and vomiting (Fuchs *et al.*, 1980), and insomnia (Goldman, 1990). Treatment of these conditions would involve the previously discussed conditioned response. Of these, perhaps the treatment of insomnia, by instigating the ability to switch off in response to a stimulus, is the most valuable in the postnatal period when 'snatched' sleep is at a premium.

During the antenatal period, mothers undergo a range of investigations. Kohen (1980) describes the use of relaxation, distraction and disassociation in the treatment of women undergoing gynaecological examinations. Hypnosis really comes into its own in the treatment of previous bad obstetric experiences which may result in considerable mental and physical trauma. Some of the trauma is the result of a previous stillbirth or insensitive handling during labour or unanticipated medical intervention of the type already discussed under Bach Flower Remedies. Hypnosis is a valuable tool in enabling the client to lay aside the previous bad experiences and separate her feelings about it from the present pregnancy and help her to experience the present pregnancy as a separate, uncontaminated episode. This can be achieved by reviewing the previous events as a mental video, in which the client can rewind and rerun the 'tape' as often as necessary until she feels she is able to turn it off for ever. Posthypnotic suggestion would include suggestions that the experiences are 'in the past' and are 'over and done with'. The mother will not forget the experiences, but they will not be able to cause any more emotional distress.

Because hypnosis involves a level of relaxation, it is particularly good at reducing the tension/pain cycle of labour which enables the mother to retain control of her body. The advantage of hypnosis is that it has no adverse effects on the fetus and will not depress maternal effort. On the contrary, it can shorten the first stage of labour (Jenkins and Pritchard, 1993), and mothers need less conventional analgesia

(Connelly, 1989). Barber (1986) suggests that often the perception of pain is the first step towards dealing with it and it is the shift in consciousness of hypnosis which allows this to happen.

Postnatal hypnotherapy

The emotional upheavals of childbirth have already been discussed under Bach Flower Remedies and many of the same problems will respond very well to hypnosis. The key at this stage is the concept of ego strengthening, a technique propounded by Hartland (1982) which includes positive suggestions of strength, calmness and control and confidence. This is particularly valuable to a new mother who is unsure of herself and is prey to the advice and influence of other people. Conditioned responses can be cued-in to facilitate lactation and if, after the best efforts of all concerned, this fails, posthypnotic suggestions to ameliorate any guilt feelings can be used.

Summary

This chapter has offered a brief overview of five complementary therapies which physiotherapists may easily incorporate into their professional practice. When used by a suitably qualified professional the therapies can generally be considered to be safe. Reported problems have arisen from the incompetence of the practitioner, rather than the therapy itself. The other question which needs to be addressed is whether it is acceptable, from both a philosophical as well as professional standpoint, to incorporate techniques from the therapies by taking an eclectic approach to problems, or whether the therapies should only be used if the practitioner is fully qualified in the therapy. Bay (1995) suggests that this could be dangerous to patients, since complementary practitioners must undergo a long training course. However, compared with the medical education undergone by physiotherapists and other professionals allied to medicine, some complementary therapy courses, bearing in mind that they purport to treat medical conditions, can be considered quite inadequate. Nurses, for example, have a long history of borrowing techniques from a variety of professions (including physiotherapy!) and incorporating them safely into their care, and are increasingly using relevant aspects of complementary therapies to enhance their range of therapeutic interventions. Physiotherapists, under their scope of professional practice, would find themselves in a similar situation.

References

Barber, J. (1986) Hypnotic analgesia. In *A Handbook of Psychological Treatments* (Holtzman, A. and Turk, D. eds). New York: Academic Press.

Bay, F. (1995) Complementary therapies – just another task? *Complement. Ther. Nurs. Midwif.*, 1(2), 34–40.

BMA (1993) *Complementary Medicine: New Approaches to Good Practice*. Oxford: Oxford University Press.

Buchbauer, G., Jirovetz, L. and Jager, W. (1991) Aromatherapy: evidence for sedative effects of the essential oil of lavender after inhalation. *Z. Naturforsch.*, **46**(C), 1067–72.

Connelly, D. (1989) A comparison of drug usage between mothers who have been trained in self hypnosis and those who have no hypnosis training. Presentation to the Irish Branch of the British Society of Experimental and Clinical Hypnosis, Belfast.

Dale, A., Cornwell, S. (1994) The role of lavender oil in relieving perineal discomfort following childbirth: a blind randomised clinical trial. *J. Advan. Nurs.*, **19**(1), 89–96.

Dantas, F. and Fisher, P. (1998) A systematic review of homoeopathic pathogenetic trials (provings) published in the United Kingdom from 1945–1995. In *Homeopathy: A Critical Appraisal* (Ernst, E. and Hahn, E., eds). Oxford: Butterworth-Heinemann.

Davis, P. (1996) *Aromatherapy: An A–Z*. Saffron Walden: C.W. Daniel.

Doyle, C. (1993) Reaching out for an alternative. *Daily Telegraph*, 6 April.

Department of Health (1993) *Changing Childbirth*. London: HMSO.

English, J. (1987) Pertussen 30 preventative for whooping cough? A pilot study. *Br. Homeopath. J.*, **76**, 61–65.

English, J. (1992) The issue of immunisation. *Br. Homeopath. J.*, **81**, 161–63.

Field, T., Morrow, C., Valdeon, D. *et al.* (1992) Massage reduces anxiety in child and adolescent psychiatric patients. *J. Am. Acad. Child Adolesc. Psychol.*, **31**(1), 125–31.

Field, T., Schalanberg, S. and Scarfidi, F. (1986) Tactile/kinesthetic stimulation effects on pre-term neonates. *Pediatrics*, **77**(5), 654–58.

Fisher, P. (1998) Is homoeopathic prescribing reliable? In *Examining Complementary Medicine* (Vickers, A., ed.). Cheltenham: Stanley Thornes.

Foundation for Integrated Medicine (1997) *Integrated Healthcare: A Way Forward for the Next Five Years? A Discussion Document*. London.

Fuchs, K., Paldi, H., Abramovici, H. *et al.* (1980) Treatment of hyperemesis gravidarum by hypnosis. *Int. J. Clin. Exp. Hypnosis*, **28**, 313.

Fulder, S. (1996) *The Handbook of Alternative and Complementary Medicine: The Essential Health Companion*, 3rd edn. Oxford: Oxford University Press.

Gemmell, D. (1997) *Everyday Homoeopathy*. Beaconsfield: Beaconsfield Publications.

Goldman, L. (1990) Control of hyperemesis. In *Handbook of Hypnotic Suggestions and Metaphors* (Hammond, D., ed.). New York: Norton.

Harlow, H. and Suomi, S. (1979) Nature of love simplified. *Am. Psychol.*, **25**(88), 161–68.

Hartland, J. (1982) *Medical and Dental Hypnosis and its Clinical Applications*. London: Baillière Tindall.

Heap, M. (1996) Hypnosis is not a separate state of mind. *Psychologist*, **9**(11), 498.

Howard, J. (1992) *Bach Flower Remedies for Women*. Saffron Walden: C.W. Daniel.

Jager, W., Buchbauer, G. and Jirovetz, L. (1992) Evidence for the sedative effect of neroli oil, citronellal and phenylethyl acetate on mice. *J. Essential Oils*, **4**, 387–94.

Jenkins, M. and Pritchard, M. (1993) Hypnosis: practical applications and theoretical considerations in normal labour. *Br. J. Obstet. Gynaecol.*, **100**, 221.

Kleijnen, J., Knipschild, P. and ter Riet, G. (1991) Clinical trials of homoeopathy. *Br. Med. J.*, **302**, 316–23.

Kohen, D. (1980) Relaxation/mental imagery (self hypnosis) and pelvic examinations in adolescents. *Develop. Behav. Paediat.*, **1**, 180.

Lockie, A. (1990) *The Family Guide to Homeopathy: The Safe Form of Medicine for the Future*. London: Hamish Hamilton.

McClure, V. (1989) *Infant Massage*, 2nd edn. New York: Bantam.

NAHAT (1993) *Complementary Therapies in the NHS*, Research Paper No. 10. London: National Association of Health Authorities and Trusts.

Porter, S. (1996) The use of massage for neonates requiring special care. *Complement. Ther. Nurs. Midwif.*, **2**(4), 93–96.

Price, S. (1991) *Aromatherapy for Common Ailments*. London: Gaia Books.

Price, S. (1993) *Aromatherapy Workbook*. London: Thorsons.

Russell, J. (1993) Touch and infant massage. *Paediat. Nurs.*, **5**(3), 8–11.

Ryman, D. (1989) *The Aromatherapy Handbook*. Saffron Walden: C.W. Daniel.

Scarfidi, F., Field, T. and Schanber, S. (1993) Factors which predict which pre-term infants benefit from massage therapy. *J. Develop. Behav. Paediat.*, **14**(3), 3–8.

Sharma, U. (1992) *Complementary Medicine Today: Practitioners and Patients*. London: Tavistock/Routledge.

Stapleton, H. (1995) The use of herbal medicine in pregnancy and labour Part II: Events after birth including those affecting the health of babies. *Complement. Ther. Nurs. Midwif.*, **1**(6), 165–67.

Stein, C. (1963) The clenched fist technique as a hypnotic procedure in clinical psychotherapy. *Am. J. Clin. Hypnosis*, **6**, 113–19.

Stevensen, C. (1994) The psychophysiological effects of aromatherapy massage following cardiac surgery. *Complement. Ther. Med.*, **2**(1), 27–35.

Swayne, J. (1998) *Homeopathic Method: Implications for Clinical Practice and Medical Science*. London: Churchill Livingstone.

Thomas, M. (1989) Fancy footwork. *Nursing Times*, **85**(41), 42–44.

Tiran, D. (1996) *Aromatherapy in Midwifery Practice*. London: Baillière Tindall.

Tiran, D. and Mack, S. (1995) *Complementary Therapies for Pregnancy and Childbirth*. London: Baillière Tindall.

Vincent, C. and Furnham, A. (1997) *Complementary Medicine: A Research Perspective*. Chichester: Wiley.

Walach, H. (1992) *Wissenschaftliche homoopathische Arzneimittlelprufing*. Heidelberg: Haug.

Wieland, F. (1998) Is a homeopathic drug proving just a clinical trial phase one? *Homeopath. Links*, **9**, 39–40.

Wilkinson, S. (1995) Aromatherapy and massage in palliative care. *Int. J. Palliative Nurs.*, **1**(1), 21–23.

Recommended reading

Downey, P. (1997) *Homeopathy for the Primary Health Care Team*. Oxford: Butterworth-Heinemann.

Ernst, E. and Hahn, E. (eds) (1996) *Homeopathy: A Critical Appraisal*. Oxford: Butterworth-Heinemann.

Gemmell, D. (1997) *Everyday Homoeopathy*. Beaconsfield: Beaconsfield Publications.

Howard, J. (1990) *The Bach Flower Remedies Step by Step*. Saffron Walden: C.W. Daniel.

Howard, J. (1994) *Growing Up with the Bach Flower Remedies*. Saffron Walden: C.W. Daniel.

Vickers, A. (1996) *Massage and Aromatherapy: A Guide for Health Care Professionals*. London: Chapman and Hall.

23 Holistic care for the dying, the bereaved and their carers

Richard Reoch

Introduction

Few other experiences have the potential to be so tender, so direct and so intense as the time devoted to caring for a dying person. The lessons of 'natural childbirth' have been learned. We are only now starting to apply that wisdom to dying well.

What makes a birth unhappy and painful can be just as true for the experience of a dying person, their loved ones and carers. Both are moments of supreme vulnerability. Yet by understanding more about these opening and closing passages of our lives, and the steps that can be taken to affect them, it is possible for great pain to coexist with – and even be transformed by – tenderness, compassion and insight.

Physical contact and touch are among the most powerful forms of support that can be given to those faced with uncertainty, fear and pain. Touch is part of our natural response to human suffering. Our sense of touch is one of the first to develop and one of the last to go. Touching meets an instinctive need. Therapeutic touching, massage and holding have been termed the 'anchor in the stormy sea of labour'. This is also the experience of those working with the dying, who recognize in these forms of human contact a way of saying to the dying: 'I care about you. You mean far more to me than I can express.'

Human contact

Recent research into the use of therapeutic massage on dying patients has opened up wonderful possibilities for people working with the dying. The results are already being put to use in more and more hospitals and hospices and by palliative care teams in the community.

Illness tends to create a spiral of pain, anxiety and tension. The cycle feeds on itself, with the anxiety and tension creating or intensifying painful sensations. This vicious cycle is common in people with terminal conditions. Even if there is little physical trauma, the fear and anxiety often associated with dying may cause intense pain. As the pain increases, so does the stress. The stress causes poor sleep and results in fatigue. The more enervated the person is, the more irritable. This leaves them more isolated, since people tend to avoid others when they are irritable. Without the diversion of human contact, the person is left with little to distract them from their pain.

The effects of this cycle can be reduced without relying solely on drugs. Therapeutic massage techniques can be used to reduce muscular and other pains and to induce relaxation. Medical research into the Gate Theory of pain has shown that nerve impulses triggered by massage travel faster than pain signals. The result is that massage actually alters the transmission of pain messages to the brain. Massage not only reduces the overall level of tension, but activates the release of endorphins, the body's own pain-killers. Doctors report that massage has the additional advantage of helping people deal with the sense of hopelessness and despair to which they often succumb.

While the full range of techniques for massage and other physical therapies can be applied by professional bodyworkers, certain simple methods can also be taught to the relatives and other carers of the dying person. Instead of sitting helplessly round in hospital or at home, they can bring great comfort to the patient – and also learn to share massage with each other as a form of mutual support. The benefits are incalculable. The massage becomes an act of loving tenderness that can be expressed and shared when words fail.

In a recent study, a cancer patient described her experience of massage provided in hospital:

> I wasn't aware of feeling sad or even sorry
> for myself, but was suddenly tired and
> weary with the effort of pretending I was
> OK. The touch was so accepting and
> compassionate, the image that went through
> my mind was that of being a child again,
> comforted by my mother. The massage itself
> was good – relaxing and so gentle that I
> began to think of other things. I cried at the
> end when the massage therapist covered me
> with a towel – it was done so lovingly and
> caringly. The whole experience made me feel
> I was worth caring about.

Complementary therapies

Massage is only one of a range of therapies being explored in the care of the dying. The spectrum of complementary treatments is now seen as particularly relevant since these systems seek internal balance and respect natural processes, including ageing and dying. Rather than preventing nature from taking its course, they offer support to the person so that nature's way is eased.

The use of complementary therapies in the care of a dying person does not, of itself, guarantee a convenient, pain-free death. Nor should such therapies be mistaken for miracle cures.

The treatments are supplements to professional medical care and are not meant to contradict or replace conventional medical treatments.

Among the most common of the therapies being used are aromatherapy and Shiatsu, herbal and flower remedies and systems such as homoeopathy, acupuncture and Chi Kung. An increasing number of support and self-help groups include such therapies in their services or directories. Hospices are offering them to dying people and carers – and many of the techniques can be used safely in the home by friends and family.

One reason for this trend is the growing attention being given to the psychological, emotional and spiritual needs of dying people. Complementary therapies act as an antidote to stress and anxiety, resulting in better sleep and better tolerance of medical procedures. In particular, because of the unconditional acceptance of the therapist or carer, the treatments help patients acknowledge and accept their changing circumstances.

Another reason that causes people to turn to complementary therapies is the fact that they are perceived to offer a form of patient autonomy, often in the face of certain types of hierarchical medical practice. This, in itself, may be a vital ingredient in sustaining a sense of quality of life in the midst of dying.

In most of the complementary therapies now being used in the care of the terminally ill, the mind–body relationship is regarded as supremely important. This recognition leads to the possibility of using multiple techniques to achieve a holistic result. Relaxation and visualization exercises can be used to ease physical distress. Bodywork such as massage, Shiatsu and aromatherapy can be used to address mental anguish.

Underlying the use of these centuries-old remedies is a profound message for the dying and those responsible for their care. Death has been with us from the dawn of life on the planet. It is part of the cycle. It is as natural as the herbs used to ease its passage.

The spectrum of care

There are many aspects to the care of the dying person. The full spectrum of care extends far beyond medical treatment and affects the entire experience of the person who is ill. Relatives commonly ask that 'everything possible' be done for their loved ones. Fortunately, the horizon of possibilities now available both before and during protracted illness is expanding.

Pain and suffering are not automatic, nor are they consistent. They are subject to considerable variation, depending on many factors. One central element is the precise nature of the illness and the response of the body and nervous system to it. But people's responses can be affected by many other elements. In recent years this has led to the development of a team approach to the care of the dying – so that a range of disciplines and influences can be considered and brought to bear in the best interests of the patient. While it may not be the direct responsibility of the physical therapist to intervene in other aspects of the person's care, it is wise to be alert to the broader context in which the person is being cared for, particularly if physical therapy is being introduced as part of a team effort.

Of particular relevance are the following questions. Is the person being cared for at home, in a hospital, a hospice, a nursing home? What freedom do they have to choose that setting? What information are they getting about their condition? How open and satisfactory is communication with their carers? What other therapies are being used to deal with the cycle of anxiety, tension and pain?

These questions, and issues linked to them, may well emerge in apparently casual conversation between the physical therapist and the patient. Indeed, the supportive and unconditional quality of the treatment offered by such therapies may well serve as a positive encouragement to the patient to raise such matters – which they may be reluctant to do in other settings.

An appropriate death

It is important to remember that each person's death is unique. It is intensely personal to them and yet, at the same time, it is a stranger, both to the person who is ill and to those caring for them. Predictions may be wildly inaccurate. Some people outlive their expected deaths by years; others die far sooner than expected. The

person's emotional reaction to their illness may have at least as dramatic effect on the outcome as any medication or other treatment.

The idea of 'a good death' is sometimes mistaken for dying in our sleep, slipping away under heavy sedation or lying back and feeling good while the body gives up the ghost. These might be some people's ideals, but dying well involves a fuller understanding of death, a conscious application of its lessons in our lives, and the cultivation of those attitudes and feelings by which both the dying person and all involved are available to each other in the fullness of their humanity.

More helpful than the notion of 'a good death' is the concept of an 'appropriate death'. This is a way of dying that reflects, as far as possible, the person's own personality and values. What matters, from this viewpoint, is not other people's stereotyped views of good and bad deaths, but the nature of each person's own experience. The psychiatrist Avery Weisman wrote:

> Obviously, appropriate death for one person might be unsuitable for another. What might seem appropriate from the outside might be utterly meaningless to the dying person himself. Conversely, deaths that seem unacceptable to an outsider, might be desirable from the inner viewpoint of the patient. (Weisman, 1972)

Any approach to the care of the dying that aims to be holistic, or that aims to contribute to the work of a team employing holistic methods, needs to bear the concept of an 'appropriate death' very firmly in mind. Without it, decisions on patient care and the subtle messages conveyed by the therapists in the course of their work, may unwittingly deny to the dying person the dignity that is their right at the end of life.

Symptom relief

Research into patients with advanced cancer has shown that most people suffer from a cluster of common symptoms. These are thought to be associated to a greater or lesser extent with many other terminal illnesses. Although not everyone experiences these symptoms, the care team should be aware that they might arise; that medication and advice from palliative care specialists will help; and that alternative remedies are available.

Retaining mobility

Most dying people find that they are losing strength. Coming to terms with this can be extremely stressful, both for the person and their carers. Intense weariness and boredom are common. Physiotherapists aim to encourage a scheme of exercises to prevent weak people becoming bedbound and to help them retain a degree of mobility and independence. At this stage in the person's life, such support can have a powerful effect, not only on their physical well-being, but on their self-image and self-respect. This is an indispensable factor in achieving the goal in the World Health Organisation's definition of palliative care: 'The best quality of life for them and their families.'

Easing the breath

Many patients are affected by breathlessness. The feeling of being unable to breathe is so disturbing, it is literally like drowning. The cause may be physical, but it can also result from being overwhelmed with anxiety.

Most forms of therapeutic touch are likely to have a beneficial effect on a person's breathing because they are so wonderfully relaxing. If the person tends to breathe in a very rapid and shallow manner, slightly slower and deeper breathing can be encouraged during a massage. This may be the natural outcome of the relaxing effect of the massage, or it may be deliberately encouraged by the therapist. The therapist can emphasize this aspect of the massage by synchronizing his or her own own breathing with the massage strokes, allowing the breathing to be slightly audible. A natural interaction often follows, enabling the patient to relax into a less distressed breathing pattern. This is best done without words, relying entirely on the interactive effect of the combined stroking and breathing.

Other possible treatments include the use of aromatherapy. The essential oils which are especially recommended for the relief of breathlessness include *Sweet Marjoram* or *Frankincense* used in a bath, as inhalations or in a vaporizer.

The successful use of herbs in the treatment of breathlessness requires diagnosis of the underlying causes by a trained herbalist. If the root problem is weakness of the heart or poor circulation, *Garlic* and *Hawthorn* may be recommended. If there is fluid retention in the lungs, a Dandelion decoction may be used. If the illness involves other chest problems, *Garlic*, *Thyme* or *Hissop* may prove beneficial.

Calming the stomach

Constant nausea and vomiting, which are both distressing and debilitating, can result from the patient's disease, but also from some medical treatments. They may also signal powerful emotional disturbance. Massive weight loss can be caused by the disease or its side-effects, but it may also reflect the fact that some people near death lose interest in food, or may develop a profound distaste for themselves. The dying person may suffer intensely from the fact that their self-image is being assaulted. They may loathe the progressively disabled, incontinent or decaying body in which they are forced to spend their days.

Visualization and relaxation exercises can be used to meet the person's need to be centred, stable and cared for and can sometimes be used very effectively to calm the disorder expressed by the stomach. Progressive relaxation techniques are often helpful and have the advantage that they can be shared by carers and receivers.

A number of herbs contain properties which are beneficial in the treatment of nausea and vomiting, including: *Camomile*, *Cinnamon*, *Dill*, *Fennel*, *Ginger*, *Peppermint* and *Rosemary*. Medication taken to counteract the side-effects of chemotherapy may adversely affect the stomach lining. The herb *Slippery Elm* is extremely useful in protecting the lining of the stomach during the period of chemotherapy and also in dealing with other irritations of the gut.

Aromatherapy for nausea and vomiting includes the use of *Peppermint*, *Ginger*, *Lemon*, *Caraway* or *Sandalwood* in a bath or massage, as an inhalation or in a vaporizer.

Relieving constipation

Often ignored, constipation is one of the most common problems that dying people face. It can contribute to many other conditions and be a source of much unexpressed, deep distress. Constipation is often related to the weakness of the energy associated with all forms of release and letting go, whether on a physical, mental or emotional level.

Abdominal massage is often extremely helpful. The person must be willing to accept the massage and not have lesions on the belly caused by operations. The technique can be used as a form of self-massage or by a carer. Studies with elderly patients who frequently suffered constipation have shown an increase in the number of bowel motions after a period of gentle massage and, in some instances, the number of enemas needed was substantially reduced.

Herbal treatments can also be used to counteract constipation. A recommended mixture uses *Psyllium* seed or *Linseed* to bulk the bowel contents and help push them along. *Licorice* is a natural laxative that can be taken either in the form of licorice root or in licorice sweets. *Yellow Dock* and *Burdock* are more powerful laxatives and can be taken in an infusion, along with equal amounts of *Licorice*, *Ginger* and *Dandelion* root.

Aromatherapy treatments recommend the use of one of several essential oils: *Bitter Orange*, *Black Pepper*, *Ginger* or *Rosemary* – in a bath or massage.

Most people are troubled if they soil themselves and find it humiliating to have to rely on someone else to enable them to go to the toilet. One way to improve the situation is to help the person retain even limited mobility for as long as possible. Physiotherapy can be of great help in prolonging the person's ability to move sufficiently to use a commode near the bed.

Pain management

The management of pain requires careful attention to all possible factors, including the person's physical, emotional, spiritual and social needs. Medication alone may not be sufficient. In most forms of complementary medicine, pain is understood to be the result of a blockage in the natural circulation of vital energy in the body. This can be a localized blockage, often causing a specific pain, or the whole system of energy circulation can be weakened, causing a wide range of symptoms. Because our fundamental energy is the basis of both our minds and our bodies, treatments which unblock or strengthen the flow of that energy address both emotional and physical manifestations of pain.

Herbal treatments can provide natural pain relief through their impact on the nervous system. They can be an excellent complement to other medication that may be prescribed. For the relief of intense pain, *Black Cohosh* is often recommended, as it is anti-inflammatory and has a powerful relaxing effect. *Camomile* is often used by people who have a great sensitivity to pain and get easily irritated even by small pains. For sustained, immovable pain, a herbalist may recommend the use of *Jamaica Dogwood* or *Pasque Flower*, after examination. Dosages will depend on whether the person is experiencing acute or chronic pain.

To deal with any form of pain and illness, it is important to strengthen the circulation of energy throughout the body. There is a range of natural remedies which can help. This includes *Cinnamon*, *Garlic*, *Ginger*, *Ginseng*, *Watercress* and *Wild Oats*. They can be added to the diet and drinks or used as infusions. Low energy can lead to depression, for which *Lemon Balm*, *Rosemary*, *St John's Wort*, *Skullcap*, *Vervain* and *Wild Oats* are often recommended. If poor circulation results in confused states of mind, *Gingko*, *Ginseng*, *Hawthorn*, *Rosemary* or *Wood Betony* may be used.

Aromatherapy for pain relief involves the use of *Lavender*, *Sweet Marjoram*, *Black Pepper*, or *Niaouli* – in a bath or massage.

Our experience of pain is influenced by many factors. Sometimes, if we choose to, we are prepared to bear very high levels of pain. On the other hand, we many find much more minor pains unbearable. A great deal depends on our underlying beliefs about the meaning of pain and our mental and emotional reactions to specific pains. There are therefore many approaches to pain relief, in addition to chemical painkillers.

Some people find that their minds can be successfully distracted from dull, chronic pain for relatively long periods by listening to music, performing gentle exercises or getting involved in intricate handicrafts. Often people benefit from massage, acupuncture and the use of TENS which counteract the flow of pain signals in the nervous system. For other people, skilled counselling can help ease their pain by reducing the stress levels which are part of the vicious pain–anxiety cycle.

Other approaches to pain relief place the emphasis on breath work, relaxation and meditation. Our mental power can be deployed in the fight against pain: sharp pain can be visualized as spikes of ice which we are slowly dissolving, dull pain can be imagined as pressure which we are slowly releasing, deep pain can be seen as an intense red light which gradually changes to a pain-free white. An ancient technique for pain relief is literally to smile into the area of the body where we think the pain is located. If we can learn to do this wholeheartedly, as if we were welcoming and befriending the pain unreservedly, remarkable changes are known to occur.

Lifting the spirit

The dispersal of the body's energies can leave a person weak, exhausted and depressed. Sometimes this happens gradually, sometimes spasmodically. The result can be a state of great weariness. It may manifest itself physically, with the person simply lying back and drifting off to sleep, or mentally and emotionally, with a loss of interest in the people and events around them. Sometimes, there is much restlessness and fitfulness, reflecting the energetic imbalances in the body and nervous system. When this happens, the carers too may be sapped of vitality and succumb to deep depression.

There is increasing interest in the use of flower remedies and flower essences in the treatment of conditions whose roots may lie in the psyche rather than in the physical make-up of the body. In the case of the Bach Flower Remedies, important distinctions are made between different manifestations of depression. If the person's depression is the result of physical exhaustion, *Olive* is recommended. If the root of the problem is mental exhaustion, a sense that the person simply cannot face the day ahead, then *Hornbeam* is suggested.

There are other flower remedies associated with the relief of depression, depending on the nature of the person's suffering. *Gentian* helps to dispel negative thinking and is useful for temporary despondency brought on by setbacks such as an unsuccessful round of treatment. *Gorse* is recommended for those whose depression is deeper: they have given up hope and have no wish to carry on. In the most extreme cases of people experiencing desperate mental anguish, *Sweet Chestnut* is advised. It helps to restore faith and is used when people can see no way out of their inner darkness. They may feel so desolate and heartbroken that they physically hurt inside from the emotional pain.

To lift the spirit, herbalists often recommend trying *St. John's Wort*, *Vervain*, *Rosemary*, *Lemon Balm*, *Skullcap*, *Wild Oats* or *Thyme*. Aromatherapists tend to recommend using one of *Bergamot*, *Roman Chamomile*, *Clary Sage*, *Frankincense*, *Lavender* or *Sandalwood* in a bath or massage, as an inhalation or in a vaporizer.

Supporting the bereaved

We are often anxious to do something for people in deep grief, to ease their pain, to show how much we care. However, just as with the dying, it is important not to impose our assumptions on the bereaved. We may have trouble witnessing their grief because of the unresolved pain it reflects in our own lives. At times we risk trivializing the importance of their grief by encouraging them 'to get over it'. Although we often speak of the need to heal the wounds of grief, we may fail to understand that some deaths change a bereaved person for ever and that the measure of our love is our willingness to be open fully to that change.

Applied with this perspective in mind, many complementary therapies can be quietly and powerfully supportive of people caught in the grip of grief and bereavement. Most forms of human contact, such as massage and therapeutic touch, if expressly consented to by the person, can work silent wonders. If the person is experiencing paralysing grief, the massage can be enhanced with the use of aromatherapy oils. Among those recommended are one or more of *Bergamot, Frankincense, Lavender, Sweet Marjoram, Melissa* or *Ylang Ylang*. These can also be used in a bath, as an inhalation or in a vaporizer. From among the Bach Flower remedies, *Star of Bethlehem* is advised for easing the effects of grief and sorrow. It can also be helpful if the person has difficulty expressing their grief.

Our bodies and minds have a remarkable ability to respond to startling and extreme events. However, at such times we often find ourselves in environments and social settings where our innate ability to restore equilibrium is seriously impaired. If you are called upon to help someone trying to cope with the intense distress caused by the sudden or violent death of someone they love, or find yourself in extreme circumstances, there are natural remedies that you may find extremely helpful.

Some practitioners of complementary therapies carry a small bottle of Bach Flower Rescue Remedy with them at all times. It is a combination of *Cherry Plum, Clematis, Impatiens, Rock Rose* and *Star of Bethlehem* which is an all-purpose emergency composite for the effects of anguish. It is used for those who have been seriously distressed and risk falling into a numbed state of mind. It has a calming, comforting and reassuring effect on the nervous system, allowing the natural healing energies within the person to work without hindrance. Place four drops of the liquid in a cup of water to be sipped at intervals.

In the event of a sudden crisis, the nervous system tends to respond positively to inhaling 4 drops of *Lavender* oil on a tissue. You can also add the following blend of essential oil, such as *Geranium, Lavender, Sandalwood* and *Ylang Ylang* to a warm bath to help relieve tension and encourage a good night's sleep.

It must always be borne in mind, however, that grief is intensely personal, does not conform to theoretical models and can be fully integrated into human life without either fear or shame. Seventeen years after the death of her small son, Simon, Dee Cooper wrote movingly of her feelings. Her words are a powerful reminder of this truth:

After many years of bewilderment I have come to the conclusion that the feelings that result from the death of a child are not resolvable. They continue, are painful, are re-experienced at intervals, and this is the normal pattern. The death of a child changes your life irrevocably. There is no going back. My feelings about Simon are part of my life. The initially fearful recognition that literally anything could happen to me or those I love at any moment has been enriching. I live more in the present. I experience each moment at a deeper level than I would previously have thought possible. Experiencing and feeling are enhanced. I am both sadder and happier than I was before. If you have the courage to be confronted by reality – the reality that the world is not a safe place, the reality that children can die, the reality that the pain of grief can be lasting – then do ask me how I am. I think that the quality of my life has been enhanced by this knowledge; perhaps yours could be.

Caring for each other

In addition to the various therapeutic interventions, whether orthodox or complementary, the human atmosphere created around a person who is suffering great distress or who is dying has an unquestionable impact. Relatives and carers may experience acute inner anguish because of the uncertainty and pain. Their normal lives are disrupted, creating conflicting pressures of both a practical and emotional nature. They may have to endure sheer exhaustion and exasperation at the seemingly endless time that is involved; they are then lacerated with guilt because of those feelings.

Caring for a dying person can be stressful, exhausting and relentless. It is an open-ended commitment and can literally extend for years. Carers can break down under the never-ending pressure. Relationships may be stretched to the breaking point. Carers' lifestyles may be altered beyond recognition. They may be beset with every conceivable worry, from financial to emotional. Some feel helpless in the face of the resentment that wells up in them. Others are obsessed with feelings of incompetence, inadequacy and frustration. To that is added the grief they feel at the impending death and their fear that they may not be able to cope.

Even in the face of these pressures, countless people find caring to be deeply rewarding, full of meaning and purpose, and the ultimate fulfilment of their love for the other person. Carers are one of the most important resources available to the dying person. They need to look after themselves in the best possible way so that they can be of maximum benefit when the dying person most needs quality care.

It is important to remember that the state of being of everyone involved in the care of the dying person has an effect on them. If someone is anxious and run down, they will communicate a sense of unease to the person they are caring for, no matter how loving or professional they are trying to be. It is in precisely this context that complementary therapies can be of help in supporting everyone involved through the unpredictability and anxiety at all stages of the death process. Relaxation and stress reduction treatments can be used to sustain the carers as well as the dying person, and thereby increase the quality of care. Indeed, health professionals often notice that the carer may be experiencing more anxiety than the patient and be in desperate need of attention, reassurance and energizing support.

People with long-term illnesses need considerable care, but there is still much they may be able to contribute – depending on their varying state of health. A distinctive feature of many of the exercises and treatments from the world of complementary therapies is that in certain instances they can be used or directed by the dying person to care for the caregivers. For example, they can often help their carers relax: giving some simple hand massage, guiding them through stress reduction exercises or reminding them of the relaxation advice that carers need, but all too often overlook. This sort of mutual

support, as long as it is possible, can be extraordinarily rewarding for all involved and transform the experience of dying.

It is sometimes wrongly assumed that children in the household are merely an additional burden on the carers. There is even the fear that children may be disturbed by the presence of a dying person in the family. But many of the massage and other techniques can be learned and used by children and may open up to them extremely useful and powerful ways of communicating with and supporting the dying person and the carers. This will depend very much on the circumstances in each family and the emotional openness of all the adults involved.

Genuine presence

It is often thought that the spiritual needs of the dying are the unique province of priests, psychologists, death counsellors or other specialists. Not so. Those who work with dying people find that neat, professional, intellectual or religious answers are often not what is being sought.

The spiritual care of the dying is a shared task. At its heart is the person who is dying. They share their work with all those to whom they have been close in life and eventually with all those who come into contact with them and assist them in dying.

As Cicely Saunders, the founder of the Hospice Movement, wrote:

The dying have shed the masks and
superficialities of everyday living and they
are all the more open and sensitive because
of this. They see through all unreality.
I remember one man saying: 'No, no
reading. I only want what is in your mind
and in your heart.'

By their presence, by their suffering, through their silences and their utterances, the dying invite us to encounters of complete honesty and openness. It is our willingness to enter into those encounters that constitutes authentic spiritual care. These are the encounters of unfettered human energy. They embrace our anger, our fears and hopes, our depression, our denial and our acceptance. Nothing is excluded, nothing is regarded as less than human or less than sacred.

If you are asked about life's meaning and have no answer, say so. If you have an answer, give it freely. What matters is the willingness to open fully to that person and to accept them, as they are, unconditionally. To the extent that we are willing to respond in that way, to that extent are they able to complete their life's work and to enrich us by the power of their death.

Listening power

A very common first reaction among people confronted with death or a dying person is: 'I don't know what to say.' The truth is that not only may you have nothing to say, but what you say is not the real entry point for the journey. The first question to ask yourself is: 'Do I know how to listen?'

A dying person often goes through phases, alternating between speech and silence. Visitors and carers may be so obsessed with doing or saying something nice that they end up trying to have a conversation when the person needs tranquillity. Or the visitor or health worker may be bustling around when the person actually just needs someone to stop and listen to them.

Tuning in to the dying person is the key to preventing this mismatch. It requires a willingness to go beyond one's own agenda and timetable and even one's own compulsive desire to be helpful. You start to create open space by simply spending time with the person with no other purpose in mind. You are just there.

Our conventional response is to rush into any vacuum, to give the person our own thoughts to comfort them. That is helpful if specifically asked for, but a far richer dialogue flows from the effort to draw the other person out and to understand the significance of what they are saying. Their insights are unique and may be of inestimable worth to those who listen. In the words of an old saying: 'When you speak you say only what you already know; when you listen, you learn.'

Those who work with the dying emphasize the importance of letting the person control the pace and content of communication. The rush of our own reactions often gets in the way. 'What is needed is the space to explore the dimensions of the situation that arises when one is confronted with a life-threatening situation', advises one worker, 'to explore the meaning, the confusion about life and death and what lies beyond, if anything.'

People with a terminal illness sometimes find other people treat them as if they were in mental quarantine. Why assume that the person has lost their natural interest in the world around them, doesn't want to know the latest news or gossip, and doesn't have views on what is happening? An essential part of good caring is to avoid making assumptions about what is or is not important to the person, and to be sensitive to their changing needs.

Everyone involved in working with the dying lives in an environment characterized by extreme uncertainty. Normally we are able to create and cling to apparent certainties – even if these are only illusions. But death strips them away. Even the effort to establish some certainties in the face of death creates additional anxiety.

It is best to face up to this reality. The advice for therapists, relatives and patients alike is to realize from the outset that literally everything can change from moment to moment, from day to day. Don't frustrate yourself by demanding consistency. Ask open-ended questions and probe the meaning of the answers. Don't overlay questions and answers with your own assumptions. Be willing to accept 'I don't really know' as an answer and to accept the fact that this may be your own answer to many questions. Be open about the uncertainty of the situation with others. Don't assume you must carry any burden on your own. Seek advice and support openly. Always remember that a dying person is a living person in a crucial phase of their existence. Respect their individuality, their experience and their autonomy.

The dying person may no longer be able to converse. But that is not the end of communication. A man sitting at the bedside of his silent, dying mother later wrote these words:

I felt powerless, small and helpless, but also peaceful, strong and quiet. I was seeing and feeling something I had never seen or felt before, an experience that to be described would require words that have not yet been found: powerless, yet strong, sad yet peaceful, broken yet whole. Everything was truthful. We experienced the privilege of being close to her suffering, intimately connected with her pain. I have never felt so strongly that the truth can make us free.

Death with dignity

Doctors often argue that 'death with dignity' is a fantasy that simply does not fit the facts. 'Dying is a series of destructive events that involve by their very nature the disintegration of the dying person's humanity' would be a typical expression of this point of view. The intention behind such remarks is often deep compassion. It is important to prevent individuals and their relatives pinning their hopes on an idealized 'happy death' and thereby setting themselves up for feeling guilty, angry and vengeful when the physical decay of the body sets in.

Studies of patients' final moments, however, do not suggest that our humanity is necessarily destroyed. A survey of over 35 000 observations by doctors and nurses, conducted by Karlis Osis, found that 10% of patients appeared conscious in the hour before death, that fear was not dominant and that 1 in 20 showed signs of elation.

Fiona Ann Monsell told the Institute for Social Inventions in London:

I have done years of nursing, often with terminal patients, and have seen many deaths. I have never seen anyone die in panic. Quite often patients will rally around within three days of death to say goodbye to their loved ones, some have said they've seen relatives that have gone before them, but at the end none has ever been afraid.

When my mother died, some 15 months ago, I was at her bedside and held her hand, and the moment she passed on I felt her leaving and pass through me on her way. I can only describe it as a beautiful experience that I shall never forget. It was like she gave me a small part of her energy to keep with me always.

Energetic interactions

Like everything that lives, each of us is a field of energy. The more sensitive we are, the more we can feel the immediate effect that other people's energy has on us. This is particularly true of people who are ill and those who are dying. Most dying people are particularly sensitive to the authentic, living presence of someone who is fully attentive to them. Making yourself available to the dying person in this way does not require special expertise or knowing 'what to say'. It is, quite literally, the interaction of two energy fields. It requires simply being there, fully present with complete acceptance, regardless of what is happening.

Normally, the energy pattern we project outwards in times of stress is disturbing to others, but we are often unaware of it ourselves. There are telltale signs: tense neck and shoulder muscles, pressure in the chest area or head, frequent blinking and rapid eye movements. This is usually because our energy constantly rushes upwards when we are under stress, causing tension, headaches and restlessness.

Rediscovering how to be genuinely present and relaxed may at first seem difficult and anything but natural. We are swept away by constant agitation and by the intensity of the emotions we feel. We need to anchor ourselves in the midst of that, be fully aware of all the disturbances around us and yet not be incapacitated by them. Once we have that anchor, and have returned to a sense of equilibrium in ourselves, nature takes over: we stop babbling and regain the innate ability to express ourselves simply and straightforwardly when needed.

Our presence begins with the way we relate to ourselves. So while we begin with the desire to be helpful to the other person, in reality we have to begin with assessing ourselves. An ancient method for anchoring ourselves is to listen to our bodies. The exercise presented in the next section to help you relax can prove extremely useful at various times. Therapists and carers can practise this quietly and unobtrusively. Simple as it appears, it affects and can transform their energy field. It can be practised before working with the dying person, while sitting beside them or while talking to them. Your relaxed presence will also have a healing effect on those around you.

The body of wisdom

The human body is a body of wisdom. It lies at the basis of our sense of being alive and enables us to know what is happening to us and around us. This wisdom continues to be available to us throughout our lives and through the process of dying. In many spiritual traditions great emphasis is laid on giving up the body at the time of death, but that cannot be done by neglecting or abusing the body. It must be loved and listened to.

Unfortunately, many of us become disconnected from our bodies as a result of the culture in which we live and so, in a very real sense, we are never fully present. Being present lies at the heart of dying well, both for the dying person and for anyone who wishes to support them in that.

The exercise below, drawn from the Chinese tradition of Chi Kung, is designed to rekindle your awareness of your body and, hence, the ground of your being. It makes use of the power of your central nervous system and the energy pathways associated with your spine. You rebalance the flow of your internal energy, lower your centre of gravity and make your nervous system more stable. You connect with the strength and nurturing energy of the earth beneath you. This ability empowers any other practice associated with dying or helping the dying.

This is of particular benefit for therapists and carers who may be under a great deal of stress. Your energy may be depleted or unsettled. Before you massage or attempt any hands-on therapy, therefore, you can balance your own energy using this exercise. Otherwise you will simply be passing on your anxiety to the person. You can practise the exercise on your own or use the instructions to guide another therapist or carer (Figure 23.1).

1. Sit comfortably, trying if possible to have a straight back. Rest your feet flat on the floor.
2. Lower your gaze.
3. Relax your shoulders and chest and breathe naturally.
4. Bring your mind to bear on the fact that you are sitting. Try to feel the weight of your entire upper body resting on your sitting

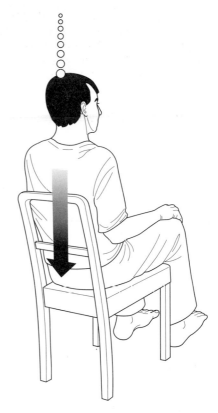

Figure 23.1 A relaxation exercise to rekindle awareness of one's body (see text for details)

bones and the bones themselves feeling the pressure of that weight.

5. Focus your awareness on the bottom of your spine. Try to feel the strength of the base of the spine as it supports the full weight of your spinal cord and skull.
6. As you become more aware of the sense of strength at the base of your spine, allow your neck, shoulders and chest to relax further, as if they were allowing the spine to bear their weight fully.
7. Then, without losing that feeling, let your mind also be aware of the very top of your head. Imagine your head being very gently supported, as if suspended from above by a fine cord.
8. Then let your attention move slowly down from the top of your head, down your neck and slowly down your spine. Imagine each of the vertebrae in your neck and back and

as you call each one to mind, imagine it is relaxing and becoming warm. It is almost as if a warm current were starting to travel from the top of your spine slowly down to the very bottom.

Repeat the eight steps of the exercise at least three times, pausing at the end each time to experience the relaxation of the muscles in the upper body and the sense of weight and strength at the base of the spine.

To conclude, simply transfer your attention to the rising and falling of your breath. Rest calmly for a minute before ending the exercise.

If you have trouble imagining the vertebrae in your spine, imagine your whole back is covered in thick, caked mud. Imagine you are under a warm shower and 'feel' the rushing water loosen the mud and gradually wash it away, so that the softened mud and warm water run slowly down your back, until your entire back is cleansed and warmed.

Conclusion

This simple, yet profound, practice is of inestimable benefit. It brings you fully into the present moment and, therefore, fully into the presence of the person you are working with. That authentic presence is at the heart of all forms of caring for the dying. In the words of a chaplain to people suffering from HIV and AIDS:

> Just knowing that someone else is there is the greatest gift you can offer . . . to make the space, to provide an environment where the person can go into their own journey more fully.

Reference

Weisman, A.D. (1972) *On Dying and Denying*. New York: Behavioural Publications.

Recommended reading

Albery, N. (1993) *The Natural Death Handbook*. London: Virgin Books.
Buckman, R. (1992) *How to Break Bad News*. London: Pan Macmillan.
Feinstein, D. and Mayo, P.E. (1993) *Mortal Acts*. New York: HarperCollins.
Levine, S. (1988) *Who Dies?* Bath: Gateway Books.
Reoch, R. (1997) *Dying Well: A Holistic Guide for the Dying and Their Carers*. London: Gaia Books.

Appendix: A short guide to UK based organizations

Bioenergy Profiling
The Centre for the Study of Alternative
Therapies, 51 Bedford Place, Southampton,
Hants SO1 2DG

Naturopathy
British College of Naturopathy. Secretary,
6 Netherhall Gardens, London NW3 6RR

British Naturopathic and Osteopathic
Association, Frazer House, 6 Netherhall
Gardens, London NW3 5RR

Healing
British Association of Therapeutic Touch.
Secretary, 33 Grange Thorpe Drive, Burnage,
Manchester M19 2LR

Chakra Energy System. John R. Cross MCSP
Dr Ac. 24 The Chequers, Castlethorpe, Bucks
MR19 7HG

Confederation of Healing Organizations.
Secretary, 113 High Street, Berkhamsted, Herts
HP4 2DJ (Represents some 15 organizations)

National Federation of Spiritual Healers
(NFSH). Secretary, The Old Manor Farm
Studio, Church Street, Sunbury-upon-Thames,
Middlesex TW16 6RG

The Reiki Association of Great Britain,
Cornbrook Bridge House, Clee Hill, Ludlow,
Shropshire SY8 3QQ

Bodywork Therapies

Acupuncture
Acupuncture Association of Chartered
Physiotherapists. Contact Vibeke Dawson,
Abbey View Complementary Health Clinic,
The Medical Centre, Shaftesbury, Dorset
SP7 8DU

The British Acupuncture Council, Park House,
206–208 Latimer Road, London W10 6RE
(Represents five professional organizations)

Applied Kinesiology
The Academy and Association of Systematic
Kinesology. Brian Butler, 39 Browns Road,
Surbiton, Surrey KT5 8ST

Ann Holdway, 78 Castlewood Drive, Eltham,
London SE9 1NG (Booklist and UK Directory)

The Kinesiology National Occupational
Standards (KNOS). Ann Parker, 11a Ripon,
North Yorks HG4 2AT (Includes the
Association of Systematic Kinesiology and the
Kinesiology Federation. Accreditation through
the Open College Network)

The Bowen Technique
The Bowen Association (UK). The Secretary,
122 High Street, Earl Shilton, Leicester
LE9 7LQ

Craniosacral Therapy
Craniosacral Therapy Association of Chartered Physiotherapists (CTACP). Marilyn Lennon MCSP, Chairman, 44 Sherwell Lane, Chelston, Torquay, Devon TQ2 6BD

The Upledger Institute (UK). Secretary, 2 Marshall Place, Perth PH2 7HB

The Feldenkrais Method
The Feldenkrais Guild UK. PO Box 370, London N10 3XA

The Feldenkrais Professional Training Programme. PO Box 1207, Hove BN3 2GG

Metamorphic Technique
The Midland School of Reflextherapy and Associated Studies. Director, Christine Jones FCSP Grad Dip Phys. 5 Church Street, Warwick, Warks CV34 4AB

The Metamorphic Association. Director, Gaston Saint-Pierre, 67 Ritherdon Road, Tooting, London SW17 8QE

Polarity Therapy
Healing by Touch. Director, Anthony Deavin, 11 The Orchard, Ashurst Drive, Tadworth, Surrey KT20 7LP

International School of Polarity Therapy. Director, Rosamund Webster, 7 Nunney Close, Cheltenham GL51 0TU

International Society of Polarity Therapists. Secretary, 54 Ashford Road, Topsham, Exeter, Devon EX3 0LA

Reflexology/Reflextherapy
International Institute of Reflexology. Secretary, 15 Hatfield Close, Tonbridge, Kent TN10 4JP

The Midland School of Reflextherapy and Associated Studies. Director, Christine Jones FCSP Grad Dip Phys. 5 Church Street, Warwick, Warks CV34 4AB

Scottish Institute of Reflexology. Secretary, 14 Tyney Road, Paisley PA1 3EY

Shiatsu
The European Shiatsu School. Central Office, Highbanks, Lockeridge, Marlborough, Wilts SN8 4EQ

Shiatsu College, Edinburgh. Principal, Andrea Battermann MCSP MRSS, 13 Scone Gardens, Edinburgh EH8 7DQ (Shiatsu Colleges also in Brighton, Bristol, London, Newcastle, Norwich)

The Shiatsu Society, Barber House, Storey's Bar Road, Fengate, Peterborough, PE1 5YN

Zero Balancing
Zero Balancing Association (ZBA). Secretary, 10 Victoria Grove, Bridport, Dorset DT6 3AA (For details of ZB workshops)

Mind-Body Therapies

Emotional Therapy
Foundation of Emotional Therapy. Secretary, Jane Rochfort, 20 Caldicott Gardens, Cheltenham Road, Evesham, Worcs WR11 6JR

Process Work
Research Society for Process Oriented Psychology UK. Secretary, 34 Narcissus Road, West Hampstead, London NW6 1TH

Stress Counselling
Centre for Stress Management. Secretary, 156 Westcombe Hill, Blackheath, London SE3 7DH

Qigong and Tai Chi
The Association for Traditional Chinese Medicine. Secretary, 78 Haverstock Hill, London NW3 2BE

Essential Oils and Fragrancies
Aromatherapy Organizations Council. Secretary, 3 Latymer Close, Braybrooke, Market Harborough, Leicestershire LE16 8NL (represents 10 organizations)

Association of Chartered Physiotherapists in Massage (ACPIM), Aromatherapy Sub Committee. Contact Elisabeth Jones MCSP 13 Fairview, Hungerford, Berks RG17 0BB (also Director of IFA, ISPA, ITEC recognized Diploma course in Aromatherapy)

International Federation of Aromatherapists, Stamford House, 2/4 Chiswick High Road, London W4 1TH

International Society of Aromatherapists, ISPA House, 82 Ashby Road, Hinckley, Leics LE10 1SN

Vibrational Medicine

Aura-Soma
Aura-Soma UK. Dev Aura, Little London, Tetford, Nr Horncastle, Lincolnshire LN9 6QL

Flower Essences
Bach Flower Remedies. Secretary, Broad Heath House, 83 Parkside, London SW19 5LP (Seminars and two day courses)

The Bach Centre, Mount Vernon, Sotwell, Wallingford, Oxon OX10 OPZ (Quarterly Newsletter, Study days and training)

Healing Herbs. PO Box 65, Hereford HR2 0UW (Study days and research)

The Living Tree, Milland, Liphook, Hants GU30 7JS (Mail order flower essences)

Vita Fons, 11 Combe Castle, Elworthy, Taunton, Somerset TA4 3PX

ElectroCrystal Therapy
School of ElectroCrystal Therapy. Director, Harry Oldfield, 117 Long Drive, South Ruislip, Middlesex HA4 0HL

Index

Reflex therapy, 190
Reflexology, 188–90
Reflextherapy, 186–95
Reiki for animals, 118–19
Relaxation techniques
   Qigong, 220, 226
   stress counselling, 211–12
   terminal illness, 286
Rescue Remedy, 248–9, 274, 289

Sacral chakra, 83, 90–1, 92
Sandalwood oil, 237
Scalar waves, 30–2
Scanning, 102
Schumann resonance, 26
Sciatica and acupuncture, 140–1
Science of Unitary Human Beings, 101
Scoliosis: craniosacral therapy, 152
Segmental acupuncture, 135–6
Sensory environment therapy, 259–68
Shiatsu, 196–205
Skin, epidermal-dermal continuum, 11
Skin wounds: therapeutic touch research, 59–62
Skull diagnosis, 45–6
Smell therapy *see* Aromatherapy
Snoezlen rooms, 260–1
Solid state
   biochemistry, 12–13
   molecular arrays, 15–16
Solar plexus chakra, 82, 89–90, 91
Soliton waves, 18–19
Soma, 171–2
Sound
   and chakras, 84
   sound therapy, 263–4
Spectroscopy, 23
Sphenoid and craniosacral therapy, 147
Spina bifida: Qigong, 228
Spinal diagnosis, 49–50
Spiritual healing, 94–9, 112
Spontaneous healing, 6–7
Stress management
   aromatherapy, 243, 244
   Qigong, 222–3
   stress counselling, 209–16
Stress mapping, 215

Stretching, dynamic, 184
Subtle bodies, 78–9
Sutures, cranial, 146
Synergetic systems, 19

Tactile stimulation, 266
Taichi, 221–2
prevention of falls, 224–5
Taste stimulation, 266
Tea tree oil, 233, 235
Tellington-Jones Equine Awareness Method, 117–19
Temperosphenoidal line, 44–5
Tensegrity, 19–21
Terminal illness, 281, 284–5, 290–2
   massage, 281–2
   relatives and carers, 288–90
   symptom relief, 285–8
Therapeutic Touch, 100–7
   biomagnetic fields, 25–6
   skin wound studies, 59–62
Thixotropy, 180
Throat chakra, 82, 87–8, 89
Tissue memory, 151
Tissue repair, 5
Tongue diagnosis, 42–3
Traditional Chinese Medicine, 39–40, 128–9
   diagnosis, 129–31
Transcendental meditation, 69–71, 73
Transcutaneous nerve stimulation (TENS), 138, 140
Trigger point acupuncture, 136
T Touch, 117–19
Tuberous sclerosis: metamorphosis, 168

V-spread craniosacral technique, 150
Vibration therapy, 266
Visual sensory stimulation, 261–3
Vita Fons II, 251
Vortices, rotating, 85–6

Water and information conduction, 16
Waves, scalar, 30–2

Yarrow Special Formula, 251
Yin and Yang, 39–40, 128–9

Now you've read the book, remember to visit our website at

http://www.bh.com/companions/0750640790

to access the associated web chapters.

Butterworth-Heinemann are delighted to offer you this extra information resource on emerging concepts in energy medicine, as well as coverage of some of the lesser-known therapies that are becoming more widely used by physical therapists worldwide. By linking the book and the web chapters we have attempted to provide you with comprehensive yet practical coverage of all the alternative therapies used by physical therapists today. We hope that you will find both types of presentation enjoyable and of practical use.

If you have any suggestions about other therapies on which you would like information we would be delighted to explore the possibility of also making them available through this medium.

Please contact Mary Seager, Senior Commissioning Editor, Medical Books Division
Tel: +(0)1865 314469; email: mary.seager@repp.co.uk